国学经典外译丛书（第一辑）

黄帝外经英译

Yellow Emperor's External Canon of Medicine

〔远古〕岐伯天师 ◎ 论述　　（明）陈士铎 ◎ 评述

刘希茹 ◎ 今译　　李照国 ◎ 英译

SJPC

上海三联书店

"十三五"国家重点图书出版规划项目

国家出版基金资助项目

译 者 赘 言

《黄帝内经》者,古人知之,今人晓之,夷人明之。其精气神韵,若日月叠璧,以应人之阴阳表里;其理法方药,似山川焕绮,以合人之寒热虚实。其传承者,千秋万代而不绝;其传扬者,天高地厚而不竭。

善哉乎? 尽善也! 至哉乎? 止至也!

然则矣,其不善者,有之;其不至者,亦有之。何以言之?《汉书·艺文志》曰:"黄帝内经十八卷,外经三十七卷;扁鹊内经九卷,外经十二卷;白氏内经三十八卷,外经三十六卷;旁篇二十五卷。右医经七家。"然自秦汉以降,《黄帝外经》《白氏内经》《白氏外经》《扁鹊内经》《扁鹊外经》,皆亡矣。如此绝圣之经,何以亡之? 天地翻覆乎? 乾坤倒转乎? 无人知之,无人晓之。

鄙人幼时学国语,习国学,童子之功虽弱,炎黄基因尚强。弱冠之年,入长安夷学之府,学夷文,习夷语,方知夷之夷者也。四度春秋,夷学终矣,夷业成矣。随之赴秦都,入国医学府,教夷语,学国医,习译理。此时之国人,虽重工商,亦重文理。故而国医之传承,依如往昔,无争无异。鄙人既学国医,亦译国医,尤以《内经》之学而时译之为重。可谓"学而时译之,不亦说乎!"

学国医、译《内经》之时,鄙人即知《外经》之亡矣,且无可觅之。虽感诧异,亦无可奈何。某日寻觅《针灸释难》,偶遇中医古籍社所刊之国医典籍,名曰《外经微言》,即《黄帝外经》是也,惊诧之至!

此《外经微言》,乃天师岐伯所传也,明人陈士铎所述也。古籍社刊本云,20世纪中叶,《外经微言》偶现天津某书馆,近年始得问世。然《外经》问世至今,皆若秋风落叶,无人问津。医界皆云其"伪者是也",故而几无学者,亦无习者。鄙人译释《内经》之余,亦研读《外经》,感触可谓至深。以医者言之,则《内经》重治已病,《外经》重治未病,两向合一,则天人相应也。其理法之意,不言而喻。

　　然以史学观之，则《外经微言》之疑，确非风言风语也。《汉书·艺文志》曰："黄帝内经十八卷，外经三十七卷"。然陈公所述之《外经》，仅九卷而已，非三十七卷。由此观之，则医界所谓之"伪者是也"，确非妄言。然以医理观之，则陈公所述之《外经》亦具"东方生风，风生木，木生酸，酸生肝"之佳径。若实为陈公之托名，其所论所道，亦为明时医家之卓见卓识，可补《内经》之理法，可充《内经》之方药。其医理医哲，自不待言。鄙人欲译《外经》，其意何为？亦不待言矣！

　　鄙人译《内经》之时，时疑时惑，时茫时困。然译《外经》之时，则时定时静，时安时虑。历经三载，《外经》之释译，今晨毕矣。回望三春三秋，悟感可谓多矣！

　　今之国人，皆欲传中土文化于泰西，时而宣之，时而论之，且言且幻，如日升天。然仰观天文，俯察地理，确乎传入泰西者，惟国医是也。而《内经》，则为国医外传之坦途、国学外扬之蹊径。此行此势，夷人明之，国人异之；夷人求之，国人厌之。此情此景，天知地晓，无须赘言。所期期以待者，惟《外经》之传是也。此乃鄙人释《外经》之意也，译《外经》之趣也，传《外经》之志也。

李照国

丙申年六月廿六夜述于华亭馨园

陈 士 铎 列 传

陈士铎,字敬之,号远公,别号朱华子,又号莲公,自号大雅堂主人,浙江山阴人。明天启年间生,清康熙年间卒。据《山阴县志》载:"陈士铎,邑诸生,治病多奇中,医药不受人谢,年八十卒。"

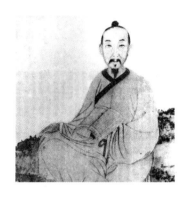

陈氏幼习儒道,欲继往圣之绝学,以开万世之太平,后因仕途之困,则以岐黄之道为本,以"良医济世"为志。平生好学,精研国医典籍之理法,博采历朝医家之方药,故而医理精深,诊疗卓异,实乃精诚之大医者。研习之余,诊治之后,则善著书立说,以惠后人。

其著甚丰,可谓等身,惜多已亡矣。据史料载,其所亡者,若《内经素问尚论》《灵枢新编》《本草新编》《脏腑精鉴》《脉诀阐微》《石室秘录》《辨证录》《辨证玉函》《六气新编》《外科洞天》《伤寒四条辨》《婴孺证治》《伤风指迷》《历代医史》《琼笈秘录》《黄庭经注》《梅花易数》。

今存者,唯《石室秘录》《洞天奥旨》《本草新编》《辨证录》《辨证玉函》《脉诀阐微》《外经微言》是也。存者虽少,然《外经微言》之存,可谓多之多者也。自汉代始,《黄帝外经》即亡矣。《外经微言》,即《黄帝外经》是也。实传抑或托名,皆有传承。陈氏之功,尤显于此。

李照国述

目 录

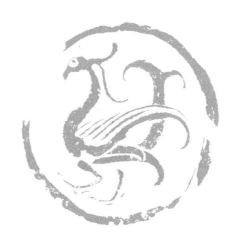

卷一

阴阳颠倒篇第一

【原文】

黄帝闻广成子窈窈冥冥之旨,叹广成子之谓天也。退而夜思,尚有未获,遣鬼臾区问于岐伯天师曰:"帝闻至道于广成子,广成子曰:'至道之精,窈窈冥冥。至道之极,昏昏默默。无视无听,抱神以静,形将自正。必静必清,无劳汝形,无摇汝精,无思虑营营,乃可以长生。目无所视,耳无所闻,心无所知,汝神将守汝形,形乃长生。慎汝内,闭汝外,多知为败,我为汝遂于大明之上矣,至彼至阳之原也。为汝入于窈冥之门矣,至被至阴之原也。天地有官,阴阳有藏。慎守汝身,物将自壮。我其守一,以处其和,故身可以不老也。天师必知厥义?幸明晰之!'。"

岐伯稽首奏曰:"大哉言乎!非吾圣帝,安克闻至道哉!帝明知故问,岂欲传旨于万祀乎!何心之仁也,臣愚,何足知之。然,仁圣明问,敢备述以闻:窈冥者,阴阳之谓也。昏默者,内外之词也。视听者,耳目之语也。至道无形而有形,有形而实无形。无形藏于有形之中,有形化于无形之内,始能形与神全,精与神合乎?"

鬼臾区曰:"诺。虽然,师言微,未及其妙也。"

岐伯曰:"乾坤之道,不外男女,男女之道,不外阴阳,阴阳之道,不外顺逆,顺则生,逆则死也。阴阳之原,即巅倒之术也。世人皆知顺生,

Volume 1

【英译】

Chapter 1
Reversal[1] of Yin and Yang

Yellow Emperor[2], knowing the mysterious and abstruse ideas of Guang Chengzi[3], [was so surprised that he] compared Guang Chengzi to the sky. Thinking about [these mystersious and abstruse ideas] all night, [Yellow Emperor] still could not fully understand. [He] sent Kui Yuqu[4] to ask Celestial Master Qibo[5]. [Kui Yuqu told Qibo], "Yellow Emperor has heard of the perfect Dao[6] of Guang Chengzi. Guang Chengzi said: 'The essence of perfect Dao is mysterious, complicated and abstruse. The absolute [development appears] dark and unclear. Never see nor hear [anything]. Tranquilize [yourself] with integration of spirit to rectify [your] body. Always [keep yourself] quiet and lucid, never exhausting your body, disscipating your essence and contemplating anything. [Only in such a way] can [you] live a long life. [There is] no [need] to see anything, to hear anything and to know anything. [Only in such a way] can your spirit protect your body [and enable you to enjoy] a long life. [Thus you must] take good care of [what is] inside [your body] and keep away from [what is] outside [of your body]. The more [you] know, the worse [you] suffer. I have told you the highest [level of] the great brightness[7], which is the source of Yang. [I have also] told you the gate to the mysterious and abstruse [world], which is the source of Yin. [In] the sky and [on] the earth, there are dominators [controlling the changes]; [in] Yin and Yang, there are depots [keeping the changes]. [If you

不知顺之有死；皆知逆死，不知逆之有生，故未老先衰矣。广成子之教，示帝行巅倒之术也。"

鬼臾区曰："何言之神乎！虽然，请示其原！"

岐伯曰："巅倒之术，即探阴阳之原乎！窈冥之中有神也。昏默之中有神也。视听之中有神也。探其原而守神，精不摇矣。探其原而保其精，神不驰矣。精固神全，形安敝乎？"

鬼臾区复奏帝前。帝曰："俞哉！载之《外经》，传示臣工，使共闻至道，同游于无极之野也。"

陈士铎曰："此篇帝问而天师答之，乃首篇之论也。问不止黄帝，而答止天师者，帝引天师之论也。帝非不知阴阳颠倒之术，明知故问，亦欲尽人皆知广成子之教也。"

【今译】

黄帝听说广成子窈窈冥冥的思想之后，非常赞美，将广成子视为天人。黄帝退居后，彻夜深思，但还有无法理解之处，于是派遣鬼臾区询问天师岐伯。

鬼臾区对岐伯说："黄帝从广成子处听说了至高无上的道。广成子说：'至高无上之道的精妙，可谓窈窈冥冥。至高无上之道的极致，可谓昏昏默默。没有视觉，没有听觉，精神上保持虚静，身体就会自然清正。保持了虚静和清正，无须劳累自己的形体，无须动摇自己的精气，无须有烦思杂念，才能保持长生不老。眼睛无须所视，耳朵无须所闻，心中无须所知，自己的神就可以保护守卫自己的形体了，形体就可

can] carefully protect your body, [all] the things[8] [in your body will be] strong. I have protected the one[9] and [I am now] in harmony. That is why I will not become old. ' Celestial Master must know the meaning. [I sincerely] hope [that you can] explain it [for me]."

Qibo bowed and said, "How excellent [what Guang Chengzi has] said! It's only the Great Emperor who is able to know such a perfect Dao [about life]! [In fact,] the Emperor is quite clear [about what Guang Chengzi has said]. [The reason that he] asked [me such a] question is to make it known to all the people in the world. This is perhaps what Ren (benevolence) means. As a fool, how can I understand such [great and perfect ideas]! However, since the Emperor has asked me to explain, I have to try to make a basic explanation. [The so-called] 'mystery and abstruseness' actually refer to Yin and Yang. [The so-called] 'darkness and silence' refer to the internal and external. [The so-called] 'seeing' and 'hearing' refer to the ears and eyes. The perfect Dao is either invisible or visible. [Although it appears] visible, it actually is invisible. [In fact] invisibility is kept in visibility and visibility is mixed with invisibility, [making it possible for] perfection of the body and spirit [as well as] integration of essence and spirit."

Kui Yuqu said: "Right. Although Master has described in details, the mystery and abstruseness are still not mentioned."

Qibo said, "The Dao (law) of Qian (the sky) and Kun (the earth) is no more than male and female; the Dao of male and female is no more than Yin and Yang; the Dao of Yin and Yang is no more than normal and abnormal. Normality protects life while abnormality causes death. The origin of Yin and Yang is the rule of reversal. People in this world all know [that] normality [protects] life, [but they] do not know [that] normality also causes death; [they] all know [that] abnormality [causes] death, [but they] do not know [that] abnormality [also] ensures life. That is why [they are] debilitated [when they are]

以长生不老了。要谨慎地守护好自己的内在精气，要慎重地紧闭自己外在的孔窍，知道的越多就越会耗损自己的精气神，就会导致衰败。我为你指出了大明之上的精要，那里是至阳形成的源头。为你所指出的进入玄妙之门的路径，就是至阴生化形成的源泉。天地的运化有主宰者，阴阳的变化有归藏处。谨慎地守护好自己的身体，身体中的一切都会自然强壮。我守护好我的玄妙之关，努力使自己的精气神和合交融，这样身体就不会衰老，天师自然知道其中的要义。希望能荣幸地听到您清清楚楚的解说。'"

岐伯跪拜说："多么伟大的言语啊！如果不是我们神圣的帝王，怎么可能听到如此至高无上的大道呢！黄帝显然是明知故问此事，难道不是为了将这一要旨传扬千秋万代吗？黄帝之心如此慈悲仁义，臣我愚昧，如何能知道如此至高无上的大道呢？但是，仁慈的黄帝如此明知故问，臣只好详细讲述我的所知所闻。所谓窈冥，指的是阴阳。所谓昏默，指的是内外之意。所谓视听，指的是耳目。至高无上的大道既无形而又有形，虽然是有形的，其实是无形的。无形隐藏在有形之中，有形化溶于无形之内。正因为如此，方能形与神俱，精与神合而为一。"

鬼臾区说："说得对。虽然天师讲得如此细微精深，但是还没有谈及其中的玄妙之处啊。"

岐伯说："所谓的乾坤之道，不外乎男女而已；所谓的男女之道，不外乎阴阳而已；所谓的阴阳之道，不外乎顺逆而已。顺则可生，逆则致死。阴阳的原理，即为颠倒之术。世人都知道顺可以生，但却不知顺也会导致死；世人都知道逆可以致死，但却不知逆也可以保生。这就是为

not old. What Guang Chengzi has instructed is to show the rule of reversal [suggested by] the Emperor."

Kui Yuqu said, "How excellent your explanation is! However, please tell [me] the principle."

Qibo said, "The rule of reversal is to explore the principle of Yin and Yang! In mystery and abstruseness, there is spirit. In darkness and silence, there is spirit. In seeing and hearing, there is spirit. [Only when] the principle is explored and the spirit is safeguarded [can] essence not be dissipated. [When] the principle is explored and the essence is protected, the spirit will not be loosened. [When] the essence is defended and the spirit is perfected, how could the body become debilitated?"

Kui Yuqu returned and reported [it] to the Emperor. The Emperor said, "Excellent! Record it in the External Canon [of Medicine], disseminate [it] to the ministers and doctors, let them all know the perfect Dao and enjoy travelling outside the world."

Chen Shiduo's comment, "This chapter [describes] the question [asked by] the Emperor and the answer [provided by] the Celestial Master. It is the first chapter [of Yellow Emperor's External Canon of Medicine]. [This question was] not only asked by Yellow Emperor. But the answer is only [provided by] the Celestial Master. The Emperor [has asked this question in order] to encourage the Celestial Master to talk [about the perfect Dao]. The Emperor is actually quite clear about the rule of reversal. [He] has deliberately asked such a question in order to enable all the people to know the instructions of Guang Chengzi."

Notes

[1] Reversal here means upside down.

[2] Yellow Emperor was one of the most important legendary kings in remote antiquity in China and was also the father of Chinese culture.

什么会有未老先衰的现象。广成子的教旨,就是向黄帝揭示巅倒之术。"

鬼臾区说:"天师所说,真的神奇啊!虽然如此,还是想请您说明大道的原理吧!"

岐伯说:"所谓巅倒之术,就是探索阴阳的原理啊!窈冥之中,有神主宰。昏默之中,有神主宰。视听之中,有神主宰。探索其原理而固守内在之神,精就不会摇散。探索其原理以保护其精,神就不会飘散。精得以固,神得以全,形体怎么会衰败呢?"

鬼臾区返回,禀奏黄帝。黄帝说:"很好!将这些至高无上的大道及其原理记载在《外经》上,传授给臣子和医家们,使他们能懂得至高无上的大道,一同遨游在无极的原野上。"

陈士铎评论说:"这篇的基本内容是,黄帝提问,天师回答。这是《外经》的首篇论述。本篇所提问的不仅是黄帝,但回答则只是天师岐伯,是黄帝引导天师岐伯论述。黄帝并非不知阴阳颠倒之术,之所以明知而故问,主要是为了让大家都知道广成子的教旨。"

Volume 1

His Chinese name was Huangdi（黄帝），Yellow Emperor was the English literal translation of Huangdi（黄帝）. Yellow Emperor was the son of Shaodian（少典）. His family name was Gongsun（公孙）. He used to live by the Ji River（姬水）. That was why people took Ji as another family name of him. Since Huangdi（黄帝）was born in a hill called Xuanyuan （轩辕），he was also named after the hill. He founded his kingdom in Youxiong（有熊）. So he was also called Youxiong（有熊）. Owing to his great merits and virtues，he was supported by the heads of all tribes as the king. Since his kingdom took the color of earth as the auspicious sign，he was called Huangdi（黄帝），literally Yellow Emperor，because the color of earth is yellow in the central region of China. During his reign，Huangdi（黄帝）made magnificent contributions to the civilization of the Chinese nation. That is why Huangdi（黄帝）was worshiped as the father of the Chinese nation.

［3］Guang Chengzi（广成子）：According to the legendary story of Daoism，Guang Chengzi was the true man in the remote antiquity，living in seclusion in Kongtong Mountain（崆峒山）. Nineteen years after coming to the throne，Yellow Emperor went to this mountain to visit him and talk with him about the perfect Dao.

［4］Kui Yuqu（鬼臾区）：The minister of Yellow Emperor and the student of the Celestial Master.

［5］Qibo（岐伯）：The prime minister of Yellow Emperor and the teacher and advisor of all the other ministers of Yellow Emperor. That is why he was called the Celestial Master.

［6］Perfect Dao（道）refers to the thought or doctrine that is perfect in content and at the highest level.

［7］Great brightness refers to the sun and the moon in the sky.

［8］All the things refer to all the organs in the human body.

［9］The one refers to the perfect Dao（道）.

顺逆探原篇第二

【原文】

伯高太师问于岐伯曰："天师言颠倒之术,即探阴阳之原也,其旨奈何?"

岐伯不答。

再问,曰:"唯唯。"

三问,岐伯叹曰:"吾不敢隐矣。夫阴阳之原者,即生克之道也。颠倒之术者,即顺逆之理也。知颠倒之术,即可知阴阳之原矣。"

伯高曰:"阴阳不同也。天之阴阳,地之阴阳,人身之阴阳,男女之阴阳,何以探之哉?"

岐伯曰:"知其原亦何异哉!"

伯高曰:"请显言其原。"

岐伯曰:"五行顺生不生,逆死不死。"

岐伯曰:"生而不生者,金生水而克水,水生木而克木,木生火而克火,火生土而克土,土生金而克金,此害生于恩也。死而不死者,金克木而生木,木克土而生土,土克水而生水,水克火而生火,火克金而生金,此仁生于义也。夫五行之顺相生而相克,五行之逆不克而不生。逆之至者,顺之至也。"

伯高曰:"美哉言乎。然何以逆而顺之也?"

Volume 1

【英译】

Chapter 2
Exploring the Rule of Normality and Abnormality

Master Bogao[1] asked Qibo, "Celestial Master's talk about the rule of reversal is to explore the origin of Yin and Yang. What is the implicatioin?"

Qibo did not answer.

When asked again, Qibo said, "Well. Well."

When asked for the third time, Qibo sighed, "[Sorry,] I dare not conceal [it]. The origin of Yin and Yang refers to the way of promotion and restriction. The rule of perversion refers to the principle of normality and abnormality. [When] knowing the rule of reversal, [you certainly] can understand the origin of Yin and Yang."

Bogao asked, "Yin and Yang are different. [In] the sky, [there are] Yin and Yang; [in] the earth, [there are] Yin and Yang; [in] the human body, [there are] Yin and Yang; [in] male and female, [there are] Yin and Yang. How to explore it?"

Qibo answered, "[When you have] understood the origin, how could there be difference?"

Bogao asked, "Please explain the origin."

Qibo answered, "[In terms of] five elements, normality [usually ensures] life, [but sometimes it will] not [ensure] life; abnormality [usually causes] death, [but sometimes it will] not

岐伯曰:"五行之顺,得土而化。五行之逆,得土而神。土以合之,土以成之也。"

伯高曰:"余知之矣。阴中有阳,杀之内以求生乎。阳中有阴,生之内以出死乎。余与帝同游于无极之野也。"

岐伯曰:"逆而顺之,必先顺而逆之。绝欲而毋为邪所侵也,守神而毋为境所移也,练气而毋为物所诱也,保精而毋为妖所耗也。服药饵以生其津,慎吐纳以添其液,慎劳逸以安其髓,节饮食以益其气,其庶几乎?"

伯高曰:"天师教我以原者全矣。"

岐伯曰:"未也,心死则身生,死心之道,即逆之之功也。心过死则身亦不生,生心之道又顺之之功也。顺而不顺,始成逆而不逆乎?"

伯高曰:"志之矣,敢忘秘诲哉。"

陈士铎曰:"伯高之问,亦有之问也。顺中求逆,逆处求顺,亦生死之门也。今奈何求生于顺乎?于顺处求生,不若于逆处求生之为得也。此一'逆'字,知者自知,迷者自迷。诸君自扪其心,知否?"

【今译】

伯高太师问岐伯:"天师所说的颠倒之术,就是探索阴阳的源泉,其要旨是什么呢?"

岐伯不回答。

伯高再问,岐伯说:"嗯嗯。"

伯高再三问,岐伯感慨地说:"我可不敢隐瞒啊!阴阳的原理,就

[cause] death. [The cases of normality that usually ensures] life but [sometimes does] not [ensure] life [include] metal [that usually] promotes water but [sometimes] restricts water, water [that usually] promotes wood but [sometimes] restricts wood, wood [that usually] promotes fire but [sometimes] restricts fire, fire [that usually] promotes earth but [sometimes] restricts earth, and earth [that usually] promotes metal but [sometimes] restricts metal. These [are the examples of] harm originating from kindness[2]. [The cases of abnormality that usually causes] death but [sometimes does] not [cause] death [include] metal [that usually] restricts wood but [sometimes] promotes wood, wood [that usually] restricts earth but [sometimes] promotes earth, earth [that usually] restricts water but [sometimes] promotes water, water [that usually] restricts fire but [sometimes] promotes fire, and fire [that usually] restricts metal but [sometimes] promotes metal. These [are the examples of] benevolence ensuring righteousness[3]. [Thus in] normality of five elements, [there are] mutual promotion and mutual restriction; [in] abnormality of five elements, [there is] no restriction and promotion. The acme of abnormality [indicates] appearance of normality."

Bogao asked, "Excellent explanation! But how to transform abnormality into normality?"

Qibo answered, "Normality in five elements will be transformed [when] earth is obtained. Abnormality in five elements will become ingenious [when] earth is obtained. Earth [will enable it] to concord [with what it needs]; earth [will enable it] to achieve [what it should]."

是相生相克的道理。所谓颠倒之术,就是顺逆之理。懂得了颠倒之术,就懂得了阴阳的原理。"

伯高说:"阴和阳有不同的类型。有天的阴阳,有地的阴阳,有人身的阴阳,有男女的阴阳,如何才能探索其原理呢?"

岐伯说:"知道了阴阳的原理,又有何差异呢!"

伯高说:"请解说其原理吧。"

岐伯说:"五行顺行相生而不生,逆行应死而不死。"

岐伯说:"相生而不生的,如金生水而克水,水生木而克木,木生火而克火,火生土而克土,土生金而克金,这就是'害生于恩'的道理。应死而不死的,如金克木而生木,木克土而生土,土克水而生水,水克火而生火,火克金而生金,这就是'仁生于义'的道理。五行顺行,相生中存在着相克;五行逆行,不相克也不相生。逆行至极,就是顺行了。"

伯高说:"您说得真好啊!但为什么逆行至极反而能顺行了呢?"

岐伯说:"五行的顺行,得到土就能运化。五行的逆行,得到土就会神化。土可以使其和合,土可以使其大成。"

伯高说:"我知道了。阴中有阳,从克杀中可以求得生机。阳中有阴,从生机中可以产生死因。我将与黄帝同游于无极的原野。"

岐伯说:"逆行而能顺生,必须先将顺行转化为逆行。断绝欲望而不为邪气所侵害,守神而不为外境所转移,练气而不为外物所诱惑,保精而不为色欲所耗散。服用药饵以生津,谨慎吐纳以添液,调理劳逸以安髓,节制饮食以益气,这样就可以养生全身了。"

伯高说:"天师将原理完全教给我了啊!"

Volume 1

Bogao said, "I have understood. There is Yang within Yin. Can survival be seeked from [the procedure of] killing?[4] There is Yin within Yang. [Is there any cause of] death during [the procedure of promoting] life? I will accompany the Emperor to travel outside the world."

Qibo said, "[To seek for] normality from abnormality, [you must] act normally first and then abnormally[5]. [Only when various] desires are abandoned [can] invasion of evil[6] be prevented; [only when] the spirit is safeguarded [can] transference to allopatry be avoided; [only when] Qi is [well] exercised [can] allure of materials [be] abstained; [only when] essence is protected [can] exhaustion [due to] eroticism be averted. Taking medicine can produce fluid, carefully exhaling and inhaling can enrich humor, cautiously work and rest can pacify the marrow, being moderate in eating and drinking can replenish Qi. These [are what you should do in order to seek for survival from the procedure of killing]."

Bogao said, "Celestial Master have fully taught me the principle!"

Qibo said, "Not fully yet. [Only when] the heart is dead[7] [can] the body be protected. The way to die the heart is the force of abnormality[8]. [But if] the heart dies to the extreme, [there will be] no [chance for] the body to survive. The way to vitalize the heart is the force of normality. [Thus only when] normality is not normal can abnormality be not abnormal."

Bogao said, "[I will] keep it [firmly in] mind. [I will] never forget [your] instructions."

岐伯说："还没有全部告诉你。心死则身生，心死的路径，就是逆行的功夫。但如果心死太过，身体也就没有生机了。生心的道路也是顺行的功夫。顺行而又不顺，才能逆行而不逆。"

伯高说："我一定牢记在心，永不忘记您的秘笈教诲。"

陈士铎评论说："伯高之问，也是有意之问。顺中求逆，逆中求顺，这就是生死之门。如今为何要求生于顺呢？因为大家不懂得在逆处求生比在顺处求生所获更多。这个'逆'字，懂得的人自然懂得，迷惑的人自然迷惑。各位君子应扪心自问，你懂得了吗？"

Volume 1

Chen Shiduo's comment，"Bogao's question was asked deliberately. To seek for abnormality from normality and to seek for normality from abnormality is also the way for life and death. Why [people] nowadays just seek for life from normality? Seeking for life from abnormality，[compared with] seeking for life from normality，[enables us] to achieve more. Such a character 'abnormality' clarifies [those who are] clear and confuses [those who are] perplexed. Gentlemen，[please] search your conscience to see whether you have understood."

Notes

[1] Bogao (伯高)：The minister of Yellow Emperor (黄帝).

[2] In the expression "harm originating from kindness", "harm" means restriction and "kindness" means promotion.

[3] In the expression "benevolence ensuring righteousness", "benevolence" refers to the origin of life while "righteousness" refers to necessity of life.

[4] Killing means restriction activity among the five elements.

[5] To act normally first and then abnormally，this is what "the rule of reversal" means.

[6] Evil (邪) refers to pathogenic factors in traditional Chinese medicine.

[7] The saying that "the heart is dead" or "to die the heart" means to abandon various secular desires in order to tranquilize the mind and spirit.

[8] The force of abnormality refers to refusal to follow secular customs and desires.

回天生育篇第三

【原文】

雷公问曰："人生子嗣，天命也。岂尽非人事乎？"

岐伯曰："天命居半，人事居半也。"

雷公曰："天可回乎？"

岐伯曰："天不可回，人事则可尽也。"

雷公曰："请言人事。"

岐伯曰："男子不能生子者，病有九；女子不能生子者，病有十也。"

雷公曰："请晰言之。"

岐伯曰："男子九病者：精寒也，精薄也，气馁也，痰盛也，精涩也，相火过旺也，精不能射也，气郁也，天厌也。女子十病者：胞胎寒也，脾胃冷也，带脉急也，肝气郁也，痰气盛也，相火旺也，肾水衰也，任督病也，膀胱气化不行也，气血虚而不能摄也。"

雷公曰："然则治之奈何？"

岐伯曰："精寒者，温其火乎。精薄者，益其髓乎。气馁者，壮其气乎。痰盛者，消其涎乎。精涩者，顺其水乎。火旺者，补其精乎。精不能射者，助其气乎。气郁者，舒其气乎。天厌者，增其势乎，则男子无子而可以有子矣。不可徒益其相火也。胞胎冷者，温其胞胎乎。脾胃冷者，暖其脾胃乎。带脉急者，缓其带脉乎。肝气郁者，开其肝气乎。痰

Volume 1

【英译】

Chapter 3
Retrieving the Sky to Conceive a Baby

Leigong[1] asked, "[It is said that] human beings breeding children [indicates] life [given by] the sky[2]. Does it mean [that the birth of children] has nothing to do with human beings?"

Qibo answered, "Half [of the contribution to] life [is made by] the sky and half [of the contribution to] life [is made by] human beings."

Leigong asked, "Can [the contribution made by] the sky [to life] be retrieved?"

Qibo answered, "It cannot be retrieved. But human beings can make more efforts."

Leigong asked, "Please tell me human affairs."

Qibo answered, "There are nine diseases [responsible for] failure to conceive a baby [among] men and ten diseases [responsible for] failure to conceive a baby [among] women."

Leigong asked, "Please explain in details."

Qibo said, "Nine diseases [among] men [include] cold semen, flimsy semen, weakness of Qi, exuberant phlegm, rough semen, effulgence of ministerial fire[3], failure to ejaculate semen, Qi stagnation and celestial aversion[4]. Ten diseases [among] women [include] cold uterus, cold spleen and stomach, spasm of the belt vessel, depression of liver-Qi, exuberance of phlegm-Qi, effulgence

气盛者,消其痰气乎。相火旺者,平其相火乎。肾水衰者,滋其肾水乎。任督病者,理其任督乎。膀胱气化不行者,助其肾气以益膀胱乎。气血不能摄胎者,益其气血以摄胎乎,则女子无子而可以有子矣。不可徒治其胞胎也。"

雷公曰:"天师之言,真回天之法也。然用天师法男女仍不生子奈何?"

岐伯曰:"必夫妇德行交亏也。修德以宜男,岂虚语哉。"

陈士铎曰:"男无子有九,女无子有十,似乎女多于男也。谁知男女皆一乎? 知不一而一者,大约健其脾胃为主,脾胃健而肾亦健矣! 何必分男女哉?"

【今译】

雷公问道:"人的一生,生儿育女,是上天的安排。难道全都与人力无关吗?"

岐伯说:"天命占居一半,人事占居一半。"

雷公说:"天命可以挽回吗?"

岐伯说:"天命不可挽回,人事则可尽力而为。"

雷公说:"请谈谈人事吧。"

岐伯说:"男子不能生育子女的,有九种病;女子不能生育子女的,有十种病。"

雷公说:"请详细说一说。"

岐伯说:"男子的九种病包括:精液寒冷,精液稀薄,元气虚弱,痰

of ministerial fire, decline of kidney-water, disorder of the conception vessel and governor vessel, failure of bladder-Qi to transform and failure to cultivate [the fetus due to] deficiency of Qi and blood. "

Leigong asked, "Then how to treat them?"

Qibo answered, "Cold semen [can be treated by] warming fire [in the kidney]; flimsy semen [can be treated by] replenishing the marrow; weakness of Qi [can be treated by] strengthening Qi; exuberant phlegm [can be treated by] resolving phlegm; rough semen [can be treated by] regulating water [in the kidney]; effulgence of fire [can be treated by] tonifying[5] semen; failure to ejaculate semen [can be treated by] supplementing Qi; Qi stagnation [can be treated by] freeing [the flow of] Qi; celestial aversion [can be treated by] increasing the ability [to conceive a baby which will enable] men unable to conceive a baby to have a baby. [It] cannot just try to replenish the ministerial fire. Cold uterus [can be treated by] warming the uterus; cold spleen and stomach [can be treated by] warming the spleen and stomach; spasm of the belt vessel [can be treated by] relaxing the belt vessel; depression of liver-Qi [can be treated by] opening liver-Qi; exuberance of phlegm-Qi [can be treated by] resolving phlegm-Qi; effulgence of ministerial fire [can be treated by] normalizing ministerial fire; decline of kidney-water [can be treated by] enriching kidney-water; disorder of the conception vessel and governor vessel [can be treated by] regulating the conception vessel and governor vessel; failure of bladder-Qi to transform [can be treated by] supplementing kidney-Qi to replenish the bladder;

涎壅盛,精液缺涩,相火过旺,精不能射,气机郁滞,上天厌恶。女子的十种病包括:胞胎寒冷,脾胃寒冷,带脉急拘,肝气郁滞,痰气壅盛,相火过旺,肾水衰弱,任督二脉有病,膀胱气化不行,气血虚弱不能摄养胎儿。"

雷公说:"那么该如何治疗呢?"

岐伯说:"精液寒冷的,要温热其火气。精液稀薄的,要益补其骨髓。元气虚弱的,要强壮其气机。痰涎壅盛的,要消除其痰涎。精液缺涩的,要理顺其肾水。相火过旺的,要补充其精水。精不能射的,要辅助其气势。气机郁滞的,要舒缓其气机。上天厌恶的,要增强其生育之能力,这样男子没有子女的就可以有子女了。不可只想方设法增益其相火。胞胎寒冷的,要温暖其胞胎。脾胃寒冷的,要温暖其脾胃。带脉急拘的,要舒缓其带脉。肝气郁滞的,要和缓其肝气。痰气壅盛的,要消除其痰气。相火旺盛的,要平和其相火。肾水衰弱的,要滋补其肾水。任督二脉有病的,要调理其任脉和督脉。膀胱气化不行的,要增强其肾气以补益膀胱。气血虚弱而不能摄养胎儿的。"

岐伯说:"要补益其气血以摄养其胎儿。这样女子不能生育子女的就可以生育了。遇到这样的情况时,不能只治疗其胞胎。"

雷公说:"天师的话,真是挽回天命的大法要法啊!但是,如果使用了天师所讲述的方法,男女仍不能生育子女,又该怎么办呢?"

岐伯说:"这显然是夫妇德行方面亏损而不足的缘故。修德养性是孕育和抚养子女的要务,怎么可能是假言虚语呢。"

failure of Qi and blood to cultivate fetus [can be treated by] replenishing Qi and blood to cultivate fetus [which will enable] women unable to conceive a baby to have a baby. [It] cannot just try to treat the uterus."

Leigong asked, "[What] Celestial Master have said is really the way to retrieve the sky. But if men and women still cannot conceive a baby [after they have] adopted the methods [suggested by] Celestial Master, what is the reason?"

Qibo answered, "[This] certainly [indicates that] husband and wife lack morality. To cultivate morality is beneficial to conceiving a baby. How could such a requirement be false?"

Chen Shiduo's comment, " There are nine [diseases] among men and ten[diseases] among women. [It] seems that [the diseases of] women are more than [those of] men. Who knows that men and women are the same [in terms of diseases related to conception of babies]? [Those who] know conformity in inconformity tend to fortify the spleen and stomach. [When] the spleen and stomach are fortified, the kidney is also fortified. There is no need to differentiate men and women."

Notes

[1] Leigong (雷公) was said to be the prince and minister of Yellow Emperor.

[2] The idea that life is given by the sky emphasizes the importance of adaptation to natural world.

[3] The so-called ministerial fire refers to fire in the kidney.

陈士铎评论说："男子不生育子女的有九种病,女子不生育子女的有十种病,似乎女子之病多于男子。有谁知道男女其实是一样的呢?不知道不一致中的一致,大约就知道以健其脾胃为主,脾胃强健了,肾也会强健的啊! 何必男女分而论之呢?"

[4] Celestial aversion refers to aversion to certain elements at certain period in different seasons.

[5] The verb "tonify" is a coined word in translating the Chinses concept "补", which means to nourish or improve or enrich or invigorate. The word "tonify" perhaps was coined on the basis of the word "tonic". It is unclear when this word was coined and who was the creater of this word.

天人寿夭篇第四

【原文】

伯高太师问岐伯曰："余闻形有缓急，气有盛衰，骨有大小，肉有坚脆，皮有厚薄，可分寿夭，然乎？"

岐伯曰："人有形则有气，有气则有骨，有骨则有肉，有肉则有皮。形必与气相合也，皮必与肉相称也，气血经络必与形相配也，形充而皮肤缓者寿。形充而皮肤急者夭。形充而脉坚大者，气血之顺也，顺则寿。形充而脉小弱者，气血之衰也，衰则危。形充而颧不起者，肉胜于骨也，骨大则寿。骨小则夭。形充而大，肉䐃坚有分理者，皮胜于肉也，肉疏则夭，肉坚则寿。形充而大肉无分理者，皮仅包乎肉也，肉厚寿，肉脆夭。此天生，人不可强也。故见则定人寿夭，即可测人生死矣。"

少师问曰："诚若师言，人之寿夭天定之矣，无豫于人乎？"

岐伯曰："寿夭定于天，挽回天命者，人也。寿夭听于天，戕贼其形骸，泻泄其精髓，耗散其气血，不必至天数而先夭者，天不任咎也。"

少师曰："天可回乎？"

岐伯曰："天不可回，而天可节也。节天之有余，补人之不足，不亦善全其天命乎？"

伯高太师闻之曰："岐天师真善言天也。世人贼天之不足，焉能留人之有余哉？"

Volume 1

【英译】

Chapter 4
Long Life and Short Life of Man Decided by the Sky

Master Bogao asked Qibo, "I have heard that the body is either of lentitude or of urgency, Qi is either of exuberance or of decline, the bones are either large or small, the flesh is either hard or brittle, the skin is either thick or thin. Can [such conditions] differentiate long [life] and short [life]?"

Qibo answered, "[In] human beings, [when] there is body, there is Qi; [when] there is Qi, there is bone; [when] there is bone, there is flesh; [when] there is flesh, there is skin. The body must be integrated with Qi; the skin must be combined with flesh; Qi, blood, meridians and collaterals must cooperate with the body. [Those whose] body is strong and the skin is smooth [can live a] long life. [Those whose] body is strong but the skin is spasmatic [will live a] short life. [When] the body is strong and the vessels are hard and large, [it indicates that] Qi and blood [will flow] smoothly, and smooth [flow of Qi and blood] ensures long life. [When] the body is strong but the vessels are small and weak, [it indicates that] Qi and blood will decline, and decline [of Qi and blood] threatens [life]. [When] the body is strong but the cheekbone is not protruding, [it indicates that] the flesh is stronger than the bones. [In this case, if] the bones are large, [there will be] a long life; [if] the bones are small, [there will be] a short life.

少师曰:"伯高非知在人之夭者乎? 在天之夭,难回也。在人之夭,易延也。吾亦修吾之夭,以全天命乎。"

陈士铎曰:"天之夭难延,人之夭易延,亦训世延人之夭也。伯高之论,因天师之教而推广,不可轻天师而重伯高也。"

【今译】

伯高太师问岐伯:"我听说形有缓急之分,气有盛衰之分,骨有大小之分,肉有坚脆之分,皮有厚薄之分,可否以此来区分长寿与短命呢?"

岐伯说:"人有形就会有气,人有气就会有骨,人有骨就会有肉,人有肉就会有皮。形必然与气相结合,皮必然与肉相对应,气血经络必然与形相配合,形体充盈且皮肤舒缓的人,必然长寿。形体充盈但皮肤却拘急的,则寿命短暂。形体充盈而脉象坚大的,气血就会顺畅,气血顺畅的就会长寿。形体充盈但脉象小弱的,气血就会衰弱,气血衰弱就有危急。形体充盈而颧骨不高的,说明肌肉胜过骨骼,骨骼大则长寿。骨骼小则短命。形体充盈并且壮硕的,肌肉坚实而纹理分明,皮肤胜于肌肉,肌肉松疏的寿命就短,肌肉厚实的寿命就长。形体充盈而壮硕但却没有纹理的,皮肤仅仅能包住肌肉,肌肉厚实的就会长寿,肌肉松脆的就会夭折。这是上天赋予人生的机理,人是不可强求的。所以根据人的外在表现就可以确定其寿命是长还是短,就可以预测人的生死了。"

少师问:"正如天师所说的那样,人的寿命长短是由上天决定的,这与人的预防有无关系呢?"

[When] the body is strong and large, the fleshes are sturdy and the texture of interstices is clear, [it indicates that] the skin outstrips the fleshes. [In this case, if] the fleshes are loose, life [will be] short; [if] the fleshes are sturdy, life [will be] long. [When] the body is strong but the fleshes bear no texture of interstices, [it indicates that] the skin can just encase the fleshes. [In this case, if] the fleshes are thick, life [will be] long; [if] the fleshes are brittle, life [will be] short. Such [conditions are] provided by the sky[1] and human beings cannot change. Thus [physical] manifestations [of a person can] decide [whether] his life is long or short and foretell his life and death."

Shaoshi[2] asked, "What you have said is right. Long life and short life of human beings are decided by the sky. Does it have nothing to do with prevention [made by] human beings?"

Qibo answered, "Long life and short life are decided by the sky, but it can be redeemed by human beings. [Although] long life and short life depend on [the arrangement of] the sky, damage of the body, dissipation of essence and marrow, and exhaustion of Qi and blood [made by human beings will cause] death before the age [decided by] the sky. The sky will not be responsible [for such cases]."

Shaoshi asked, "Can [life arranged by] the sky be redeemed?"

Qibo answered, "[The life arranged by] the sky cannot be redeemed, but it can be saved. To save sufficiency [offered by] the sky[3] and to supplement insufficiency of human [body], is it not the right way to protect life?"

Master Bogao said: "Celestial Master are adept at talking about the sky. People in this world damage [what] the sky [has provided

岐伯说:"人的寿命长短取决于天,但挽回其寿命则取决于人。寿命长短取决于天,但残害人的形骸,泻泄人的精髓,耗散人的气血,还没有达到天命指数就已经夭折了,这个责任却不在于天。"

少师问:"天命能挽回吗?"

岐伯说:"天命是不可挽回的,但天命却是可以节制的。天命节制了,就不会耗费,就能弥补人体的不足,这就是善于保全人的天命。"

伯高太师听后说:"岐伯天师真的精于解说天命啊!世人损害上天的不足,怎么能为人留下有余之机呢?"

少师说:"伯高不知道这取决于人的天命吗?取决于天命的夭折,是无法挽回的。取决于人的夭折,则易于延长。我也要修养我的天命,以便保全天命。"

陈士铎评论说:"因天命而导致的夭折,难以延续;因人为而造成的夭折,则易于延长。这也是在训导人们努力延长寿命。伯高的论述,是因受天师的教导而推而广之。所以不能轻视天师的教导而重视伯高的论述。"

and therefore make it]⁴ insufficient. How can [they] preserve sufficiency for human beings?"

Shaoshi said, "Does Bogao not know that [the life of] man depends on the sky? Short life originating from the sky cannot be redeemed. [But] short life caused by human beings can be redeemed. I am also cultivating [life offered by] the sky in order to fully preserve my life."

Chen Shiduo's comment, "[The idea that] short life [caused by] the sky cannot be redeemed and short life [caused by] human beings can be redeemed is to persuade people to cultivate and prolong their lives. Because of the Celestial Master's instruction, Bogao's idea is popularized. Therefore we cannot neglect the Celestial Master's instruction and just pay attention to Bogao's idea."

Notes

[1] It means that such conditions are natural and cannot be changed.

[2] Shaoshi (少师) was the minister of Yellow Emperor and also a great doctor in remote antiquity.

[3] Sufficiency offered by the sky means that natural life span is long enough. But it also depends on the improvement, cultivation and protection of human beings.

[4] Human beings in secular world usually only care about materials, neglecting life cultivation and integration with the natural world. That is why they often unconsciously damage their body and weaken their life.

命根养生篇第五

【原文】

伯高太师复问岐伯曰："养生之道,可得闻乎?"

岐伯曰："愚何足以知之?"

伯高再问,岐伯曰："人生天地之中,不能与天地并久者,不体天地之道也。天赐人以长生之命,地赐人以长生之根。天地赐人以命根者,父母予之也。合父母之精,以生人之身,则精即人之命根也。魂魄藏于精之中,魂属阳,魄属阴,魂趋生,魄趋死。夫魂魄皆神也。凡人皆有神,内存则生,外游则死。魂最善游,由于心之不寂也。广成子谓'抱神以静'者,正抱心而同寂也。"

伯高曰："夫精者,非肾中之水乎? 水性主动,心之不寂者,不由于肾之不静乎?"

岐伯曰："肾水之中,有真火在焉。水欲下而火欲升,此精之所以不静也。精一动而心摇摇矣。然而制精之不动,仍在心之寂也。"

伯高曰："吾心寂矣,肾之精欲动,奈何?"

岐伯曰："水火原相须也,无火则水不安,无水则火亦不安。制心而精动者,由于肾水之涸也。补先天之水以济心,则精不动而心易寂矣。"

Volume 1

【英译】

Chapter 5
The Root of Life in Cultivating Life

Master Bogao again asked Qibo, "Could I know the way to cultivate life?"

Qibo answered, "How can I know it?"

Bogao asked again, Qibo said, "Human beings live between the sky and earth. [If they] cannot live together with the sky and earth[1], [it indicates that they have] failed to understand Dao (law) of the sky and earth. The sky has offered long life [for human beings] and the earth has offered the root for long life [of human beings]. The root of life provided by the sky and earth is offered through parents. Integration of the essence from father and mother has constituted the body of a person. [That is to say that] the essence is the root of life. The ethereal soul and corporeal soul are stored in the essence. The ethereal soul belongs to Yang and the corporeal soul belongs to Yin. The ethereal soul tends [to promote] life while the corporeal soul tends [to cause] death. Thus both the ethereal soul and the corporeal soul are all spirit. All human beings have spirit. [When the spirit is] kept inside [the body], [it will protect] life; [when the spirit is] wandering outside [the body], [it will cause] death. The ethereal soul tends to wander [outside the body] because the heart is not calm. Guang Chengzi said, 'Keep the spirit to calm [the heart]'. [It means] to keep the heart [calm]

陈远公曰："精出于水,亦出于水中之火也。精动,由于火动;火不动,则精安能摇乎? 可见,精动由于心动也。心动之极,则水火俱动矣! 故安心为利精之法也。"

【今译】

伯高太师又问岐伯："关于养生的道理,可以讲给我听听吗?"

岐伯说："我很愚笨,怎么能知道养生的道理呢?"

伯高再次请问,岐伯说："人生于天地之间,但却不能与天地共存,是因为没有体察到天地之道啊! 上天赐予人长生之命,大地赐予人长生之根。天地赐予人以长生的命根,是通过父母赋予子女的。父母之精的交融,形成了人的身体,精就是人的命根啊。魂与魄储藏于精之中,魂属于阳,魄属于阴,魂趋向于生,魄趋向于死。但魂与魄都是神。所以凡是人都有神,神内存于体内,人就可以生存;神外游于体外,人就会死亡。魂之所以最善于出游,是由于人的心不寂静。广成子说:'只有保持神的清静,才能保持心的寂静。'"

伯高说："难道精不是肾中之水吗? 水的本性是主动,心之所以不寂静,难道不是由于肾水的不宁静吗?"

岐伯说："肾水之中有真火的存在。水趋向于下行,而火则趋向于上升,这就是精不宁静的缘故。精只要一动,心就会摇摇欲动。然而要想控制精,使其不动,仍然在于心的寂静。"

伯高说："我的心寂静了,但肾中之精又欲动,这是什么原因呢?"

岐伯说："水火原本是相辅相成的,没有火水就不能安静,没有水

together [with the ethereal soul]."

Bogao asked, "Is the essence not the water in the kidney? The water tends to move and the heart is not calm. Is it caused by kidney [-water that is] not calm?"

Qibo answered, "In kidney-water, there is true fire. Water tends to [flow] downwards while fire tends [to flame] upwards. That is why the essence is not calm. [When] the essence moves, the heart is uneasy. However to prevent the essence from moving still depends on tranquility of the heart."

Bogao asked, "My heart is calm. But why does the essence still tend to move?"

Qibo answered, "Originally water and fire are opposite and complementary. Without fire, water cannot be quiet; without water, fire cannot be quiet. [When] the heart is tranquilized but the essence still moves, [it is caused by] dryness of kidney-water. To supplement innate water [in the kidney] will cultivate the heart. [Only when] the essence is unmovable can the heart be tranquil."

Chen Yuangong's[2] comment, " The essence originates from water, and also from fire in the water. Movement of the essence is due to movement of fire. [If] fire does not move, how could the essence shake? Obviously movement of the essence is caused by uneasiness of the heart. [When] the heart is extremely uneasy, both water and fire will simultaneously move. Thus to tranquilize the heart is the way to replenish the essence."

火也不能安宁。控制了心但精却欲动的,这是由于肾水之干涸了的缘故。这就需要补益先天的肾水以辅济心内之火,这样精就不妄动,心就易于寂静。"

陈远公评论说:"精既源自于水,也出之于水中之火。精之所以动,是由于火气之动。如果火不动,精怎么能摇动呢?可见,精动是由于心动。心动到了极点,水火就会一起动。所以,安心就是有利于补精的要法。"

Volume 1

Notes

［1］To live together with the sky and earth means to live as long as that of the sky and earth.

［2］Chen Yuangong（陈远公）is another name of Chen Shiduo （陈士铎）.

救母篇第六

【原文】

容成问于岐伯曰:"天癸之水,男女皆有之,何以妇人经水谓之天癸乎?"

岐伯曰:"天癸水,壬癸之水也。壬水属阳,癸水属阴,二水者先天之水也。男为阳,女为阴,故妇人经水以天癸名之。其实壬癸未尝不合也。"

容成曰:"男子之精,不以天癸名者,又何故欤?"

岐伯曰:"精者,合水火名之。水中有火,始成其精。呼精而壬癸之义已包于内,故不以天癸名之。"

容成曰:"精与经同一水也,何必两名之?"

岐伯曰:"同中有异也。男之精,守而不溢;女之经,满而必泄也。癸水者,海水也,上应月,下应潮,月有盈亏,潮有往来,女子之经水应之,故潮汐月有信,经水亦月有期也。以天癸名之,别其水为癸水,随天运为转移耳。"

容成曰:"其色赤者何也?"

岐伯曰:"男之精,阳中之阴也,其色白。女之经,阴中之阳也,其色赤。况流于任脉,通于血海,血与经合而成浊流矣。"

容成曰:"男之精亏而不溢者,又何也?"

Volume 1

【英译】

Chapter 6
To Rescue Mother[1]

Rongcheng[2] asked Qibo, "There is water [known as] Tiangui[3] in both men and women. Why is only women's menstruation called Tiangui?"

Qibo answered, "[The so-called] Tiangui water refers to Ren[4] water and Gui[5] water. Ren water belongs to Yang and Gui water belongs to Yin, both of which are innate water. Men belong to Yang and women belong to Yin. That is why menstruation in woman is called Tiangui. Actually both Ren [water] and Gui [water] are fit in with [Tiangui water]."

Rongcheng asked, "[But] why is semen in men not called Tiangui?"

Qibo answered, "Semen [in men] is so named in combination with water and fire. There is fire in water and [that is why it can] transform into semen. [The reason to] call [the essence transformed from water] semen [is that it] contains the implication of Ren [water] and Gui [water]. That is why it is not called Taingui."

Rongcheng asked, "Semen and menstruation originate from the same water. Why are they named in two ways?"

Qibo answered, "[Although they are] the same, there is still difference. Semen in man just remains inside and will not [periodically] spill over; menstruation in woman must excrete

岐伯曰："女子阴有余阳不足,故满而必泄。男子阳有余阴不足,故守而不溢也。"

容成曰："味咸者何也?"

岐伯曰："壬癸之水,海水也。海水味咸,故天癸之味应之。"

容成曰："女子二七经行,稚女不行经何也?"

岐伯曰："女未二七则任冲未盛,阴气未动,女犹纯阳也,故不行经耳。"

容成曰："女过二七,不行经而怀孕者,又何也?"

岐伯曰："女之变者也,名为暗经,非无经也。无不足,无有余,乃女中最贵者。终身不字,行调息之功,必长生也。"

容成问曰："妇女经水,上应月,下应潮,宜月无愆期矣。何以有至有不至乎?"

岐伯曰："人事之乖违也。天癸之水,生于先天,亦长于后天也。妇女纵欲伤任督之脉,则经水不应月矣。怀抱忧郁以伤肝胆,则经水闭而不流矣。"

容成曰："其故何也?"

岐伯曰："人非水火不生,火乃肾中之真火,水乃肾中之真水也。水火盛则经盛,水火衰则经衰。任督脉通于肾,伤任督未有不伤肾者。交接时,纵欲泄精,精伤任督之脉亦伤矣。任督脉伤,不能行其气于腰脐,则带脉亦伤,经水有至有不至矣。夫经水者,火中之水也。水衰不能制火,则火炎水降,经水必先期至矣。火衰不能生水,则水寒火冷,经水必后期至矣。经水之愆期,因水火之盛衰也。"

[periodically when it is] full. Gui water is sea water, corresponding to the moon in the upper and tide in the lower. The moon either waxes or wanes and tide runs to and fro, to which menstruation in woman correspond. That is why every month there is a cycle of tide and a period of menstruation. To name [menstruation] Tiangui is to demonstrate [the fact that] this water is Gui water [which] transfers in correspondence to movement of the sky[6]."

Rongcheng asked, "Why is the color red?"

Qibo answered, "[In] semen in men, there is Yin within Yang, [that is why] its color is white; [in] menstruation in women, there is Yang within Yin, [that is why] its color is red. In addition, [menstruation] flows in the conception vessel and runs into the blood sea[7]. Combination of the blood and menstruation makes it into turbid liquid."

Rongcheng asked, "Why is semen in men often deficient rather than sufficient?"

Qibo answered, "[In] women, Yin is excessive but Yang is insufficient. That is why [menstruation] must excrete [when it is] full. [In] men, Yang is excessive but Yin is insufficient. That is why [semen usually] remains [inside the body] and seldom spill out."

Rongcheng asked, "Why does it taste salty?"

Qibo answered, "[Because] Ren [water] and Gui [water] are both sea water. Sea water is salty and that is why the taste of Tiangui [water] corresponds to it."

Rongcheng asked, "Women begin to have menstruation at the age of fourteen. Why do young girls not have menstruation?"

容成曰："肝胆伤而经闭者,谓何?"

岐伯曰："肝藏血者也,然又最喜疏泄。胆与肝为表里也,胆木气郁,肝木之气亦郁矣。木郁不达,任冲血海皆抑塞不通,久则血枯矣。"

容成曰："木郁何以使水之闭也?"

岐伯曰："心肾无暑不交者也。心肾之交接,责在胞胎,亦责在肝胆也。肝胆气郁,胞胎上交肝胆,不上交于心,则肾之气亦不交于心矣。心肾之气不交,各脏腑之气抑塞不通,肝克脾,胆克胃,脾胃受克,失其生化之司,何能资于心肾乎? 水火未济,肝胆之气愈郁矣。肝胆久郁,反现假旺之象,外若盛,内实虚。肾因子虚,转去相济涸水,而郁火焚之,木安有余波以下泄乎? 此木郁所以水闭也。"

鬼臾区问曰："气郁则血闭,血即经乎?"

岐伯曰："经水,非血也。"

鬼臾区曰："经水非血,何以血闭而经即断乎?"

岐伯曰："经水者,天一之水也,出于肾经,故以经水名之。血闭者,经水则失动生之源,故血闭经断矣。"

鬼臾区曰："水出于肾,色宜白矣,何赤乎?"

岐伯曰："经水者,至阴之精,有至阳之气存焉,故色赤耳,非色赤即血也。"

鬼臾区曰："人之肾有补无泻,安有余血乎?"

岐伯曰："经水者,肾气所化,非肾精所泄也。女子肾气有余,故变化无穷耳。"

鬼臾区曰："气能化血,各经之血不从之而泄乎?"

Qibo answered, "Before the age of fourteen in women, the conception [vessel] and thoroughfare [vessel] are not strong enough, Yin Qi is still static, and there seems to have only Yang [Qi]. That is why there is no menstruation."

Rongcheng asked, "After the age of fourteen, a woman may not have menstruation but still can be pregnant. What is the reason?"

Qibo answered, "[This is a sort of menstrual] change in woman, called latent menstruation, not absence of menstruation. [In women with latent menstruation,] there is no insufficiency and no excess, [which is a] best [condition] in women. [If such a woman] does not get married all her life and is able to exhale the stale and inhale the fresh, [she] will live a long life."

Rongcheng asked, "Menstruation in women, corresponding to the moon in the upper and tide in the lower, should not be irregular. But why is it sometimes regular and sometimes irregular?"

Qibo answered, "[This is the result of] indulging in sensual pleasures. Tiangui water is innate and develops after birth. [In] women, indulging in sensual pleasures will damage the conception vessel and governor vessel, causing irregular menstruation. [If there is] depression and anxiety [in the heart, it will] damage the liver and gallbladder, consequently resulting in amenorrhea."

Rongcheng asked, "What is the reason?"

Qibo answered, "Without water and fire, human beings cannot exist [because] fire is the true fire in the kidney and water is the true water in the kidney. [Only when] water and fire are exuberant, [can] menstruation be exuberant. [If] water and fire

44

黄帝外经英译

岐伯曰："肾化为经,经化为血,各经气血无不随之而各化矣。是以肾气通则血通,肾气闭则血闭也。"

鬼臾区曰："然则气闭宜责在肾矣,何以心肝脾之气郁而经亦闭也?"

岐伯曰："肾水之生,不由于三经。肾水之化,实关于三经也。"

鬼臾区曰："何也?"

岐伯曰："肾不通肝之气,则肾气不能开。肾不交心之气,则肾气不能上。肾不取脾之气,则肾气不能成。盖交相合而交相化也。苟一经气郁,气即不入于肾,而肾气即闭矣。况三经同郁,肾无所资,何能化气而成经乎?是以经闭者,乃肾气之郁,非止肝血之枯也。倘徒补其血,则郁不宣反生火矣。徒散其瘀,则气益微反耗精矣。非惟无益,而转害之也。"

鬼臾区曰："大哉言乎!请勒之金石,以救万世之母乎。"

陈远公曰："一篇救母之文,真有意于母者也!讲天癸无余义,由于讲水火无余义也。水火之不通,半成人气之郁。解郁之法,在于通肝胆也,肝胆通则血何闭哉?正不必又去益肾也。谁知肝胆不郁,而肾受益乎?郁之害,亦大矣!"

【今译】

容成问岐伯："天癸之水男女都有,为什么只将妇女的经水称为天癸呢?"

are debilitated, menstruation will also be debilitated. The conception vessel and the governor vessel are interlinked with the kidney. [When] the conception vessel and governor vessel are damaged, the kidney is inevitable. [In] sexual activity, indulgence in sensual pleasures will exhaust essence. [When] essence is damaged, the conception vessel and governor vessel are inevitable. [When] the conception vessel and governor vessel are damaged, Qi cannot be transferred to the waist and navel, [inevitably] resulting in damage of the belt vessel and amenorrhea. Menstruation is the water in fire. [When] water is debilitated, [it] cannot control fire. [As a result,] fire will be blazing, water will be declined, and menstruation will certainly occur in advance. [When] fire is debilitated, [it] cannot produce fire, consequently leading to chilly water and cold fire [as well as] delayed menorrhea. Irregular menstruation is the result of exuberance or debilitation of water and fire."

Rongcheng asked, "Why does damage of the liver and gallbladder lead to amenorrhea?"

Qibo answered, "The liver stores the blood and likes to soothe[8]. The gallbladder and the liver are internally and externally [related to each other]. [When] Qi in the gallbladder-wood is stagnated, Qi in the liver-wood is also stagnated[9]. [When] wood[10] is stagnated and cannot relax, the conception vessel, the thoroughfare vessel and the blood sea will be blocked, long-term blockage [of which will cause] dryness of the blood."

Rongcheng asked, "Why will stagnation of wood block water?"

Qibo answered, "The heart and the kidney never cease mutual

岐伯说:"天癸之水指的是壬癸这两种水。壬水属于阳,癸水属于阴,这两种水是先天之水。男为阳,女为阴,所以妇女的经水以天癸命名。其实称为壬癸二水,也未尝不合适。"

容成问:"男子之精不以天癸命名,又是什么原因呢?"

岐伯说:"男子之精,综合起来以水火命名之。水中有火,才能构成男子之精。将其称为'精'就已经包含了壬癸之义,所以不用天癸命名。"

容成问:"精与经同样是水,何必用两个词来命名呢?"

岐伯说:"相同之中也存在着差异。男子之精可以固守而不溢出;女子之经水一旦满了,就必须排泄出来。癸水是海水,在上应对月亮,在下应对潮水,月亮有盈亏,潮水有往来,女子的经水与之相对应。所以潮汐每月有周期,女子经水每月也有周期。用天癸命名月经,以便说明其中的水为癸水,并随着天然规律而转移。"

容成问:"为什么月经是赤色的呢?"

岐伯说:"男子的精液,阳中有阴,其颜色为白色。女子月经,阴中有阳,其颜色为红色。况且月经流行于任脉之中,贯通于血海之中,血与经气相融合,因而变成混浊的液体。"

容成问:"男子的精液因亏损而不能溢出的,又是什么原因呢?"

岐伯说:"女子阴有余而阳不足,因此血满就必然要排泄;男子阳有余而阴不足,所以只要坚守就不会溢出。"

容成问:"为什么味道是咸的呢?"

岐伯说:"壬癸之水,属于海水。海水的味道是咸的,所以天癸之

communication. The mutual communication between the heart and the kidney depends on the uterus and also relies on the liver and gallbladder. [When Qi in] the liver and gallbladder are stagnated, the uterus will communicate with the liver and gallbladder, but will not communicate with the heart, making it impossible for Qi in the kidney to communicate with the heart. Failure of Qi in the heart and kidney to communicate with each other [will result in] obstruction and blockage of Qi in all the viscera, consequently the liver restricting the spleen and the gallbladder restricting the stomach. [When] the spleen and stomach are restricted, there is no function of transformation. How can they support the heart and kidney? [When] water and fire are not supported, Qi in the liver and gallbladder tend to become stagnated. [When] the liver and gallbladder have become stagnated for a long time, there will be a phenomenon of false exuberance [characterized by] external exuberance and internal deficiency. [When] the kidney tends to support dry water due to deficiency of the liver, [it will be] burned by stagnated fire. [In this case,] how can wood have extra energy to excrete? This is the reason why water is blocked."

Gui Yuqu asked, "Qi stagnation will cause blood block. Does the blood refer to menstruation?"

Qibo answered, "[It refers to] menstrual water[11], not the blood."

Gui Yuqu asked, "If menstrual water is not the blood, why does menstruation stop [when] the blood is blocked?"

Qibo answered, "Menstruation water is the water of celestial one[12] from the kidney. That is why it is called menstrual water."

味也与之相应。"

容成问:"女子十四岁就来月经,为什么幼女不来月经呢?"

岐伯说:"女子十四岁时,冲脉和任脉没有充盛,阴气也没有启动,这些女子犹如纯阳之体,所以就不来月经。"

容成问:"女子十四岁以后,不来月经也可以怀孕,这是什么原因呢?"

岐伯说:"这是女子月经的变化,称为'暗经',并不是没有月经。这样的女子不存在'不足'的问题,也不存在'有余'的问题,这是女子中最难得的生理现象。这样的女子如果终身不嫁,并坚持练习吐纳之功,就必然会长寿。"

容成问:"妇女的经水在上对应月象,在下对应潮水,每月应当不会不准时吧,为什么有时应当来月经但反而没有来呢?"

岐伯说:"这是纵欲的后果。天癸之水,生于先天,长于后天。如果女子纵欲,就会损伤任督之脉,这样经水就不会应于月象了。如果女子心中抑郁,就会伤害了肝胆,从而导致闭经,月经就闭阻不来了。"

容成问:"原因是什么呢?"

岐伯说:"人没有了水火就不能生存。火是肾中的真火,水是肾中的真水。水火旺盛则经气就会旺盛,水火衰弱则经气就会衰弱。任督二脉通于肾脏,如果任脉和督脉遭受了损伤,肾脏也会遭受损伤。性交时纵欲,不但泄精,而且伤精,任脉和督脉也随之受到伤害。如果任脉和督脉遭受损伤,就不能将气输送到腰部和脐部,带脉也会因之而遭受损伤,这样月经就会在该出现的时候而不能出现。经水是火中之水,水

Gui Yuqu asked, "Water from the kidney should be white in color. Why is [menstrual water] red?"

Qibo answered, "Menstrual water is the essence of extreme Yin [in which] there is also Qi from extreme Yang. That is why the color is red. [Water] red in color is not necessarily the blood."

Gui Yuqu asked, "[In] human kidney, there is only in need of tonification[13], not purgation. Why is there extra blood?"

Qibo answered, "Menstrual water is transformed by kidney-Qi, not discharged by kidney essence. Kidney-Qi in women is often excessive. That is why there are always changes."

Gui Yuqu asked, "Qi can transform the blood. Does the blood from each meridian excrete in such a way?"

Qibo answered, "The kidney transforms meridians, the meridians transform the blood, Qi and blood from each meridian transform in the same way. Thus [only when] kidney-Qi is disinhibited can the blood be disinhibited, [only when] kidney-Qi is blocked can the blood be blocked."

Gui Yuqu asked, "It is the kidney [that is] responsible for Qi blockage. Why does stagnation of Qi from the heart, liver and spleen also cause amenorrhea?"

Qibo answered, "[Although] the production of kidney-water is not from these three meridians, the transformation of kidney-water is actually related to these three meridians."

Gui Yuqu asked, "What is the reason?"

Qibo answered, "[If] the kidney fails to connect with Qi in the liver, kidney-Qi cannot be open. [If] the kidney fails to communicate with Qi in the heart, kidney-Qi cannot [flow]

衰就不能制火,就会导致火炎而水降,月经必然会先期而至。火衰则不能生水,就会导致水寒火冷,月经必然会因此而迟来。经水不能按期而来,就是因水火盛衰而引起。"

容成问:"肝胆受到损伤后就会闭经,这是什么意思呢?"

岐伯说:"肝脏藏血,但又最喜欢疏泄。胆与肝互为表里,如果胆木之气抑郁了,肝木之气也会随之抑郁了。如果木气因抑郁而不能舒泄,任脉和冲脉的血海都会因郁塞而不通,久而久之就会导致经血枯竭。"

容成问:"木气抑郁为何会使水闭塞呢?"

岐伯说:"心肾无时无刻不相交。心肾之间的相互交接,主要在于胞胎,同时也在于肝胆。肝胆之气抑郁,胞胎就只能上交于肝胆,而不能上交于心,这样肾之气也不能上交于心。心肾之气不相交,各脏腑之气就会因之而郁塞不通。肝克脾,胆克胃,脾胃遭受克制,就会失去生化的职责,怎么还能得到心肾的资助呢?水火未济,肝胆之气也就会更加抑郁。肝胆抑郁时间长了,反而会出现虚假的旺盛之象,外表似乎旺盛,内部则确实虚弱。由于肝脏虚,肾脏就转而资济干涸之水,从而引起郁火的焚烧,木怎么能有余力下泄呢?这就是木郁导致水闭的原因。"

鬼臾区问道:"气郁血闭,血就是经血吗?"

岐伯说:"经水并非血液。"

鬼臾区问:"既然经水不是血液,但为什么血液闭塞就会导致月经不通呢?"

upwards. [If] the kidney fails to get Qi from the spleen, kidney-Qi cannot be formed. Only mutual communication can ensure mutual tansformation. If Qi just from one meridian is stagnated, Qi cannot enter the kidney and kidney-Qi will be blocked. If [Qi from] three meridians is all stagnated, the kidney cannot be supported. [In this case,] how can Qi be transformed into menstruation? That is why amenorrhea is caused by stagnation of kidney-Qi, not just by dryness of liver blood. If [measures are taken] only to tonify the blood, stagnation cannot be resolved. On the countrary, fire will be produced. [If measures are taken] only to dissipate [blood] stasis, Qi is just slightly replenished, but essence is seriously dissipated. [Such a way of treatment] is not just ineffective, but quite harmful.

Gui Yuqu said, "How great [your analysis] is! Please carve it on metal and stone to rescue mothers in all generations."

Chen Yuangong's comment, "This chapter about how to rescue mother is quite significant in [treating] mother. There is no extra meaning in talking about Tiangui because there is no extra meaning in talking about water and fire. Inhibition of water and fire is responsible for half of Qi stagnation. The way to resolve stagnation depends on disinhibition of the liver and gallbladder. [If] the liver and gallbladder are disinhibited, how can the blood become blocked? This is why it is unnecessary to just replenish the kidney. Who knows [that only when] the liver and gallbladder are not stagnated can the kidney be replenished? The harm [caused by] stagnation [of the liver and gallbladder] is so serious!"

岐伯说:"经水是天一之水,出自于肾经,因此以经水命名。如果血液闭塞了,经水就失去了生化之源,血液也就因此而闭塞,月经也就因此而断绝。"

鬼臾区问:"经水出自于肾脏,颜色应当是白的,但为什么是红的呢?"

岐伯说:"经水是至阴之精,其中存在着至阳之气,所以其颜色为红色。但颜色红的并不一定都是血液。"

鬼臾区问:"人的肾脏只有补没有泻,为何会有多余的血液呢?"

岐伯说:"经水是肾脏所化生的,不是肾精所排泄的。女子的肾气有余,所以其变化是无穷的。"

鬼臾区问:"气能化血,各经脉的血液不会随之而排泄吗?"

岐伯说:"肾化生为经,经化生为血,各经络中的气血无不随之而变化。所以肾气通畅血液就会流通,肾气闭塞血液也会闭塞。"

鬼臾区问:"气闭塞主要在于肾,但为什么心肝脾的气郁也会导致闭经呢?"

岐伯说:"肾水的生发,虽然不是由于心肝脾这三经,但肾水的变化,却还是与这三经相关的。"

鬼臾区问:"为什么呢?"

岐伯说:"如果肾脏不能通肝之气,肾气就不能开启;如果肾脏不与心之气相交,肾气就不能上行;如果肾脏不能资取脾之气,肾气就不能形成。这是因为只有相互交合才能引发互相之间的变化。如果只是一经之气抑郁,气就不能进入于肾脏,肾气就会因之而闭塞了!何况三

Notes

［1］This chapter discusses about how to treat woman diseases.

［2］Rongcheng（容成）was the minister of Yellow Emperor, seeming to be an expert of woman disease.

［3］Tiangui（天癸）refers to necessary element responsible for development of the body and reproductive function.

［4］Ren（壬）is number nine in Tian Gan（天干，Heavenly Stems）.

［5］Gui（癸）is number ten in Tian Gan（天干，Heavenly Stems）.

［6］Movement of the sky refers to natural law or natural changes.

［7］In traditional Chinese medicine，blood sea（血海）means three things，i. e. the thoroughfare vessel，liver and Xuehai（SP 10）.

［8］Soothe（疏泄），also translated as free coursing，referring to the function of the liver that ensures the free movement of Qi and prevents Qi stagnation.

［9］When the five zang-organs match with the five elements, the liver pertains to wood. Since the gallbladder is internally and externally related to the liver，it also pertains to wood. That is why the gallbladder and the liver are traditionally also called gallbladder-wood and liver-wood.

［10］Wood here refers to the liver and gallbladder.

［11］Menstrual water（经水）refers to menorrhea.

［12］The so-called celestial one（天一）refers to the innate water. This concept was first used in the sentence "when the sky

条经脉同时郁闭，肾脏就得不到任何的资助，怎么能化气而成经呢？所以经闭就是肾脏气的郁闭，并非仅仅为肝血的枯竭。如果单纯补血，郁气就得不到宣发，火反而会产生了！如果只是散瘀，气就会更加衰微，精也会因之而耗伤。这样做不仅无益，反而为害。"

鬼臾区说："解释得真好啊！请刻在金石之上，以便救万世之母啊！"

陈远公评论说："一篇救母之文，真的有益于母啊！讲述天癸没有其他意义，是由于讲述水火也没有其他意义。水火不通畅，一半是由于人体之气的郁闭所造成的。解除气郁的方法，在于通畅肝胆。肝胆通畅了，血液又怎么能闭塞呢？所以根本不必要单纯地去补肾。谁知道肝胆不郁，肾脏就会受益呢？肝胆郁闭所造成的危害，原来如此之大啊！"

follows the Dao to move，it will become fine and bright"（天得一则清）in *Dao De Jing*（《道德经》，*Canon of Dao and Morality*）written by Laozi（老子），in which Tian（天）refers to the sky and Yi（一）refers to the Dao that governs the constitution and movement of the sky.

[13] The word "tonification" is the noun of "tonify". Please see [5] in Chapter 3.

红铅损益篇第七

【原文】

容成问曰："方士采红铅接命，可为训乎？"

岐伯天师曰："慎欲者采之，服食延寿；纵欲者采之，服食丧躯。"

容成曰："人能慎欲，命自可延，何藉红铅乎？"

岐伯曰："红铅，延景丹也。"

容成曰："红铅者，天癸水也。虽包阴阳之水火，溢满于外则水火之气尽消矣，何以接命乎？"

岐伯曰："公之言，论天癸则可，非论首经之红铅也。经水甫出户辄色变，独首经之色不遽变者，全其阴阳之气也。男子阳在外，阴在内；女子阴在外，阳在内。首经者，坎中之阳也。以坎中之阳补离中之阴，益乎，不益乎？独补男有益，补女有损。补男者，阳以济阴也；补女者，阳以亢阳也。"

容成曰："善。"

陈远公曰："红铅何益于人，讲无益而成有益者，辨其既济之理也。谁谓方士非恃之以接命哉？"

Volume 1

【英译】

Chapter 7
Menarche: Damage and Benefit

Rongcheng asked, "Fang Shi[1] obtains menarche to prolong life. Is it necessary?"

Celestial Master Qibo answered, "[When those who are quite] careful in sexuality collect menarche and take [it], life will be prolonged; [when those who] indulge in sexuality collect menarche and take [it], life will be lost."

Rongcheng asked, "Sexual abstinence will certainly prolong life. Why is it related to menarche?"

Qibo answered, "Menarche is [a unique] bolus for prolonging life."

Rongcheng asked, "Menarche is Tiangui water. Although [it] contains both water and fire in Yin and Yang, [when it] overflows in the external, Qi from water and fire will be completely dispersed. How can it prolong life?"

Qibo answered, "What you have said can describe Tiangui, but cannot describe menarche. The color of menses changes immediately [after] discharge from the vagina, but the color of menarche will not change immediately [after discharge from the vagina because it] contains the whole of Qi from Yin and Yang. [In] men, Yang is in the external and Yin is in the internal. [But in] women, Yin is in the external and Yang is in the internal. Menarche represents Yang from Kan [Gua][2]. To use Yang from Kan [Gua] to supplement Yin in Li [Gua][3], is it

【今译】

容成请问道:"方士采取女子红铅以延长寿命,这种做法可取吗?"

岐伯说:"节欲之人,采取并服用红铅是可以延寿。纵欲之人,采取和服用红铅则会丧命。"

容成问:"人若能节制性欲,寿命自然就可延长,为何还要依靠红铅呢?"

岐伯说:"红铅是延景丹。"

容成问:"红铅是天癸之水,虽然包含有阴阳水火,但如果溢满于外,水火之气就会完全消散,为什么还能延长寿命呢?"

岐伯说:"你所谈的可以说明天癸,但却不能说明女子初潮的红铅。经水一从阴道流出就会变色,惟独初潮的红铅颜色不会随之变化,这是因为其保全了阴阳之气。男子阳在外,阴在内;女子阴在外,阳在内。首经为坎中之阳,用坎中阳补离中之阴,到底是有益还是无益呢?惟独补男子是有益的,而补女子则是有损伤的。补男子,是用阳来助阴;补女子,是以阳亢阳。

容成说:"好!"

陈远公说:"红铅对人有何好处?将无益说成有益,无非是辨明其济助之理。谁能说方士非得靠红铅来延续生命呢?"

effective or ineffective? [The fact is that it is] only effective in tonifying men [but] harmful in tonifying women. [To use it] to tonify men, Yang will support Yin; [to use it] to tonify women, Yang will stimulate Yang."

Rongcheng said, "Good!"

Chen Yuangong's comment, "How can menarche be beneficial to a man's [health]? To describe useless as useful [is just for the purpose of describing] the rule of tonification. Who has said that Fang Shi just depend on menarche to prolong their life?"[4]

Notes

[1] Fang Shi (方士): In ancient China, Fang Shi (方士) refers to people who worshiped Daoism and were familiar with various ceremonies in Daoism practice, or people who devoted themselves to the study and practice of doctrines related to astronomy, calendar, medicine, theurgy and augury, or the people who were familiar with and practiced the Dao.

[2] Kan Gua (坎卦) is the fifth diagram in Ba Gua (八卦, Eight Diagrams) created by Fu Xi (伏羲) in the remote antiquity. In Ba Gua (八卦, Eight Diagrams), Kan Gua (坎卦) represents water, the structure of which contains two Yin and one Yang: the upper level and the lower level are Yin, the middle level is Yang.

[3] Li Gua (离卦) is the sixth diagram in the Ba Gua (八卦, Eight Diagrams), representing fire.

[4] Chen Yuangong's comment shows that he was doubtful about the idea related to application of menarche in this chapter.

初生微论篇第八

【原文】

容成问曰:"人之初生,目不能睹,口不能餐,足不能履,舌不能语,三月而后见,八月而后食,期岁而后行,三年而后言,其故何也?"

岐伯曰:"人之初生,两肾水火未旺也。三月而火乃盛,故两目有光也。八月而水乃充,故两龈有力也。期岁则髓旺而膑生矣。三年则精长而囟合矣。男十六天癸通,女十四天癸化。"

容成曰:"男以八为数,女以七为数,予知之矣。天师于二八、二七之前,《内经》何未言也?"

岐伯曰:"《内经》首论天癸者,叹天癸难生易丧也。男必至十六而天癸满,年未十六皆未满之日也。女必至十四而天癸盈,年未十四皆未满之日也。既满既盈,又随年俱耗,示人宜守此天癸也。"

容成曰:"男八八之后犹存,女七七之后仍在,似乎天癸之未尽也。天师何以七七、八八之后不再言之欤?"

岐伯曰:"予论常数耳,常之数可定,变之数不可定也。予所以论常不论变耳。"

陈远公曰:"人生以天癸为主,有则生,无则死也。常变之说,惜此天癸也。二七、二八之论,亦可言而言之,非不可言而不言也。"

Volume 1

【英译】

Chapter 8
Brief Discussion About Neonate

Rongcheng asked, "[When] a baby is just born, the eyes are unable to see; the mouth is unable to eat; the feet are unable to walk; and the tongue is unable to speak. Three months after [birth], [the baby is able] to see; eight months after [birth], [the baby is able] to eat; one year after [birth], [the baby is able] to walk; three years after [birth], [the baby is able] to speak. What is the reason?"

Qibo answered, "[When] a baby is just born, water and fire in the two kidneys are not effulgent. Three months [after birth], fire becomes effulgent and the two eyes are bright. Eight months [after birth], water is sufficient and the teeth are strong. One year [after birth], the marrow is vigorous and the patella is constituted. Three years [after birth], essene is formed and fontanelle is closed. [At the age of] sixteen, Tiangui[1] in men is freeing; [at the age of] fourteen, Tiangui in women is transformed."

Rongcheng asked, "You know that number eight represents men and number seven represents women. Why did Celestial Master not mention [the time] before sixteen and fourteen in Nei Jing[2]?"

Qibo answered, "[When] first discussing Tiangui in Nei Jing, [I have] sighed that Tiangui is difficult to form but easy to lose. Only [when reaching the age of] sixteen can a man have enough

【今译】

容成问："人刚出生的时候,目不能视,口不能食,足不能行,舌不能言。三个月后眼睛才能看见,八个月后才能张口饮食,一岁之后才能举步行走,三岁才能开口讲话。这是什么原因呢?"

岐伯说："人刚出生的时候,两个肾脏中的水火还没有旺盛。三个月后火气就旺盛了,因而双目就有光彩了。八个月后水气充盈,所以两龈才会有力。一岁时骨髓旺盛,膑骨就产生了。三岁时精气长成,所以囟门就愈合了。男子十六岁时天癸畅通,女子十四岁天癸化生。"

容成问："男子以八为数,女子以七为数,我已经知道了。对于男子十六岁、女子十四岁之前,天师在《内经》中为什么没有谈到呢?"

岐伯说:"《内经》首先论述了天癸,感叹天癸难以产生但却容易丧失。必须到十六岁时,男子的天癸才会充满,没有到十六岁就没有到充满的年龄。必须到十四岁时,女子天癸才会充盈,没有到十四岁就没有到充盈的年龄。既然到了一定年龄天癸已经充满充盈,但又会随着年龄的增长而慢慢全部消耗,这就是告诉人们应谨守天癸。"

容成问:"男子八八六十四岁后依然生存,女子七七四十九岁之后也依然生存,似乎天癸并没有全部耗尽。为什么在女子七七四十九和男子八八六十四岁之后,天师就不再论述有关天癸的问题了呢?"

岐伯说:"我讲述的只是常数而已。常数是可以论定的,变数却不能论定,所以我只讲述了常数而没有讲述变数。"

陈远公评论说:"人生以天癸为主,有天癸则生,无天癸则死。常数与变数之论,就是为了珍惜天癸。二七、二八的论述,也是可继续谈论的,并不是不能再论述的。"

Volume 1

Tiangui. [Before he has reached the age of] sixteen, [Tiangui] is always insufficient. [When] a woman has reached [the age of] fourteen, Tiangui is sufficient. [Before she has reached the age of] fourteen, [Tiangui] is always insufficient. [Although after the age of sixteen in men and fourteen in women, Tiangui is] sufficient and exuberant, but [it will be] eventually consumed as time flies, indicating the necessity to appropriately keep Tiangui."

Rongcheng asked, "After [the age of] sixty-four in men and forty-nine in women, Tiangui seems to be not completely consumed. Why did Celestial Master not discuss about it after [the age of] sixty-four [in men] and forty-nine [in women in Nei Jing]?"

Qibo answered, "What I have said [in Nei Jing] is about constants. Constant is definite while variable is indefinite. That is why [in Nei Jing] I have just talked about constants, not variables."

Chen Yuangong's comment, "Human life depends on Tiangui. Existence [of Tiangui] ensures life while loss [of Tiangui] causes death. Talking about constant and variable [is actually] to emphasize [the importance of] Tiangui. The discussion about [the age of] fourteen and sixteen is necessary, not unnecessary."

Notes

[1] Tiangui is explained in [3] in Chapter 6.

[2] Nei Jing is the abbreviation of *Huang Di Nei Jing* (《黄帝内经》, *Yellow Emperor's Internal Canon of Medicine*).

骨阴篇第九

【原文】

鸟师问于岐伯曰:"婴儿初生,无膝盖骨,何也?"

岐伯曰:"婴儿初生,不止无膝盖骨也,囟骨、耳后完骨皆无之。"

鸟师曰:"何故也?"

岐伯曰:"阴气不足也。阴气者,真阴之气也。婴儿纯阳无阴,食母乳而阴乃生,阴生而囟骨,耳后完骨、膝盖骨生矣。生则儿寿,不生则夭。"

鸟师曰:"其不生何也?"

岐伯曰:"三骨属阴,得阴则生,然亦必阳旺而长也。婴儿阳气不足,食母乳而三骨不生,其先天之阳气亏也。阳气先漓,先天已居于缺陷,食母之乳,补后天而无余,此三骨之所以不生也。三骨不生,又焉能延龄乎!"

鸟师曰:"三骨缺一,亦能生乎?"

岐伯曰:"缺一则不全乎其人矣。"

鸟师曰:"请悉言之。"

岐伯曰:"囟门不合则脑髓空也;完骨不长则肾宫虚也;膝盖不生则双足软也。脑髓空则风易入矣;肾宫虚则听失聪矣;双足软则颠仆多矣。"

Volume 1

【英译】

Chapter 9
Bones and Yin

Niaoshi[1] asked Qibo, "Why does the newborn baby have no kneecap?"

Qibo answered, "The newborn baby not only has no kneecap, but also has no frontal fontanelle and Wangu (GB 12) behind the ears."

Niaoshi asked, "What is the reason?"

Qibo answered, "[Because of] deficiency of Yin Qi. Yin Qi is Qi of true Yin[2]. [In] the newborn baby, [there is only] pure Yang but no Yin. [Only after] sucking milk [from] mother [can] Yin appear. [When] Yin has appeared, frontal fontanelle, Wangu (GB 12) and kneecap begin to emerge. [When these three bones have] emerged, the [newborn] baby [will live a] long life. [If these three bones have] not emerged, [the newborn baby will] die young."

Niaoshi asked, "Why can [the newborn baby] not live [a long life]?"

Qibo answered, "These three bones belong to Yin and [only when] there is Yin [can the newborn baby] live [normally]. However, [it] also depends on exuberance and development of Yang[3]. [If there is] no sufficient Yang Qi [in the newborn] baby, the three bones cannot grow [after] sucking maternal milk [because] the innate Yang Qi is deficient. [If] Yang Qi is initially

鸟师曰："吾见三骨不全亦有延龄者,又何故欤?"

岐伯曰："三者之中,惟耳无完骨者亦有延龄,然而疾病不能无也。若囟门不合、膝盖不生,吾未见有生者。盖孤阳无阴也。"

陈远公曰："孤阳无阴,人则不生,则阴为阳之天地。无阴者,无阳也。阳生于阴之中,阴长于阳之外。有三骨者,得阴阳之全也。"

【今译】

鸟师请问岐伯："初生的婴儿为什么没有膝盖骨呢?"

岐伯说："初生的婴儿不仅没有膝盖骨,也没有囟骨和耳后的完骨。"

鸟师问："这是什么原因呢?"

岐伯说："这是因为阴气不足。阴气是真阴之气。婴儿纯阳而无阴,食母乳之后阴气才能生起。阴气生起后,囟骨、耳后完骨、膝盖骨才会长出来。这些骨生长起来了,婴儿就会长寿,否则就会夭折。"

鸟师问："如果不能生长,会是什么原因呢?"

岐伯说："这三块骨头属于阴,只有得到阴气才会生长,但也必须等到阳气旺盛的时候才能生长起来。如果婴儿阳气不足,食母乳之后这三块骨还是不能生长,这是因为这样的婴儿先天之阳气亏虚。由于阳气先亏,先天的阳气本身就缺陷了。而食母乳仅仅能弥补后天的不足,这就是这三块骨不能生长出来的原因。如果这三块骨不能生长,其寿命又怎么能够延长呢?"

weak, the innate [one will] become deficient. That is why the three bones have failed to grow. [If] the three bones have failed to grow, how can [the newborn baby] live a long life?"

Niaoshi asked, "[Among] the three bones, [if there is just] one [that] has failed [to grow], can [the newborn baby] live [normally]?"

Qibo answered, "[Even if just] one has failed [to grow], [the newborn baby] still cannot live a normal life."

Niaoshi asked, "Please explain in details."

Qibo answered, "[If] the frontal fontanelle is not closed, the brain will become empty; [if] Wangu (GB 12) does not grow, the kidney will become deficient; [if] the kneecaps have failed to emerge, the feet will become soft. [If] the brain is empty, wind tends to invade; [if] the kidney is deficient, listening [ability will be] lost; [if] the feet are soft, [there will be] frequent falling down."

Niaoshi asked, "I have seen [some people whose] three bones are not perfect, [but they] still can live a long life. What is the reason?"

Qibo answered, "[Among] these three bones, only [when] Wangu (GB 12) behind the ears has failed to grow [can the newborn baby] live [a normal life]. However, [certain] diseases cannot be prevented. I have not seen [any person who] lives [a normal life] when the frontal fontanelle and kneecaps have failed to grow. Because there is no Yin [when] Yang is isolated."

Chen Yuangong's comment, "[In] isolated Yang, [there is] no

鸟师问:"如果三块骨仅缺乏其中之一,婴儿也能生存吗?"

岐伯说:"如果缺乏其中一,也不能成为完整的健康人。"

鸟师问:"请详细予以说明。"

岐伯说:"如果囟门不合,脑髓就会空虚;如果完骨不长,肾脏就会亏虚;如果膝盖不生,双足就会发软。如果脑髓空虚,邪风就容易侵入;如果肾宫亏虚,听力就会失聪;如果双足发软,患者就会经常跌倒在地。"

鸟师问:"我见过三骨发育不全的人,但有些人也能延续寿命,这又是什么原因呢?"

岐伯说:"在这三块骨中,只有耳朵旁边没有完骨的人寿命才可以延续,但疾病却不能避免。如果有人囟门不合、膝盖不生,我还没有见过这样的人还能够继续存活下去,因为孤阳无阴。"

陈远公评论说:"如果孤阳无阴,人就不能生存,可见阴是阳之天地。所以没有阴就没有阳。阳生于阴之中,阴长于阳之外。有了这三块骨,就能得到全部的阴阳。"

Volume 1

Yin. [In this case,] man cannot exist [because] Yin is the sky and earth[4] of Yang. [If there is] no Yin, [there will be certainly] no Yang. Yang originates from the internal of Yin while Yin grows from the external of Yang. [Only when one] has all these three [important] bones can both Yin and Yang be perfect."

Notes

[1] Niaoshi (鸟师), literally a bird master, was a paleontologist in remote antiquity.

[2] True Yin refers to the spirit that controls the body.

[3] Although Yang originates from Yin, Yin alone cannot exist.

[4] Sky and earth here refer to the basic foundation of Yang.

卷二

媾精受妊篇第十

【原文】

雷公问曰："男女媾精而受妊者,何也?"

岐伯曰："肾为作强之官,故受妊而生人也。"

雷公曰："作强而何以生人也?"

岐伯曰："生人者,即肾之技巧也。"

雷公曰："技巧属肾之水乎,火乎?"

岐伯曰："水火无技巧也。"

雷公曰："离水火又何以出技巧乎?"

岐伯曰："技巧成于水火之气也。"

雷公曰："同是水火之气,何生人有男女之别乎?"

岐伯曰："水火气弱则生女,水火气强则生男。"

雷公曰："古云:女先泄精则成男,男先泄精则成女。今曰:水火气弱则生女,水火气强则生男。何也?"

岐伯曰："男女俱有水火之气也,气同至则技巧出焉,一有先后不成胎矣。男泄精,女泄气,女子泄精则气脱矣,男子泄气则精脱矣,焉能成胎!"

雷公曰："女不泄精,男不泄气,何以受妊乎?"

Volume 2

【英译】

Chapter 10
Copulation and Conception

Leigong asked, "Why copulation between men and women can conceive a baby?"

Qibo answered, "The kidney is an organ with dexterity and strength. That is why [it can promote] conception and [ensures] birth [of people]."

Leigong asked, "Why dexterity and strength can [ensure] birth [of people]?"

Qibo answered, "[Because] birth [of people] demonstrates the skills and dexterity of the kidney."

Leigong asked, "Do skills and dexterity belong to water in the kidney or fire [in the kidney]?"

Qibo answered, "There are no skills and dexterity in water and fire."

Leigong asked, "Why are there skills and dexterity apart from water and fire?"

Qibo answered, "The skills and dexterity [of the kidney] originate from Qi in water and fire."

Leigong asked, "[That means the skills and dexterity of the kidney] all originate from Qi in water and fire. But why the people born are male and female, quite different?"

岐伯曰："女气中有精，男精中有气，女泄气而交男子之精，男泄精而合女子之气，此技巧之所以出也。"

雷公曰："所生男女，有强有弱，自分于父母之气矣。但有清浊寿夭之异，何也？"

岐伯曰："气清则清，气浊则浊，气长则寿，气促则夭。皆本于父母之气也。"

雷公曰："生育本于肾中之气，余已知之矣。但此气也，豫于五脏七腑之气乎？"

岐伯曰："五脏七腑之气，一经不至，皆不成胎。"

雷公曰："媾精者，动肾中之气也。与五脏七腑何豫乎？"

岐伯曰："肾藏精，亦藏气。藏精者，藏五脏七腑之精也。藏气者，藏五脏七腑之气也。藏则俱藏，泄则俱泄。"

雷公曰："泄气者，亦泄血乎？"

岐伯曰："精即血也。气无形，血有形，无形化有形，有形不能化无形也。"

雷公曰："精非有形乎？"

岐伯曰："精虽有形，而精中之气正无形也。无形隐于有形，故能静能动。动则化耳，化则技巧出矣。"

雷公曰："微哉言乎，请传之奕祀，以彰化育焉。"

陈士铎曰："男女不媾精，断不成胎。胎成于水火之气，此气即男女之气也。气藏于精中，精虽有形而实无形也。形非气乎，故成胎即成

Volume 2

Qibo answered, "[If] Qi in water and fire is weak, [the people] born are female; [if] Qi from water and fire is strong, [the people] born are male."

Leigong asked, "[People in] ancient [times] said, '[If] a woman emits essence[1] first [when copulating with a man], a male baby will be conceived; [if] a man emits semen first [when copulating with a woman], a female baby will be conceived.' [People] nowadays say, "[If] Qi in water and fire is weak, a female baby will be conceived; [if] Qi in water and fire is strong, a male baby will be conceived.' What is the reason?"

Qibo answered, "[In] both a man and a woman, there is Qi from water and fire. [If] Qi [from water and fire in both men and women] arrives at the same time[2], skills and dexterity will be formed[3]. If there is difference, a baby cannot be conceived. [Under normal condition of copulation,] a man emits semen and a woman emits Qi [and blood]. [If] a woman emits essence [in copulation], Qi will be collapsed. [If] a man emits Qi [in copulation], essence will be collapsed. [In such a case,] how can a baby be conceived?"

Leigong asked, "[If] a woman does not emit essence and [if] a man does not emit Qi, how can a baby be conceived?"

Qibo answered, "Qi in a woman contains essence and essence in a man contains Qi. [The reason] why skills and dexterity are formed is that Qi emited from a woman mixes with semen from a man and semen emitted from a man combines with Qi from a woman."

Leigong asked, "Male and female [babies] born are either

气之谓。"

【今译】

雷公问道:"男女交媾而怀孕,这是什么原因呢?"

岐伯说:"肾脏是主管技巧的强壮器官,所以就具有怀孕和生育的功能。"

雷公问:"主管技巧的强壮器官为什么可以生育人呢?"

岐伯说:"生育人就是肾脏技巧的表现。"

雷公问:"技巧属于肾脏的水还是火?"

岐伯说:"水火本身并无技巧。"

雷公问:"离开了水火肾脏又怎么能够具有技巧呢?"

岐伯说:"技巧形成于水火之气。"

雷公问:"同样是水火之气,为什么生育的人有男女之别呢?"

岐伯说:"如果水火之气虚弱,所生育的就是女孩;如果水火之气强壮,所生育的就是男孩。"

雷公问:"古人说'如果女子先泄精,所生育的是男孩;如果男子先泄精,所生育的是女孩'。今人却说'如果水火之气虚弱,所生育的就是女孩;如果水火之气强壮,所生育的就是男孩'。为什么呢?"

岐伯说:"男女都有水火之气,水火之气同至就形成了生育的技巧。一旦有先后之别,就不能形成胎儿。男子泄出的是精,女子泄出的是气。如果女子泄出了精,气就会虚脱;如果男子泄出了气,精就会虚脱。这种情况下怎么能够成胎儿呢?"

strong or weak, [this] is related to [the condition of] Qi from the father and mother. "

Qibo answered, "[If] Qi [from the father and mother] is clear, [Qi from the baby] is also clear[4]; [if] Qi [from the father and mother] is turbid, [the baby conceived] is also turbid[5]; [if] Qi [from the father and mother] is long[6], [the baby will live] a long life; [if] Qi [from the father and mother] is short[7], [the baby will] die young. All these are related to Qi from the father and mother. "

Leigong asked, "I have known that Qi in the kidney is the foundation of conception. But is such a Qi related to Qi from the five Zang-organs and six Fu-organs?"

Qibo answered, "[In terms of] Qi from the five Zang-organs and six Fu-organs, [if it] does not flow through one meridian, conception is impossible. "

Leigong asked, "Combination of essence [from men and women][8] draws on Qi from the kidney. Does it have anything to do with the five Zang-organs and six Fu-organs?"

Qibo answered, "The kidney stores essence and Qi. To store essence [means] to store essence from the five Zang-organs and six Fu-organs. To store Qi [means] to store Qi from the five Zang-organs and six Fu-organs. [In terms of] storage, [both essence and Qi are] stored [at the same time]; [in terms of] emission, [both essence and Qi are] emitted [at the same time]. "

Leigong asked, "[When] Qi is emitted, why is the blood also emitted?"

Qibo answered, "Essence also means blood. Qi is invisible and

雷公问："如果女子不泄精，男子不泄气，又怎么能受孕呢?"

岐伯说："女子的气中有精，男子的精中有气，女子泄出的气与男子的精相交，男子泄出的精与女子的气相合，这是生育技巧形成的原因。"

雷公问："生下来的男孩和女孩，有强壮的也有虚弱的，都源自于父母之气，但也有清浊寿夭的差异，这是为什么呢?"

岐伯说："父母之气清，孩子之气也清;父母之气浊，孩子之气也浊;父母之气长，孩子则长寿;父母之气短，孩子则夭折。这些都取决于父母之气。"

雷公问："生育基于肾中之气，这我已经知道了。但是这些气与五脏七腑中的气有什么关系呢?"

岐伯说："五脏七腑之气，只要有一条经脉没运行到，都不能形成胎儿。"

雷公问："精之交媾，动用的是肾中之气，与五脏七腑又能有什么关系呢?"

岐伯说："肾藏精，但也藏气。肾所藏的精，是来自五脏七腑的精;肾所藏的气，是来自五脏七腑的气。所以精气同时隐藏，但也同时泄泻。"

雷公问："这是否意味着泄出气的同时也泄出血呢?"

岐伯说："精就是血。气无形，血有形。无形可以转化为有形，但有形却不能转化为无形。"

雷公问："精不是有形的吗?"

the blood is visible. Invisible [one] can transform into visible [one]. [But] visible [one] cannot transform into invisible [one]."

Leigong asked, "Is essence invisible?"

Qibo answered, "Although essence is visible, healthy Qi in essence is invisible. [The fact is that] the invisible [element] is hidden in the visible [element]. That is why [it] can be static and dynamic. [When it becomes] dynamic, [it begins] to transform. [When it begins] to transform, the skills and dexterity will be formed."

Leigong said, "What a brief and excellent explanation! Please let the future generations know [such an important principle] in order to show the significance of conception."

Chen Shiduo's comment, "[If] essence from the man and woman does not mix with each other, no baby can be conceived. A baby is conceived from Qi from water and fire. Such Qi actually refers to Qi from a man and a woman. Qi stores in essence. Although essence is visible, in fact [it is] invisible. Is being visible not Qi? Thus conception of a baby is actually formation of Qi."

Notes

[1] Essence here refers to the essential liquid which flows out of the vagina when a woman is copulating with a man, indicating that she is in orgasm.

[2] The saying that Qi [from water and fire in both men and women] arrives at the same time actually means copulation.

[3] The saying that skills and dexterity will be formed actually

岐伯说:"精虽然有形,但是精中之气却无形,这就是无形隐藏在有形之中的体现,所以精既能静又能动。精一运动就会有变化,精一变化就会有生育技巧的出现。"

雷公说:"这道理真微妙啊!请将其世代相传,以彰显化育的规律。"

陈士铎评论说:"男女之精血不交媾,就根本不能形成胎儿。胎儿形成于水火之气,此气就是男女之气。气藏于精中,精虽然有形但其实却是无形。形不是气吗?所以成胎就是成气的体现。"

means to conceive a baby.

[4] Clear here means pure.

[5] Turbid here means unpure.

[6] Long means strong and sufficient.

[7] Short means weak and deficient.

[8] The expression of combination of essence [from men and women] refers to copulation.

社生篇第十一

【原文】

少师问曰:"人生而白头,何也?"

岐伯曰:"社日生人,皮毛皆白,非止鬓发之白也。"

少师曰:"何故乎?"

岐伯曰:"社日者,金日也。皮毛须鬓皆白者,得金之气也。"

少师曰:"社日非金也,天师谓之金日,此余之未明也。"

岐伯曰:"社本土也,气属金,社日生人犯金之气。金气者,杀气也。"

少师曰:"人犯杀气,宜天矣,何又长年乎?"

岐伯曰:"金中有土,土乃生气也。人肺属金,皮毛亦属金,金之杀气得土则生,逢金则斗。社之金气伐人皮毛,不入人脏腑,故得长年耳。"

少师曰:"社日生人皮毛鬓发不尽白者,又何故欤?"

岐伯曰:"生时不同也。"

少师曰:"何时乎?"

岐伯曰:"非巳午时,必辰戌丑未时也。"

少师曰:"巳午火也,火能制金之气,宜矣。辰戌丑未,土也,不助金之气乎?"

Volume 2

【英译】

Chapter 11
People Born [on the Day of] She [Ri]

Shaoshi[1] asked, "Why [some] people's hair is innately white?"

Qibo answered, "[In] people born on [the day of] She Ri[2], both the skin and hair are white, not just the hair on the temples."

Shaoshi asked, "What is the reason?"

Qibo answered, "[The day of] She Ri is [the day of] metal. [If a person's] skin, hair and hair on the temples are all white, [it] originates from metal Qi."

Shaoshi asked, "[The day of] She Ri does not belong to metal. [But] Celestial Master call it metal day. This is what I am unclear."

Qibo answered, "[The day of] She Ri originally is [the day for sacrificing god of] the earth, [but] Qi [in this special day] belongs to metal. People born [on the day of] She Ri have offended metal Qi. Metal Qi [is the element that] kills Qi."

Shaoshi asked, "[If] a person has offended Qi, [he should] die young. [But] why can he still live a longer life?"

Qibo answered, "[In] metal there is earth [Qi], [in] earth [Qi] there is vital Qi. [In] human beings, the lung belongs to metal, the skin and hair also belong to metal. [The function of] metal in killing Qi is invigorated [when] obtaining earth [Qi]. [When] meeting with metal [Qi], [it] contends with [it]. Metal Qi [in the day of] She Ri attacks the skin and hair [of the concerned

岐伯曰："社本土也，喜生恶泄，得土则生，生则不克矣。"

少师曰："同是日也，何社日之凶如是乎？"

岐伯曰："岁月日时俱有神司之，社日之神与人最亲，其性最喜洁也，生产则秽矣。两气相感，儿身受之，非其煞之暴也。"

少师曰："人生有记，赤如朱，青如靛，黑如锅，白如雪，终身不散，何也？岂亦社日之故乎？"

岐伯曰："父母交媾，偶犯游神，为神所指，志父母之过也。"

少师曰："色不同者，何欤？"

岐伯曰："随神之气异也。"

少师曰："记无黄色者，何也？"

岐伯曰："黄乃正色，人犯正神，不相校也，故亦不相指，不相指，故罔所记耳。"

陈远公曰："社日生人，说来有源有委，非孟浪成文者可比。"

【今译】

少师问道："有的人生下来头发就是白的，这是什么原因呢？"

岐伯说："社日生下来的人，皮肤和毛发都是白的，并不是只有鬓发才是白的。"

少师问："这是什么原因呢？"

岐伯说："社日属于金日。皮肤、毛发、胡须、鬓发都是白的，因为得到了金气的影响。"

people], [but] has not entered the viscera. That is why [these people still] can live a longer life."

Shaoshi asked, "Why are the skin, hair and hair on the temples of the people born on [the day of] She Ri not completely white?"

Qibo answered, "[Because the time of their] birth is not the same."

Shaoshi asked, "What is the time?"

Qibo answered, "[If they were] not born in Si (9: 00 – 11: 00) and Wu (11: 00 – 13: 00), [they were] surely [born] in Chen (7: 00 – 9: 00), Xu (19: 00 – 21: 00), Chou (1: 00 – 3: 00) and Wei (13: 00 – 15: 00).[3]"

Shaoshi asked, "[The time of] Si (9: 00 – 11: 00) and Wu (11: 00 – 13: 00) [pertains to] fire and fire can control metal Qi, quite appropriately. [But the time of] Chen (7: 00 – 9: 00), Xu (19: 00 – 21: 00), Chou (1: 00 – 3: 00) and Wei (13: 00 – 15: 00) [pertains to] earth. Does it not assist metal Qi?"

Qibo answered, "[The day of] She Ri originally [belongs to] earth, liking to grow and disliking to emit. [When] obtaining earth [Qi], [it will] grow and growth will not be restricted."

Shaoshi asked, "Day and day are the same. [But] why is [the day of] She Ri so ferocious?"

Qibo answered, "[Every] day, [every] month and [every] year is controlled by god. God of She Ri is intimate to people and loves cleanness and purity. [But women appear] filthy [when they] deliver babies [on the day of She Ri]. Both Qi[4] interact with each other [on this special day]. [It is such an interaction that has] affected the baby. [It does] not indicate that [this special day is] ferocious."

少师问："社日并非属于金，天师却说属于金日，对此我不明白。"

岐伯说："社日本来属于土，但其气则属于金。属于社日生人则触犯了金气。金气是杀气。"

少师问："人触犯了杀气，应当导致夭折。但为什么又能延长生命呢？"

岐伯说："金中有土，土为生气。人体中的肺属金，皮毛也属金。金的杀气遇到了土气就能生发，但遇到了金气就会争斗。社日的金气只是克伐人的皮毛，并未克伐人的脏腑，所以相关的人就可以延长生命。"

少师问："社日出生的人，其皮毛鬓发并不全部变白，这又是什么原因呢？"

岐伯说："这是因为出生的时辰不同。"

少师问："什么时辰呢？"

岐伯说："如果不是出生在巳、午之时，就一定出生在辰、戌、丑、未这四个时辰。"

少师问："巳、午属于火，火能制约金气，这是很适宜的。辰、戌、丑、未这四个时辰属于土，难道土岂不能助长金气吗？"

岐伯说："社日本来属土，喜生厌泄，得到土气就能生，能生就不会受到克制。"

少师问："同样是日子，为什么社日如此凶暴呢？"

岐伯说："年月日之时都有神司管，司管社日的神与人最亲，其本性最喜清洁之气，但是生育时则有污秽之气。清洁之气与污秽之气相

Volume 2

Shaoshi asked, "[In some] babies, there are [various] imprintings, [some are] as red as cinnabar, [some are] as blue as indigo, [some are] as black as pan, [some are] as white as snow, [which will] not disperse all the life. What is the reason? Is it also due to [the day of] She Ri?"

Qibo answered, "[When] the father and mother [of a baby] are copulating, [they may] have accidentally offended a god passing by. To record the errors made by the father and mother, the god has left a mark [on the body of the baby]."

Shaoshi asked, "Why are the colors different?"

Qibo answered, "[Because] Qi of gods differs [from each other]."

Shaoshi asked, "Why is there no yellow [imprinting]?"

Qibo answered, "Yellow is the color of the orthodoxy [gods]. [If] a person has offended the orthodoxy gods, [the orthodoxy gods do] not care about it and [will not] record anything. [Since the orthodoxy gods do] not record anything [done by the father and mother of a baby], [they will] not leave any imprintings [on the body of the baby]."

Chen Yuangong's comment, "People born on [the day of] She Ri have certain causes and effects, [but] not as what described randomly in this article.[5]"

Notes

[1] Shaoshi (少师) was the title of an official responsible for teaching princes.

感,则影响了婴儿的身体,并不是因为该日为凶暴之日。"

少师问:"有些婴儿出生时身上有印记,红的像朱砂,青的像靛蓝,黑的像铁锅,白的像雪花,为什么这些印记终身都不会消散?难道也是因为社日的原因吗?"

岐伯说:"父母交媾时,偶然会触犯到过往之神,过往之神会对其有所指点,因此在婴儿身体上就留下了印记,以记录父母的过失。"

少师问:"为什么印记的颜色不同呢?"

岐伯说:"因为神之气不同,印记便有了差异。"

少师问:"为什么印记没有黄色的呢?"

岐伯说:"黄色是正色。人若触犯了正神,正神不会在意,因此也不会指责,因此就没有留下任何印记了。"

陈远公评论说:"社日出生的人,说起来肯定是有原委的,并非随意写成的文字就可以与之相比。"

Volume 2

[2] She Ri（社日）was a sacrifice day for god of the earth in ancient China.

[3] In ancient China，one day was divided into 12 periods and each period contains two hours，namely Zi（子），Chou（丑），Yin（寅），Mao（卯），Chen（辰），Si（巳），Wu（午），Wei（未），Shen（申），You（酉），Xu（戌）and Hai（亥）.

[4] Both Qi here refers to Qi of purity and Qi of filth.

[5] Chen Yuangong's comment indicates that he did not agree with the ideas described in this chapter.

天厌火衰篇第十二

【原文】

容成问曰："世有天生男子音声如女子，外势如婴儿，此何故欤？"

岐伯曰："天厌之也。"

容成曰："天何以厌之乎？"

岐伯曰："天地有缺陷，安得人尽皆全乎？"

容成曰："天未尝厌人，奈何以天厌名之。"

岐伯曰："天不厌而人必厌也，天人一道，人厌即天厌矣。"

容成曰："人何不幸成天厌也？"

岐伯曰："父母之咎也。人道交感，先火动而后水济之，火盛者生子必强，火衰者生子必弱，水盛者生子必肥，水衰者生子必瘦。天厌之人，乃先天之火微也。"

容成曰："水火衰盛分强弱肥瘦，宜也，不宜外阳之细小。"

岐伯曰："肾中之火，先天之火，无形之火也。肾中之水，先天之水，无形之水也。火得水而生，水得火而长，言肾内之阴阳也。水长火，则水为火之母；火生水，则火为水之母也。人得水火之气以生身，则水火即人之父母也。天下有形不能生无形也，无形实生有形。外阳之生，实内阳之长也。内阳旺而外阳必伸，内阳旺者得火气之全也。内阳衰矣，外阳亦何得壮大哉？"

Volume 2

【英译】

Chapter 12
Celestial Dislike and Faint Fire

Rongcheng asked, "[In] this world, there are some men [whose] sound [is] like [that of] women, [whose] external force[1] [is] like [that of] a baby. What is the reason?"

Qibo answered, "[Because] the sky dislikes them[2]."

Rongcheng asked, "Why does the sky dislike them?"

Qibo answered, "[Even] the sky and earth have certain defects, how can human beings all be perfect?"

Rongcheng asked, "The sky has never disliked any people. Why [do you] use [the term of] sky dislike to name such a problem?"

Qibo answered, "[It is true that] the sky never dislikes [any people], but [among human beings, there] must [be some] people [who] dislike [others]. [Since] the sky and human beings [follow] the same Dao (law), [that is why] human beings' dislike is equal to the sky's dislike."

Rongcheng asked, "Why do [some] people unfortunately become the disliked [objects of] the sky?"

Qibo answered, "[It is] the fault of parents. [When] parents are copulating [with each other], fire stirs first and then water promotes. [If] fire is exuberant, the baby to be conceived must be strong; [if] fire is waned, the baby to be conceived must be weak.

容成曰："火既不全,何以生身乎?"

岐伯曰："孤阴不生,孤阳不长。天厌之人,但火不全耳,未尝无阴阳也;偏于火者,阳有余而阴不足,偏于水者,阴有余而阳不足也。阳既不足,即不能生厥阴之宗筋,此外阳之所以屈而不伸也,毋论刚大矣。"

容成曰："善。"

陈远公评论曰："外阳之大小,视水火之偏全,不视阴阳之有无耳,说来可听。"

【今译】

容成问道："世上有些天生的男人,声音像女子一样,阴茎像婴儿一样,这又是什么造成的呢?"

岐伯说："这是上天厌弃他们的缘故。"

容成问："上天为什么会厌弃他们呢?"

岐伯说："天地尚且有缺陷,人又怎么能够十全十美呢?"

容成问："上天并没有嫌弃人类呀,为什么要用'天厌'来称呼此类情况呢?"

岐伯说："上天虽然并没有嫌弃人,但人必然有自身厌弃。天与人同道,人自身所厌弃的也就是天所厌弃的。"

容成问："有的人为何不幸为上天所厌弃呢?"

岐伯说："这都与父母有关。人性交时,先是火动,然后是水济。如果火气旺盛,生下来的孩子必然强壮;如果火气衰弱,生下来的孩子必然

Volume 2

[If] water is exuberant, the baby to be conceived must be fat; [if] water is waned, the baby to be conceived must be emaciated. [In] those [who are] disliked by the sky, the innate fire is faint."

Rongcheng asked, "To differentiate strength and weakness [as well as] obesity and emaciation [according to] wane and exuberance of water and fire, [it is] appropriate. [But is it] inappropriate [to explain] thin and small external Yang[3] [in such a way]?"

Qibo answered, "Fire in the kidney [is] innate fire and invisible fire. Water in the kidney is innate water and invisible water. [When] meeting with water, fire will flame; [when] meeting with fire, water will increase. [Such an analysis about fire and water is actually a] description about Yin and Yang in the kidney. [When] water promotes fire, water is the mother of fire; [when] fire increases water, fire is the mother of water. [When] a person has obtained Qi from water and fire, [his] body [will be] constituted, and water and fire will be his parents. [In] this world, [the one that is] visible cannot produce [the one that is] invisible, [but the one that is] invisible certainly can produce [the one that is] visible. The development of external Yang actually [depends on] the development of internal Yang. [When] internal Yang is exuberant, external Yang must be erect. [Why] internal Yang is exuberant? [Because it has] got perfect Qi from fire. [If] internal Yang is in wane, how could external Yang become strong and large?"

Rongcheng asked, "Since fire is not perfect, [but] why is the body formed?"

Qibo answered, "Isolated Yin cannot exist and isolated Yang

虚弱。如果水气旺盛,生下来的孩子必然肥壮;如果水气衰弱,生下来的孩子必然瘦弱。所谓上天厌弃的人,是因为先天火气衰微的缘故。"

容成说:"水火的虚弱与旺盛,适宜用来区分人体的强、弱、肥、瘦,但阴茎不应当也细小如此。"

岐伯说:"肾中的火为先天之火,也是无形之火;肾中的水为先天之水,也是无形之水。火气得到水气才能资生,水气得到火气才能资长,这是说肾脏中的阴阳。水生火时水是火之母,火生水时火是水之母,人得到水火之气才能形成身体,所以水火就是人的父母。天下有形的不能生无形的,但无形的却可以生有形的。外阳的生长其实就是内阳的生长。如果内阳旺盛,外阳(即阴茎)就必然会坚挺。内阳之所以旺盛,是因为得到了所有的火气。如果内阳衰弱,外阳(即阴茎)又怎么能够壮大呢?"

容成问:"火气既然不全,又怎么能够形成身体呢?"

岐伯说:"孤单的阴气不能生发,孤单的阳气不会成长。上天厌弃的人,只是火气不全的缘故,并非没有阴阳。偏于火气的,则阳气有余而阴气不足;偏于水气的,则阴气有余而阳气不足。阳气既然不足,就无法生成厥阴的宗筋,这就是为什么外阳(即阴茎)软弱不挺。正因为如此,就更不必论其刚劲强壮了!"

容成说:"好!"

陈远公评论说:"外阳(即阴茎)的大小,与水火之气的偏全有关,并非仅仅与阴阳的有无相关。这方面的情况说说还是可以听听的。"

cannot grow. [In] the people disliked by the sky, only fire is not perfect, [it is] impossible to have no Yin and Yang. [If a person's physique is] inclined to fire, [it indicates that] there is excessive Yang and insufficient Yin; [if a person's physique is] inclined to water, [it indicates that] there is excessive Yin and insufficient Yang. [If] Yang is insufficient, all sinews of Jueyin cannot be formed. That is why the external Yang is feeble and cannot erect, let alone being strong and firm."

Rongcheng said, "Good!"

Chen Yuangong's comment, "The size of external Yang [should be examined] according to the perfect or imperfect [condition of] water and fire, not only according to existence or non-existence of Yin and Yang. [However, such] an analysis is worth listening."

Notes

[1] External force here is an euphemism about penis.

[2] The expression that the sky dislikes actually refers to innate defects in the body of certain people.

[3] External Yang here is also an euphemism about penis.

经脉相行篇第十三

【原文】

雷公问曰："帝问脉行之逆顺若何，余无以奏也。愿天师明教以闻。"

岐伯曰："十二经脉有自上行下者，有自下行上者，各不同也。"

雷公曰："请悉言之。"

岐伯曰："手之三阴从脏走手，手之三阳从手走头，足之三阳从头走足，足之三阴从足走腹，此上下相行之数也。"

雷公曰："尚未明也。"

岐伯曰："手之三阴：太阴肺，少阴心，厥阴包络也。手太阴从中府走大指之少商，手少阴从极泉走小指之少冲，手厥阴从天池走中指之中冲。皆从脏走手也。手之三阳：阳明大肠，太阳小肠，少阳三焦也。手阳明从次指商阳走头之迎香，手太阳从小指少泽走头之听宫，手少阳从四指关冲走头之丝竹空，皆从手走头也。足之三阳：太阳膀胱，阳明胃，少阳胆也。足太阳从头睛明走足小指之至阴，足阳明胃从头头维走足次指之厉兑，足少阳从头前关走四指之窍阴，皆从头走足也。足之三阴：太阴脾，少阴肾，厥阴肝也。足太阴从足大指内侧隐白走腹之大包，足少阴从足心涌泉走腹之俞府，足厥阴从足大指外侧大敦走腹之期门，皆从足走腹也。"

Volume 2

【英译】

Chapter 13
Circulation of Meridians

Leigong asked, "The Emperor[1] has asked [me] about the reverse and normal circulations of meridians. I do not know how to reply. [I] hope [that] Celestial Master can teach [me]."

Qibo answered, "[Among] the twelve meridians, some circulate from the upper to the lower and some circulate from the lower to the upper, quite different."

Leigong asked, "Please tell [me] in detail."

Qibo answered, "The three Yin meridians of hand circulate from the Zang-organs to the hand; the three Yang meridians of hand circulate from the hand to the head; the three Yang meridians of foot circulate from the head to the foot; the three Yin meridians of foot circulate from the foot to the abdomen. These are the situations [about how the meridians] circulate from the upper and lower."

Leigong asked, "[I am] still unclear."

Qibo answered, "The three Yin [meridians of] hand [include] the lung [meridian of] hand-Taiyin, the heart [meridian of] hand-Shaoyin and the pericardium [meridian of] hand-Jueyin. [The lung meridian of] hand-Taiyin runs from Zhongfu (LU 1) to Shaoshang (LU 11) [located on] the thumb; [the heart meridian of] hand-Shaoyin runs from Jiquan (HT 1) to Shaochong (HT 9) [located

雷公曰："逆顺若何?"

岐伯曰："手之阴经,走手为顺,走脏为逆也;手之阳经,走头为顺,走手为逆也;足之阴经,走腹为顺,走足为逆也;足之阳经,走足为顺,走头为逆也。"

雷公曰："足之三阴,皆走于腹,独少阴之脉下行,何也? 岂少阴经易逆难顺乎?"

岐伯曰："不然,夫冲脉者,五脏六腑之海也。五脏六腑皆禀焉。其上者,出于颃颡,渗诸阳,灌诸精,下注少阴之大络,出于气冲,循阴阳内廉入腘中,伏行骭骨内,下至内踝之后,属而别。其下者,并由少阴经渗三阴,其在前者,伏行出跗属,下循跗入大指间,渗诸络而温肌肉,故别络邪结则跗上脉不动,不动则厥,厥则足寒矣。此足少阴之脉少异于三阴,而走腹则一也。"

雷公曰："其少异于三阴者为何?"

岐伯曰："少阴肾经中藏水火,不可不曲折以行,其脉不若肝脾之可直行于腹也。"

雷公曰："其走腹则一者何?"

岐伯曰："肾之性喜逆行,故由下而上,盖以逆为顺也。"

雷公曰;"逆行宜病矣。"

岐伯曰："逆而顺,故不病,若顺走是违其性矣,反生病也。"

雷公曰："当尽奏之。"

岐伯曰："帝问何以明之,公奏曰以言导之,切而验之,其髁必动。乃可以验逆顺之行也。"

on] the small finger; [the pericardium meridian of] hand-Jueyin runs from Tianchi (PC 1) to Zhongchong (PC 9) [located on] the middle finger. The three Yang [meridians of] hand [include] the large intestine [meridian of hand-] Yangming; the small intestine [meridian of hand-] Taiyang; and the triple energizer [meridian of hand-] Shaoyang. [The large intestine meridian of] hand-Yangming runs from Shangyang (LI 1) [located on] the second finger to Yingxiang (LI 20); [the small intestine meridian of] hand-Taiyang runs from Shaoze (SI 1) [located on] the small finger to Tinggong (SI 19); [the triple energizer meridian of] hand-Shaoyang runs from Guanchong (TE 1) [located on] the fourth finger to Sizhukong (TE 23) [located on] the head. All [these meridians] run from the hand to the head. The three Yang [meridians of] foot [include] the bladder [meridian of foot-] Taiyang, the stomach [meridian of foot-] Yangming and the gallbladder [meridian of foot-] Shaoyang. [The bladder meridian of] foot-Taiyang runs from Jingming (BL 1) to Zhiyin (BL 67) [located on] the small toe of foot; [the stomach meridian of] foot-Yangming runs from Touwei (ST 8) [located on] the head to Lidui (ST 45) [located on] the second toe of foot; [the gallbladder meridian of] foot-Shaoyang runs from Qianguan[2] [located on] the head to Qiaoyin (GB 44) [located on] the fourth toe. All [these meridians] run from the head to the foot. The three Yin [meridians of] foot [include] the spleen [meridian of foot-] Taiyin, the kidney [meridian of foot-] Shaoyin and the liver [meridian of foot-] Jueyin. [The spleen meridian of] foot-Taiyin runs from Yinbai (SP 1) [located on] the medial side of the big toe of foot to Dabao (SP 21) [located on] the

雷公曰:"谨奉教以闻。"

陈远公曰:"十二经脉,有走手、走足、走头、走腹之异,各讲得凿凿。其讲顺逆不同处,何人敢措一辞。"

【今译】

雷公问道:"黄帝问经脉循行的逆顺如何,我无法回奏,请天师予以指教。"

岐伯说:"十二经脉,有自上向下循行的,也有自下向上循行的,各有不同。"

雷公说:"请详细说明。"

岐伯说:"手三阴经从脏循行到手,手三阳经从手循行到头部,足三阳经从头循行到足,足三阴经从足部循行到腹,这就是经脉的上下循行。"

雷公问:"但我还是不清楚。"

岐伯说:"手三阴经包括手太阴肺经、手少阴心经和手厥阴心包经。手太阴肺经从中府穴循行到大指的少商穴,手少阴心经从极泉穴循行到小指的少冲穴,手厥阴心包经从天池穴循行到中指的中冲穴,这些经脉都是从脏循行到手部。手三阳经包括手阳明大肠经、手太阳小肠经和手少阳三焦经。手阳明大肠经从次指的商阳穴循行到头部的迎香穴,手太阳小肠经从小指的少泽穴循行到头部的听宫穴,手少阳三焦经从第四指的关冲穴循行到头部的丝竹空穴,这些经脉都是从手循行

abdomen; [the kidney meridian of] foot-Shaoyin runs from Yongquan (KI 1) [located on] the sole to Yufu (KI 27) [located on] the abdomen; [the liver meridian of] foot-Jueyin runs from Dadun (LR 1) [located on] lateral side of the big toe of foot to Qimen (LR 14). All [these meridians] run from the foot to the abdomen."

Leigong asked, "How about reverse and normal [circulation]?"

Qibo answered, "The Yin meridians of hand that run towards the hand are normal while run towards the viscera are reverse; the Yang meridians of hand that run towards the head are normal while run towards the hand are reverse; the Yin meridians of foot that run towards the abdomen are normal while run towards the foot are reverse; the Yang meridians of foot that run towards the foot are normal while run towards the head are reverse."

Leigong asked, "The three Yin [meridians of] foot all run towards the abdomen, only [the kidney meridian of foot-] Shaoyin runs downwards. Why? Does it mean that [the kidney meridian of foot-] Shaoyin is easy [to run] reversely and difficult [to run] normally?"

Qibo answered, "No. The thoroughfare vessel [is] the sea of the five Zang-organs and six Fu-organs. All the five Zang-organs and six Fu-organs receive [Qi from it]. [The thoroughfare vessel] runs upwards from Hangsang[3] [located on the head] towards all the Yang [meridians], spreading [innate] essence to all [areas], pouring [it] downwards to the large collateral of [the kidney meridian of foot] Shaoyin, running out from Qichong (ST 30), entering the popliteal fossa along the medial side of the Yin and

到头。足三阳经包括足太阳膀胱经、足阳明胃经和足少阳胆经。足太阳膀胱经从头的睛明穴循行到足小指的至阴穴,足阳明胃经从头的头维穴循行到足次指的厉兑穴,足少阳胆经从头的前关穴循行到足四指的窍阴穴,这些经脉都是从头循行到足部。足三阴经包括足太阴脾经、足少阴肾经和足厥阴肝经。足太阴脾经从足大指内侧的隐白穴循行到腹部的大包穴,足少阴肾经从足心的涌泉穴循行到腹部的俞府穴,足厥阴肝经从足大指外侧的大敦穴循行到腹部的期门穴,这些经脉都是从足部循行到腹部。"

雷公问:"逆顺是怎样的呢?"

岐伯说:"手三阴经循行到手为顺行,循行到脏腑为逆行;手三阳经循行到头部为顺行,循行到手为逆行;足三阴经循行到腹部为顺行,循行到足部为逆行;足三阳经循行到足部为顺行,循行到头部为逆行。"

雷公问:"足三阴经都是从足部循行到腹部,惟独足少阴肾经向下循行,这是为什么呢?难道是足少阴肾经易于逆行而难于顺行吗?"

岐伯说:"不是这样的。冲脉是五脏六腑之海,五脏六腑都禀受其气。冲脉上行,由头部的颃颡穴出,然后渗入各条阳经,灌输其精,又下注于足少阴肾经的大络,从气街穴而出,循阴阳内臁而进入腘中,伏行在胻骨之内,下行到内踝之后,与其他的经脉相通。下行时,冲脉则同时由足少阴肾经渗入足三阴经。循行于身体前面的冲脉,隐伏循行到跗属的络脉而出,向下循行到跗部,进入足大指之间,渗入各条经脉以温养肌肉。所以邪气滞结则跗上之脉不动,跗上之脉不动就会造成厥逆,出现厥逆时足部就会寒冷。这就是足少阴肾经的循行与足三阴经

Yang [meridians], sneaking in the fibula and descending behind the medial ankle, enabling [it to communicate with] other [meridians and collaterals]. [When] running downwards, [the thoroughfare vessel] penetrates into the three Yin [meridians of foot] through [the kidney meridian of foot-] Shaoyin. [When circulating] along the front [of the body], [it] sneaks, runs out from [the collaterals in] the dorsum of foot and enters the interval of the big toe from the dorsum of foot, penetrating into the collaterals [of different meridians] to warm fleshes. Thus [when] evil Qi is stagnated in the collaterals in the dorsum of foot, the meridian is unable to move. [If the meridian is] unable to move, reversal [flow of Qi will be caused]. [If there is] reversal [flow of Qi], [there will be] cold in the foot. So [the kidney] meridian of foot-Shaoyin is different from the three Yin [meridians of foot]. [However it also] circulates towards the abdomen [as that of the other Yin meridians of foot]. "

Leigong asked, " Why does it differ from the three Yin [meridians of foot]?"

Qibo answered, "There is water and fire in the kidney meridian [of foot] Shaoyin. [Thus it] has to circulate in a zigzag way. [That is why] this meridian cannot circulate like the liver [meridian] and spleen [meridian] directly towards the abomen.

Leigong asked, "Why does it move to the abdomen in the same way?"

Qibo answered, "The kidney tends to move reversely. That is why it runs from the lower to the upper, taking reverse [circulation] as normal [circulation]. "

Leigong said, "Reverse circulation tends [to cause] disease. "

略有差异的缘故,但其循行到腹部则是一致的。"

雷公问:"为什么足少阴肾经的循行与足三阴经略有差异?"

岐伯说:"足少阴肾经中隐藏着水火,其经脉不能不曲折地循行,其经脉不像肝经和脾经那样,可以直行到腹部。"

雷公问:"为什么其循行到腹部则是一致的呢?"

岐伯说:"肾经喜逆行,所以由下向上循行,这就是以逆为顺的原因。"

雷公说:"经脉逆行,就应引发疾病。"

岐伯说:"由下向上逆行为顺,所以就不会生病。如果由上往下顺行,就会违背其循行的本性,反而会引发疾病。"

雷公说:"应当全部奏报黄帝。"

岐伯说:"黄帝会问如何才能证明吗? 你可以奏报说:以上面的论述为引导,通过切脉加以验证,踝部之脉必然会动,这样就可以验证逆顺之行了。"

雷公说:"一定遵照您的指教向黄帝奏报。"

陈远公评论说:"十二经脉的循行,有循行到手的、有循行到足的、有循行到头的、有循行到腹的,这就是其差异,分别讲述的可谓言之凿凿。其中所谈到的顺逆不同之处,谁还敢随意地再论一番?"

Qibo said, "Reverse [circulation is proved to be] normal [circulation in the kidney meridian], that is why [it will] not [cause] disease. If normal circulation[4] runs counter to its property, [it] will cause disease."

Leigong said, "All these should be reported [to Yellow Emperor]."

Qibo said, "[If] the Emperor asked about how to prove it, you can tell [the Emperor that] taking [pulse] can prove it [because the pulse of the kidney meridian located in] the ankle must beat. Thus [it] can prove the reverse and normal circulation [of the kidney meridian]."

Leigong said,"[I will] seriously follow [what I have] heard and learned."

Chen Yuangong's comment, "[Among] the twelve meridians, [some] circulate to the hand, [some] to the foot, [some] to the head, [some] to the abdomen, [quite] differing [from each other]. The analysis [about the circulation of] each [meridian] is well-founded. Who dare to doubt about the difference of normal [circulation] and reverse [circulation] mentioned [in this chapter]?"

Notes

[1] Emperor here refers to Yellow Emperor.

[2] Qianguan（前关）refers to Tongziliao（瞳子髎，GB1）.

[3] Hangsang（颃颡）refers to the region between the upper jaw and the nose.

[4] Normal circulation here refers to the circulation from the upper to the lower.

经脉终始篇第十四

【原文】

雷公问于岐伯曰："十二经之脉既有终始,《灵》《素》详言之。而走头、走腹、走足、走手之义,尚未明也,愿毕其辞。"

岐伯曰："手三阳从手走头,足三阳从头走足,乃高之接下也。足三阴从足走腹,手三阴从腹走手,乃卑之趋上也。阴阳无间,故上下相迎,高卑相迓,与昼夜循环同流而不定耳。夫阴阳者,人身之夫妇也;气血者,人身之阴阳也。夫倡则妇随,气行则血赴,气主煦之,血主濡之。乾作天门,大肠司其事也。巽作地户,胆持其权也。泰居艮,小肠之昌也。否居坤,胃之殃也。"

雷公曰:"善,请言顺逆之别。"

岐伯曰:"足三阴自足走腹,顺也;自腹走足,逆也。足三阳自头走足,顺也;自足走头,逆也。手三阴自脏走手,顺也;自手走脏,逆也。手三阳自手走头,顺也;自头走手,逆也。夫足之三阴从足走腹,惟足少阴肾脉绕而下行,与肝脾直行者,以冲脉与之并行也,是以逆为顺也。"

陈远公曰:"十二经,有头腹手足之殊,有顺中之逆,有逆中之顺,

Volume 2

【英译】

Chapter 14
Ending and Beginning of Meridians

Leigong asked Qibo, "[In] *Ling* [*Shu*] (*Spiritual Pivot*) and *Su* [*Wen*] (*Plain Conversation*)[1], there is thorough discussion about the ending and beginning of the twelve meridians [in circulation]. But [the procedure about how] to move to the head, to the abdomen, to the foot and to the hand is not clearly mentioned. Please explain it thoroughly."

Qibo answered, "The three Yang [meridians of] hand run from the hand to the head and the three Yang [meridians of] foot run from the head to the foot, indicating reception of the lower from the upper. The three Yin [meridians of] foot run from the foot to the abdomen and the three Yin [meridians of] hand run from the abdomen to the hand, indicating intension to move from the lower to the upper. [There is] no opposition [between] Yin and Yang, that is why [there is] reception [between] the upper and lower, [there is] communication [between] the high and the low and [the meridians] circulate in accordance with daytime and night without any unchangeability. Yin and Yang [are just like] the husband and wife in the human body; Qi and blood [are just like] Yin and Yang in the human body. [When] the husband has proposed [something], the wife [must] follow. [When] Qi moves [to a certain place], the blood [must] reach [it because] Qi is responsible for warming and the blood is responsible for moistening. Qian[2] serves as the celestial gate and the large intestine is responsible for things related to it.

说得更为明白。"

【今译】

雷公请问岐伯:"十二经脉的循行有始有终,《灵枢》和《素问》已有详细论述。但对于经脉循行到头、循行到腹、循行到足、循行到手的含义,还没有明确的论述,请予以明确的解释。"

岐伯说:"手三阳经从手部循行到头,足三阳经从头部循行到足,这是从高处衔接低处;足三阴经从足循行到腹,手三阴经从腹循行到手部,这是从下部向上部循行。阴与阳没有间隔,所以上下相迎,高与低相接,与昼夜一起循环流行,而不是固定不变。阴阳就是人身之夫妇,气血就是人身之阴阳。夫倡导则妇跟随,气运行则血随行。气主温煦,血主濡养。乾卦是天门,大肠主管其事务;巽卦是地户,胆腑主持其权力;泰卦位于艮位,是小肠昌盛之处;否卦位居坤位,是胃所辖之处。"

雷公说:"好!请解说顺逆之别。"

岐伯说:"足三阴经从足循行到腹,这就是顺行;从腹循行到足,这就是逆行。足三阳经从头部循行到足,这就是顺行;从足部循行到头,这就是逆行。手三阴经,从脏器循行到手,这就是顺行;自手循行到脏器,这就是逆行。手三阳经从手循行到头部,这就是顺行;从头循行到手部,这就是逆行。足三阴经从足循行到腹,这只有足少阴肾经环绕向下循行,与肝和脾一起直行,由于冲脉与之并行,这就是以逆为顺的

Volume 2

Xun[3] serves as the door of the earth and the gallbladder controls its power. Tai[4] is located [in the position of] Gen[5], [where] the small intestine is prosperous. Pi[6] is located [in the position of] Kun[7], [which is the place that] the stomach governs."

Leigong said, "Good! Please tell [me] the difference [between] reverse [circulation] and normal [circulation]."

Qibo answered, "The three Yin [meridians] of foot run from the foot to the abdomen, it is normal [circulation]; [if they] run from the abdomen to the foot, [it is] reverse [circulation]. The three Yang [meridians] of foot run from the head to the foot, [it is] normal [circulation]; [if they] run from the foot to the head, [it is] reverse [circulation]. The three Yin [meridians of] hand run from the viscera to the hand, [it is] normal [circulation]; [if they] run from the hand to the viscera, [it is] reverse [circulation]. The three Yang [meridians of] hand run from the hand to the head, [it is] normal [circulation]; [if they] run from the head to the hand, [it is] reverse [circulation]. [Among] the three Yin [meridians of] foot that run from the foot to the abdomen, only the kidney meridian of foot-Shaoyin moves round downwards. [Besides, it also] runs directly with the liver [meridian] and spleen [meridian] because the thoroughfare vessel runs together with it. That is why reverse [circulation] is actually the normal [circulation in the movement of the kidney meridian of foot-Shaoyin]."

Chen Yuangong's comment, "[Among] the twelve meridians, there is difference [in terms of moving towards] the head, abdomen, hand and foot, there is reverse [circulation] in normal [circulation] and there is normal [circulation] in reverse

含义。"

陈远公评论说："十二经脉有头、腹、手和足的差别,有顺中之逆的现象,也有逆中之顺的现象,这里解说得更加明白了。"

[*circulation*]. [*All these problems are*] *quite clearly explained*."

Notes

[1] In this Chapter，*Ling* (《灵》) and *Su* (《素》) are the abbreviated titles of *Ling Shu* (《灵枢》, *Spiritual Pivot*) and *Su Wen* (《素问》, *Plain Conversation*)，two fascicles of *Huang Di Nei Jing* (《黄帝内经》，*Yellow Emperor's Internal Canon of Medicine*).

[2] Qian (乾) refers to Qian Gua (乾卦, Qian Diagram)，representing the sky. Qian Gua (乾卦, Qian Diagram) is the first diagram in the *Yi Jing* (《易经》, the *Book of Change*). The Chinese character 易 in *Yi Jing* (《易经》, *the Book of Change*) is usually translated as "Change" in English. In fact 易 traditionally means three things，i.e. simplication (简易), change (变易) and no change (不易).

[3] Xun (巽) refers to Xun Gua (巽卦, Xun Diagram)，the fourth diagram in the *Yi Jing* (《易经》, the *Book of Change*)，representing wind.

[4] Tai (泰) refers to Tai Gua (泰卦, Tai Diagram)，the eleventh diagram in the *Yi Jing* (《易经》, the *Book of Change*)，representing the earth and the sky. In its structure，the earth is in the upper and the sky is in the lower.

[5] Gen (艮) refers to Gen Gua (艮卦，Gen Diagram)，the fifty-two diagram in the *Yi Jing* (《易经》, the *Book of Change*)，representing double mountain.

[6] Pi (否) refers to Pi Gua (否卦，Pi Diagram)，the twelfth diagram in the *Yi Jing* (《易经》, the *Book of Change*)，representing the sky and earth. In its structure，the sky is in the upper and the earth is in the lower.

[7] Kun (坤) refers to Kun Gua (坤卦，Kun Diagram)，the second diagrm in the *Yi Jing* (《易经》, the *Book of Change*)，representing the earth. Its structure is composed of double earth.

经气本标篇第十五

【原文】

雷公问于岐伯曰："十二经气有标本乎?"

岐伯曰："有之。"

雷公曰："请言标本之所在。"

岐伯曰："足太阳之本在跟以上五寸中,标在两络命门。足少阳之本在窍阴之间,标在窗笼之前。足少阴之本在内踝下三寸中,标在背腧。足厥阴之本在行间上五寸所,标在背腧。足阳明之本在厉兑,标在人迎,颊挟颃颡。足太阴之本在中封前上四寸中,标在舌本乎。足太阳之本在外踝之后,标在命门之上一寸。手少阳之本在小指次指之间上二寸,标在耳后上角下外眦。手阳明之本在肘骨中上至别阳,标在颜下合钳上。手太阴之本在寸口中,标在腋内动脉。手少阴之本在锐骨之端,标在背腧。手心主之本在掌后两筋之间二寸中,标在腋下三寸。此标本之所在也。"

雷公曰："标本皆可刺乎?"

岐伯曰："气之标本皆不可刺也。"

雷公曰;"其不可刺,何也?"

岐伯曰;"气各有冲,冲不可刺也。"

雷公曰:"请言气冲。"

Volume 2

【英译】

Chapter 15
Root and Tip of Meridian Qi

Leigong asked Qibo, "Are there root and tip of Qi in the twelve meridians?"

Qibo answered, "Yes."

Leigong asked, "Please tell [me about] the place [where] the root and tip [of meridian Qi are located]."

Qibo answered, "[In the bladder meridian of] foot-Taiyang, the root [is located] five *Cun* above the heel and the tip [is located] in Mingmen (GV 4) [between] two collaterals; [in the gallbladder meridian of] foot-Shaoyang, the root [is located] between Qiaoyin (GB 44) and the tip [is located] in front of Chuanglong (ear); [in the kidney meridian of] foot-Shaoyin, the root [is located] three *Cun* below the medial ankle and the tip [is located] in an acupoint on the back; [in the liver meridian of] foot-Jueyin, the root [is located] five *Cun* above Xingjian (LR 2) and the tip [is located] in an acupoint on the back; [in the stomach meridian of] foot-Yangming, the root [is located] in Lidui (ST 45) and the tip [is located] in Renying (ST 9) and Hangsang (the region between the upper jaw and nose) in the cheek; [in the spleen meridian of] foot-Taiyin, the root [is located] four *Cun* before Zhongfeng (LR 4) and the tip [is located] in the tongue root; [in the bladder meridian of foot-] Taiyang, the root [is located] behind the external ankle

岐伯曰:"胃气有冲,腹气有冲,头气有冲,胫气有冲,皆不可刺也。"

雷公曰:"头之冲何所乎?"

岐伯曰:"头之冲,脑也。"

雷公曰:"胸之冲何所乎?"

岐伯曰:"胸之冲,膺与背腧也。亦不可刺也。"

雷公曰:"腹之冲何所乎?"

岐伯曰:"腹之冲,背腧与冲脉及左右之动脉也。"

雷公曰:"胫之冲何所乎?"

岐伯曰:"胫之冲,即脐之气街及承山踝上以下。此皆不可刺也。"

雷公曰:"不可刺止此乎?"

岐伯曰:"大气之抟而不行者,积于胸中,藏于气海,出于肺,循咽喉,呼吸而出入也。是气海犹气街也,应天地之大数,出三入一,皆不可刺也。"

陈远公曰:"十二经气,各有标本,各不可刺。不可刺者,以冲脉之不可刺也。不知冲脉,即不知刺法也。"

【今译】

雷公请问岐伯:"十二经气有标本吗?"

岐伯说:"有的。"

雷公问:"请解释标本位于何处。"

and the tip [is located] one *Cun* above Mingmen (GV 4); [in the triple energizer meridian of] hand-Shaoyang, the root [is located] two *Cun* between the small finger and the second finger and the tip [is located in between] the upper angle of the ear and lateral angle of the eye; [in the large intestine meridian of] hand-Yangming, the root [is located] above the middle of the elbow to Bieyang[1] and the tip [is located] in the middle below the cheeks; [in the lung meridian of] hand-Taiyin, the root [is located] in Cunkou[2] and the tip [is located] in the artery inside the armpit; [in the heart meridian of] hand-Shaoyin, the root [is located in] the top of the styloid process of radius, and the tip [is located] in an acupoint on the back; [in] the pericardium [meridian of hand-Jueyin], the root [is located in the region] two *Cun* between two sinews behind the palm, and the tip [is located] three *Cun* below the armpit. These are the places [where] the root and tip [of these twelve meridians are] located. "

Leigong asked,"Can all the roots and tips be needled?"

Qibo answered, "The root and tip of Qi all cannot be needled. "

Leigong asked,"Why can they not be needled?"

Qibo answered, "[Both the root and tip of] Qi may surge [under certain condition]. [When] surging, [they] cannot be needled. "

Leigong asked,"Please tell [me] about [what kind of] Qi [that may]surge. "

Qibo answered, "Qi [from] the stomach may surge, Qi [from] the abdomen may surge, Qi [from] the head may surge and Qi [from] the shank may surge. [The root and tip of meridians in

岐伯说:"足太阳经之本在足跟以上五寸中,标在两络的命门穴处;足少阳经之本在足窍阴穴之间,标在窗笼穴之前;足少阴经之本在内踝下三寸之中,标在背腧穴之中;足厥阴经之本在行间之上五寸之处,标在背腧穴之中;足阳明经之本在厉兑穴之中,标在人迎穴和面颊部的颃颡穴中;足太阴经之本在中封穴前上四寸之中,标在舌根之中;足太阳经之本在足外踝之后,标在命门穴上一寸处;手少阳经之本在小指与次指之间上二寸处,标在耳后上角之下的外眦穴中;手阳明经之本在肘骨中上至别阳穴位,标在面部下的合钳穴上;手太阴经之本在寸口穴中,标在腋内的动脉中;手少阴经之本在掌后的锐骨之端,标在背腧穴中;手少阴心经之本在掌后两筋之间二寸中,标在腋下三寸中,这是标和本的所在之处。"

雷公问:"标和本都可以针刺吗?"

岐伯说:"标和本都不能针刺。"

雷公问:"标本为什么不能针刺呢?"

岐伯说:"标本之气均有气冲,气冲不能针刺。"

雷公问:"请说明气冲。"

岐伯说:"胃气有冲,腹气有冲,头气有冲,胫气有冲,都不能针刺。"

雷公问:"头部的气冲在何处?"

岐伯说:"头部的气冲在脑。"

雷公问:"胸部的气冲在何处?"

岐伯说:"胸部的气冲在胸膺与背腧处,背腧穴也不可针刺。"

these places] all cannot be needled. "

Leigong asked, "Where does [Qi from] the head surge?"

Qibo answered, "[Qi from] the head surges to the brains. "

Leigong asked, "Where does [Qi] from the chest surge?"

Qibo answered, "[Qi from] the chest surges to the chest and the acupoint on the back. [The acupoint on the back] also cannot be needled. "

Leigong asked, "Where does [Qi from] the abdomen surge? "

Qibo answered, "[Qi from] the abdomen surges to the acupoint on the back, the thoroughfare vessel and the arteries at the right and left [sides]. "

Leigong asked, "Where does [Qi from] the shank surge?"

Qibo answered, "[Qi from] the shank surges to Qijie[3] at the navel and Chengshan (BL 57) below the ankle. These [regions] cannot be needled. "

Leigong asked, "Only these [regions] cannot be needled?"

Qibo answered, "Great Qi may just gather and does not move. [In this case, Qi] accumulates in the chest, conceals in Qihai (CV 6), emerges from the lung, circulates in and out along the throat with respiration. [In this way,] Qihai (CV 6) is the same as Qijie, corresponding to the big number of the sky and earth with three outflows and one inflow. All [these regions] cannot be needled. "

Chen Yuangong's comment, " There are roots and tips of Qi [in] the twelve meridians, all [of which] cannot be needled. [The reason that they] cannot be needled is the thoroughfare vessel [which] cannot be needled. [If one is] unclear about the

雷公问："腹部的气冲在何处?"

岐伯说："腹部的气冲在背腧与冲脉以及左右的动脉处。"

雷公问："足胫的气冲在何处?"

岐伯说："足胫的气冲在脐部的气街及足踝之下的承山穴,这些都不能针刺。"

雷公问："不可针刺的只有这些地方吗?"

岐伯说："大气聚集而不能循行,就积累在胸中,隐藏在气海中,从肺部出来,沿着咽喉呼吸而出入,所以气海正如气街一样,应于对天地的大数,出三入一,都不能针刺。"

陈远公评论说："十二经之气,分别有标本之分,都不能针刺。这些部分之所以不能针刺,是因为冲脉不能针刺。如果不知道冲脉,就不知道如何使用刺法了。"

thoroughfare vessel，［*he is certainly*］ *unclear about needling techniques*."

Notes

［1］Bieyang（别阳）refers to either Yangchi（阳池，TE 4）or Yangjiao（阳交，GB 35）.

［2］Cunkou（寸口）refers to the radial artery in the medial side of the radius.

［3］Qijie（气街）here refers to Qichong（气冲，ST 30）.

脏腑阐微篇第十六

【原文】

雷公问于岐伯曰:"脏止五乎? 腑止六乎?"

岐伯曰:"脏六腑七也。"

雷公曰:"脏六何以名五也?"

岐伯曰:"心肝脾肺肾五行之正也,故名五脏。胞胎非五行之正也,虽脏不以脏名之。"

雷公曰:"胞胎何以非五脏之正也?"

岐伯曰:"心火也,肝木也,脾土也,肺金也,肾水也,一脏各属一行。胞胎处水火之歧,非正也,故不可称六脏也。"

雷公曰:"肾中有火,亦水火之歧也,何肾称脏乎?"

岐伯曰:"肾中之火,先天火也,居两肾中,而肾专司水也。胞胎上系心,下连肾,往来心肾,接续于水火之际,可名为火,亦可名为水,非水火之正也。"

雷公曰:"然则胞胎何以为脏乎?"

岐伯曰:"胞胎处水火之两歧,心肾之交,非胞胎之系不能通达上下,宁独妇人有之,男子未尝无也。吾因其两歧置于五脏之外,非胞胎之不为脏也。"

雷公曰:"男女各有之,亦有异乎?"

Volume 2

【英译】

Chapter 16
Brief Discussion About the Viscera

Leigong asked Qibo, "Are there just five Zang-organs and six Fu-organs?"

Qibo answered, "[In fact there are] six Zang-organs and seven Fu-organs."

Leigong asked, "[There are] six Zang-organs. [But why] is the nomenclature five Zang-organs?"

Qibo answered, "The heart, liver, spleen, lung and kidney are five authentic [organs according to] the five elements. That is why [they are] named five Zang-organs. Uterus is not the authentic [organ] in the five elements. [That is why it is] a Zang-organ, [but it is] not named Zang-organ."

Leigong asked, "Why is the uterus not authentic in the five Zang-organs?"

Qibo answered, "The heart [corresponds to] fire, the liver [to] wood, the spleen [to] earth, the lung [to] metal and the kidney [to] water, one organ corresponding to one element [in the five elements]. The uterus is located [in the region where] water and fire interact [with each other], not in the authentic [position]. That is why [these six Zang-organs are] not called six Zang-organs."

Leigong asked, "There is fire in the kidney, [indicating that it

岐伯曰:"系同而口异也。男女无此系,则水火不交,受病同也。女系无口,则不能受妊。是胞胎者,生生之机,属阴而藏于阳,非脏而何?"

雷公曰:"胞胎之口又何以异?"

岐伯曰:"胞胎之系,上出于心之膜膈,下连两肾,此男女之同也。惟女下大而上细,上无口而下有口,故能纳精以受妊。"

雷公曰:"腑七而名六何也?"

岐伯曰:"大小肠、膀胱、胆、胃、三焦、包络,此七腑也。遗包络不称腑者,尊帝耳。"

雷公曰;"包络可遗乎?"

岐伯曰:"不可遗也。包络为脾胃之母,土非火不生。五脏六腑之气咸仰于心君。心火无为,必藉包络有为,往来宣布胃气,能入脾气,能出各脏腑之气,始能变化也。"

雷公曰:"包络既为一腑,奈何尊帝遗之? 尊心为君火,称包络为相火,可乎?"

岐伯曰:"请登之《外经》咸以为则。"

陈远公曰:"脏六而言五者,言脏之正也;腑七而言六者,言腑之偏也。举五而略六,非不知胞胎也;举六而略七,非不知包络也。有雷公之问,而胞胎、包络,昭于古今矣!"

【今译】

雷公请问岐伯:"脏只有五个,腑只有六个,是这样的吗?"

is⌉ also ⌈located in the region where⌉ water and fire interact ⌈with each other⌉. ⌈But⌉ why is the kidney named Zang-organ?"

Qibo answered, "Fire in the kidney is innate fire and located between the two kidneys. And the kidney mainly controls water. The uterus is connected with the heart in the upper and the kidney in the lower, acting to and fro ⌈between⌉ the heart and kidney, communicating ⌈with the region where⌉ water and fire interact ⌈with each other⌉. ⌈For this reason, it⌉ can be named fire, and also be named water ⌈because it is⌉ not the authentic ⌈position of⌉ water and fire."

Leigong asked, "Why can the uterus be called Zang-organ?"

Qibo answered, "The uterus is located ⌈in the place where⌉ water and fire interact ⌈with each other⌉ and the heart and kidney communicate ⌈with each other⌉. Without connection of the uterus, ⌈it⌉ cannot penetrate the upper and lower. ⌈It is⌉ not only located in women, but also in men. Since it bears two properties ⌈of water and fire⌉, I do not involve it into the five Zang-organs. ⌈But it does⌉ not ⌈mean that⌉ the uterus is not a Zang-organ."

Leigong asked, "Both men and women have uterus. Is there any difference?"

Qibo answered, "The connection is the same, but the opening is different. ⌈If there is⌉ no such a connection ⌈of the uterus⌉ in men and women, water and fire cannot interact ⌈with each other⌉, ⌈and therefore⌉ suffering from the same disease. ⌈If there is only connection but⌉ no opening in women, ⌈it is⌉ impossible to conceive a baby. Thus the uterus ⌈is⌉ an organ ⌈responsible for⌉ life and growth. ⌈It⌉ belongs to Yin ⌈in nature⌉, but still contains Yang.

岐伯说:"其实脏有六个,腑有七个。"

雷公问:"既然脏有六个,但为什么将其命名为五脏呢?"

岐伯说:"心、肝、脾、肺、肾,是五行之正,因此将其命名为五脏。胞胎不是五行之正,虽然是脏,但却不以脏命名。"

雷公问:"胞胎为什么不是五脏之正呢?"

岐伯说:"心是火,肝是木,脾是土,肺是金,肾是水,这五脏分别属于五行中的一行。胞胎为水火交互之处,不是五脏的正位,所以不能将其称为六脏。"

雷公问:"肾中有火,也是水火交互之处,但为什么将肾称为脏呢?"

岐伯说:"肾中的火,是先天之火,位于两肾之中,而肾则专门司管水液。胞胎向上连接到心,向下连接到肾,往来于心肾之间,接续于水火交互之处,可以命名为火,也可以命名为水,但却不是水火之正位。"

雷公问:"但为什么胞胎也可称为脏呢?"

岐伯说:"胞胎位于水火交互之处,心肾之间的相交,如果没有胞胎的联系,就不能上通下达,这并不只有女子才有,男子也并不是没有。我因为觉得胞胎具有水火两性,所以将置于五脏之外,这并不是说胞胎不能成为脏器。"

雷公问:"男女各有胞胎,之间存在差异吗?"

岐伯说:"虽然其联系渠道相同,但是其开口却是有差异的。如果男女之间没有这样的联系性,水火就会不交,所患之病也就相同了。女子如果只有联系而没有胞胎口,就不能受孕。所以胞胎是生生不息的

Why is it not a Zang-organ?"

Leigong asked, "Why is the opening of the uterus different?"

Qibo answered, "The system of the uterus emerges upwards from the membrane of the heart and connects downwards with the two kidneys. This is the same in men and women. Only [in] women, [the uterus is] large in the lower with opening and small in the upper without opening. That is why [the uterus in women] can receive semen to conceive a baby."

Leigong asked, "[There are] seven Fu-organs, [but] why is the nomenclature six [Fu-organs]?"

Qibo answered, "The seven Fu-organs [include] large intestine, small intestine, bladder, gallbladder, stomach, triple energizer and Baoluo (elliptic collateral). [The reason that] Baoluo (elliptic collateral) is neglected and not named Fu-organ is to respect [it as] the Emperor."

Leigong asked: "Why can Baoluo (elliptic collateral) be neglected?"

Qibo answered, "[It] cannot be neglected. Baoluo (elliptic collateral) is the mother of the spleen and stomach. Without fire, earth cannot exist. Qi in the five Zang-organs and six Fu-organs all depends on the heart [emphasized as a] monarch. Fire in the heart governs by noninterference and depends on the activities of Baoluo (elliptic collateral), emitting and spreading stomach-Qi to and fro, promoting spleen-Qi and invigorating Qi in every Zang-organ and Fu-organ, [consequently] leading to transformation [of Qi in the viscera]."

Leigong asked, "Since Baoluo (elliptic collateral) is a Fu-organ,

机制,本性属阴而藏于阳中,这如果不是脏又会是什么呢?"

雷公问:"胞胎的开口,又有什么差异呢?"

岐伯说:"胞胎的连接,在上从心脏的膈膜出来,在下联系着两肾,这在男女中是相同的。但在联系中,惟独女子的下端大而上端小,上端没有开口,下端有开口,所以可以受精怀孕。"

雷公问:"腑有七个,但为什么将其命名为六呢?"

岐伯说:"大小肠、膀胱、胆、胃、三焦、包络,这是七腑。遗漏了包络而不称其为腑这是尊其为帝的缘故。"

雷公问:"包络可以遗漏吗?"

岐伯说:"包络不可遗漏。包络是脾胃之母,如果没有了火土就不能生发,五脏六腑之气都依赖于心主。心火虽然无为而治,但却必须依靠包络的有为,通过其往来宣精布气,胃气才能入,脾气才会出,各脏腑之气才会发生变化。"

雷公问:"包络既然是一腑,为什么要尊称其为帝而遗漏呢? 可以尊称心为君火,称呼包络为相火吗?"

岐伯说:"请刊登在《外经》上,令大家都以此为原则。"

陈远公评论说:"脏有六个,但却称为五个,是说明脏居于正位;腑有七个,但却称为六个,是说明腑处于偏位。称呼五脏而忽略了第六个脏,并不是不知道有胞胎的存在;称呼六腑而忽略了第七个腑,也不是不知道有心包络的存在。有雷公的询问,经过岐伯的解释说明,胞胎和心包络的问题从古到今就大白于天下了!"

why [do you just] respect the Emperor and neglect it? Is it necessary to respectfully call the heart as monarch-fire and Baoluo (elliptic collateral) ministerial fire? "

Qibo answered, "Please record it in [*Yellow Emperor's*] *External Canon* [*of Medicine*] to publicize this principle."

Chen Yuangong's comment, " The six Zang-organs [that are] named five [Zang-organs is for the purpose of] discussing the authentic [position] of the Zang-organs; the seven Fu-organ [that are] named six [Fu-organs is for the purpose of] discussing the non-authentic [position] of the Fu-organs. To list the five [Zang-organs] and neglect the sixth [one] does not mean [that the Celestial Master is] unclear about the uterus; to list the six [Fu-organs] and neglect the seventh [one] does not mean [that the Celestial Master is] unclear about Baoluo (elliptic collateral). [Because of the question] asked by Leigong, [the positions and functions of] the uterus and Baoluo (elliptic collateral) are very clear now!"

考订经脉篇第十七

【原文】

雷公问于岐伯曰："十二经脉天师详之,而所以往来相通之故,尚来尽也。幸宣明奥义,传诸奕祀可乎?"

岐伯曰："可。肺属手太阴,太阴者,月之象也,月属金,肺亦属金。肺之脉走于手,故曰手太阴也。起于中焦胃脘之上,胃属土,土能生金,是胃乃肺之母也。下络大肠者,以大肠亦属金,为胃之庶子,而肺为大肠之兄,兄能包弟,足以网罗之也。络即网罗包举之义。循于胃口者,以胃为肺之母,自必游熙于母家,省受胃土之气也。肺脉又上于鬲,胃之气多,必分气以给其子,肺得胃母之气,上归肺宫,必由膈而升。肺受胃之气肺自成家,于是由中焦而脉乃行,横出腋下,畏心而不敢犯也。然而肺之系实通于心,以心为肺之君,而肺乃臣也,臣必朝于君,此述职之路也。下循臑内,行少阴心主之前者,又谒相之门也。心主即心包络,为心君之相,包络代君以行事。心克肺金,必借心主之气以相刑,呼吸相通,全在此系之相联也。肺禀天王之尊,必奉宰辅之令,所以行于少阴心主之前而不敢缓也。自此而下干肘中,乃走于臂,由臂而走于寸口、鱼际,皆肺脉相通之道。循鱼际出大指之端,为肺脉之尽。经脉尽,复行,从腕后直出次指内廉,乃旁出之脉也。"

Volume 2

【英译】

Chapter 17
To Examine and Correct Meridians and Vessels

Leigong asked Qibo, "[You], the Celestial Master, have thoroughly [described] the twelve meridians. [However,] the circulation [of the twelve meridians] to and fro still needs to explain. [I sincerely] hope [that you can] clearly explain [its] profound significance and keep [it] for the future generations. Could [you] explain [it]?"

Qibo answered, "Yes. The lung belongs to [the meridian of] hand-Taiyin. Taiyin is the image of the moon. The moon belongs to metal [in nature] and so does the lung. The lung meridian circulates along the hand. That is why [it is] called hand-Taiyin. [The lung meridian] originates from above the stomach in the middle energizer. The stomach belongs to the earth [in nature] and the earth can produce metal. Thus the stomach is the mother of the lung. [The lung meridian runs] downwards to the large intestine and the large intestine also belongs to metal [in nature]. [For this reason, the large intestine] is the collateral son of the stomach while the lung is the elder brother of the large intestine. Elder brother can protect and get together with younger brother. Collateral indicates the significance of getting together. [The lung meridian] circulates around the opening of the stomach because the stomach is the mother of the lung. [As the son of the stomach, the lung meridian]

雷公曰："脾经若何?"

岐伯曰："脾乃土脏,其性湿,以足太阴名之。太阴之月,夜照于土,月乃阴象,脾属土,得月之阴气,故以太阴名之。

其脉起于足大指之端,故又曰足太阴也。脾脉既起于足下,下必升上,由足大指内侧肉际,过横骨后,上内踝前廉,上踹内,循胫骨后,交出厥阴之前,乃入肝经之路也。

夫肝木克脾,宜为脾之所畏,何故脉反通于肝? 不知肝虽克土,而木亦能成土,土无木气之通,则土少发生之气,所以畏肝而又未尝不喜肝也。交出足厥阴之前,图合于肝木耳。上膝股内前廉入腹者,归于脾经之本脏也。盖腹脾之正宫,脾属土,居于中州,中州为天下之腹,脾乃人一身之腹也。

脾与胃为表里,脾内而胃外,脾为胃所包,故络于胃。脾得胃气则脾之气始能上升,故脉亦随之上鬲,趋喉咙而至舌本,以舌本为心之苗,而脾为心之子,子母之气自相通而不隔也。

然而舌为心之外窍,非心之内廷也,脾之脉虽至于舌,而终未至于心,故其支又行,借胃之气,从胃中中脘之外上鬲,而脉通于膻中之分,上交于手少阴心经,子亲母之象也。"

雷公曰："心经若何?"

岐伯曰："心为火脏,以手少阴名之者,盖心火乃后天也。后天者,有形之火也。星应荧惑,虽属火而实属阴,且脉走于手,故以手少阴名之。

他脏腑之脉皆起于手足,心脉独起于心,不与众脉同者,以心为君

certainly travels freely in the place of the mother to receive Qi from stomach-earth[1]. The lung meridian circulates upwards to the diaphragm. [When] Qi in the stomach is sufficient, [it] will certainly give some to its son. [When] the lung has received Qi from the stomach, the mother, [it will] return to the lung, rising up from the diaphragm. [When] the lung has received Qi from the stomach, [it becomes] an independent organ and its meridian begins to circulate from the middle energizer, transversely flowing out below the armpit and daring not to offend the heart. But the system of the lung actually communicates with the heart [because] the heart is respected as the monarch of the lung and the lung is [respected as] the minister [of the heart]. [As a] minister, [the lung] must worship the monarch and this is the way to accomplish [its] duty. [The lung meridian] circulates downwards to the medial side of the forearm, flowing before the heart [meridian of hand-] Shaoyin and the pericardium [meridian of hand-Jueyin] to pay homage [to the monarch]. The heart defender is the pericardium [which] is the prime minister of the heart and works for the monarch. The heart restricts lung-metal and controls it with the aid of Qi from the pericardium. [Therefore,] the connection [between] respiration [and the heart] depends on the communication of this system. The lung worships the monarch[2] and certainly execute the order of the prime minister[3], therefore moving before the heart [meridian of hand-] Shaoyin and the pericardium [meridian of hand-Jueyin] and daring not to be sluggish. Then [the lung meridian circulates] downwards to the elbow, moving to [the medial side of] the forearm and reaching

主,总揽权纲,不寄其任于四末也。心之系,五脏七腑无不相通,尤通者,小肠也。

小肠为心之表,而心实络于小肠,下通任脉,故任脉即借小肠之气以上通于心,为朝君之象也。

心之系又上与肺相通,挟咽喉而入于目,以发其文明之彩也。复从心系上肺,下出腋下,循臑内后廉,行手厥阴经心主之后,下肘,循臂至小指之内出其端,此心脉系之直行也。又由肺曲折而后,并脊直下,与肾相贯串,当命门之中,此心肾既济之路也。

夫心为火脏,惧畏水克,何故系通于肾,使肾有路以相犯乎?不知心火与命门之火,原不可一日不相通也,心得命门之火则心火有根,心非肾水之滋则心火不旺。盖心火必得肾中水火以相养,是以克为生也。既有肾火肾水之相生,而后心之系各通脏腑,无扞格之忧矣。

由是而左通于肝,肝本属木,为生心之母也。心火虽生于命门先天之火,而非后天肝木培之,则先天之火气亦不旺,故心之系通于肝者,亦欲得肝木相生之气也。肝气既通,而胆在肝之旁,通肝即通于胆,又势之甚便者,况胆又为心之父,同本之亲尤无阻隔也。

由是而通于脾,脾乃心之子也,虽脾土不藉心火之生,然胃为心之爱子,胃土非心火不生,心既生胃,生胃必生脾,此脾胃之系所以相接而无间也。由是而通于肺,火性炎上,而肺叶当之,得母有伤。然而顽金非火不柔,克中亦有生之象,倘肺金无火则金寒水冷,胃与膀胱之化源

Volume 2

Cunkou (pulse in the wrist) and thenar eminence from the forearm, [which are] the ways [that] the lung meridian communicates and connects [with other meridians and regions]. Circulating from the thenar eminence to the tip of the thumb, the lung meridian has reached the terminal [of its circulation]. [When the circulation of] meridian has reached the terminal, [it begins] to restart, circulating directly from the back of the wrist to the medial side of the second finger. This is a branch [of the lung meridian] stemming from the lateral side [of it]."

Leigong asked,"How does the spleen meridian [circulate]?"

Qibo answered, "The spleen is a Zang-organ [related to] earth and its nature is dampness. [That is why it is] named foot-Taiyin. The moonshine of Taiyin[2] lights the earth at night. The moon is the image of Yin and the spleen belongs to earth [in matching with the five elements] and receives Yin Qi from the moon. That is why [the spleen is] named Taiyin. The meridian [of the spleen] originates from the top of the big toe. That is why [it is] also named foot-Taiyin. Since the spleen meridian starts from the lower of the foot, [it] must run to the upper from the lower. From the medial side of the big toe, [the spleen meridian] runs over the transverse bone, circulating upwards to the front of the medial ankle, the medial side of the shank and posterior side of the tibia, interacting [with the liver meridian of] foot-Jueyin in the front, and finally entering the path [along which] the liver meridian [circulates].

The liver-wood restricts the spleen [and is the organ that] the spleen fears. But why can [the spleen] meridian enter [the path

绝矣，何以温肾而传化于大肠乎？

由是而通于心主，心主即膻中包络也，为心君之相臣，奉心君以司化。其出入之经，较五脏六腑更近，真有心喜亦喜，心忧亦忧之象，呼吸相通，代君司化以使令夫三焦，俾上中下之气无不毕达，实心之系通之也。”

雷公曰：“肾经若何？”

岐伯曰：“肾属水，少阴正水之象。海水者，少阴水也，随月为盈虚，而肾应之。名之为足少阴者，脉起于足少阴之下也，由足心而上，循内踝之后，别入跟中，上腨出腘，上股贯脊，乃河车之路，即任督之路也。

然俱属于肾，有肾水而河车之路通，无肾水而河车之路塞，有肾水而督脉之路行，无肾水而督脉之路断，是二经之相通相行，全责于肾，故河车之路、督脉之路，即肾经之路也。

由是而行于肝，母入于子舍之义也。由是而行于脾，水行于地中之义也。过肝脾二经而络于膀胱者，以肾为膀胱之里，而膀胱为肾之表，膀胱得肾气而始化，正同此路之相通，气得以往来之耳。

其络于膀胱也，贯脊会督而还出于脐之前，通任脉始得达于膀胱，虽气化可至，实有经可通而通之也。其直行者，又由肝以入肺，子归母之家也。由肺而上循喉咙，挟舌本而终，是欲朝君先通于喉舌也。

夫肾与心虽若相克，而实相生，故其系别出而绕于心，又未敢遽朝于心君，注胸之膻中包络，而后肾经之精上奉，化为心之液矣，此君王下

along which] the liver [meridian] circulates? [One may know that] the liver restricts earth, but may not know [that] wood can promote [the formation of] earth. Without communication with wood, earth will lack production of Qi. For this reason, [the spleen] fears the liver, but also loves the liver. Before communicating with [the liver meridian of] foot-Jueyin, [it] tends to combine with [Qi in] the liver-wood. [When circulating] upwards to the kneecap and the front of the medial side of the thigh, [it] enters the abdomen, returning to the source organ of the spleen meridian. In the abdomen, the spleen is the authentic palace. The spleen belongs to the earth and is located in the central plains. The central plains is the abdomen of this world. [In the human body,] the spleen is the abdomen.

The spleen and the stomach are internally and externally [related to each other]. [In terms of the human body,] the spleen is in the internal and the stomach is in the external. That is why the collateral [belongs to] the stomach. [When] receiving Qi from the stomach, Qi in the spleen begins to rise and accordingly the meridian starts to circulate upwards to the diaphragm, and finally to the throat and tongue root. The tongue root is the sprout of the heart and the spleen is the son of the heart. Qi from the son and mother certainly connects [with each other] naturally without any intervals.

However, the tongue is the external orifice of the heart, not the internal court. Although the spleen meridian reaches at the tongue, [it] finally fails to reach the heart. That is why the branches [of the spleen meridian] continue to circulate. With the

取于民之义,亦草野上贡于国之谊也。

各脏止有一而肾有二者,两仪之象也。两仪者,日月也。月主阴,日主阳,似肾乃水脏,宜应月不宜应日,然而月之中未尝无阳之气,日之中未尝无阴之气,肾配日月正以其中之有阴阳也。阴藏于阳之中,阳隐于阴之内,叠相为用,不啻日月之照临也。盖五脏七腑各有水火,独肾脏之水火处于无形,乃先天之水火,非若各脏腑之水火俱属后天也。

夫同是水火,肾独属之先天,实有主以存乎两肾之间也。主者,命门也。命门为小心,若太极之象能生先天之水火,因以生后天之水火也。于是裁成夫五脏七腑,各安于诸宫,享其奠定之福,化生于无穷耳。"

雷公曰:"肝经若何?"

岐伯曰:"肝属足厥阴。厥阴者,逆阴也。上应雷火,脉起足大指丛毛之际,故以足厥阴名之。

雷火皆从地起,腾于天之上,其性急,不可制抑,肝之性亦急,乃阴经中之最逆者,少拂其意,则厥逆而不可止。循跗上,上踝,交出太阴脾土之后,上腘内廉,循腹入阴毛中,过阴器,以抵于小腹,虽趋肝之路,亦趋脾之路也。

既趋于脾,必趋于胃矣。肝之系既通于脾胃,凡有所逆,必先犯于脾胃矣,亦其途路之熟也。虽然,肝之系通于脾胃,而肝之气必归于本宫,故其系又走于肝叶之中,肝叶之旁有胆附焉,胆为肝之兄,肝为胆之弟,胆不络肝而肝反络胆者,弟强于兄之义也。

aid of Qi from the stomach, [it circulates] upwards to the diaphragm from the middle of the gastric cavity, and finally reaching the external of Danzhong (CV 17) and communicating with the heart meridian of hand-Shaoyin, [which demonstrates the fact that] the son loves the mother."

Leigong asked, "How does the heart meridian circulate?"

Qibo answered, "The heart is a Zang-organ [pertaining to] fire. [The reason that it is] named hand-Shaoyin [is that] heart-fire is acquired postnatally. Postnatally acquired [fire] is visible fire, corresponding to the dazzling and puzzling star. Although [the heart] belongs to fire, [it] actually belongs to Yin. Since [the heart] meridian circulates along the hand, [it is] named hand-Shaoyin.

The meridians of other Zang-organs and Fu-organs all start from the hand and foot. [But] the heart meridian starts from the heart, differing from [the origination of] other meridians. [This is due to the fact that] the heart is the monarch [in the human body] and wields all the power [and controls] all the rules, never empowering any of the four limbs. [The parts that] the heart communicates with are all connected with the five Zang-organs and seven Fu-organs, especially the small intestine.

The small intestine is the external [image] of the heart and the heart is actually connected with the small intestine. Downwards [it] communicates with the conception vessel. Therefore the conception vessel, with the aid of Qi from the small intestine, circulates upwards to communicate with the heart, demonstrating the manifestation [of a minister] paying respect to the monarch.

上贯膈者,趋心之路也。肝性急,宜直走于心之宫矣,乃不直走于心,反走膜鬲,布于胁肋之间者,母慈之义也。慈母怜子,必为子多方曲折,以厚其藏,胁肋正心宫之仓库也,然而其性正急,不能久安于胁肋之间,循喉咙之后,上入颃颡,连于目系,上出额间而会督脉于巅项,乃木火升上之路也。

其支者,从目系下颊,环唇,欲随口舌之窍以泄肝木之郁火也。其支者,又从肝别贯膈,上注肺中,畏肺金之克木,通此经为侦探之途也。"

雷公曰:"五脏已知其旨矣。请详言七腑。"

岐伯曰:"胃经亦称阳明者,以其脉接大肠手阳明之脉,由鼻頞而下走于足也。然而胃经属阳明者,又非同大肠之谓。

胃乃多气多血之腑,实有日月并明之象,乃纯阳之腑,主受而又主化也。阳主上升,由额而游行于齿口唇吻,循颐颊耳前而会于额颅,以显其阳之无不到也。

其支别者,从颐后下人迎,循喉咙入缺盆,行足少阴之外,下隔,通肾与心包之气。盖胃为肾之关,又为心包之用,得气于二经,胃始能蒸腐水谷,以化精微也。胃既得二经之气,必归于胃中,故仍属胃也。

胃之旁络于脾,胃为脾之夫,脾为胃之妇,脾听胃使,以行其运化者也。其直行者,从缺盆下乳内廉,挟脐而入气街。气街者,气冲之穴也,乃生气之源,探源而后,气充于乳房,始能散布各经络也。其支者,起于胃口,循腹过足少阴肾经之外,本经之里,下至气街而合,仍是取气于肾,以助其生气之源也。

The lateral [parts of] the heart [meridian] are also connected with the lung in the upper, reaching the eyes along the throat to demonstrate the brightness of the heart. From the heart system [it circulates] upwards to the lung again, emerging downwards below the armpit, along the medial side of the forearm running to [the region] behind the pericardium meridian [of hand-Jueyin], descending to the elbow, reaching the medial side of the small finger along the forearm and finally emerging from the top [of the small finger]. This is the direct circulation of the heart meridian system. Again from the lung [the heart meridian circulates] tortuously downwards, descending directly along the spine, connecting with the kidney [and finally reaching] the center of Mingmen (GV 4). This is how [that] the heart and the kidney support each other.

The heart is a fire Zang-organ and fears restriction by water. [But] why [is it] connected with the kidney? Does it try to pave the way for the kidney to invade [it]? [Some people may] not know [that] fire in the heart and fire in the life gate[3] communicate with each other every day. [When] receiving fire from the life gate, heart-fire will have its root. Without the moisturization of kidney-water, heart-fire is unable to become effulgent, indicating that heart-fire must be nourished by water and fire in the kidney. Therefore restriction actually functions as promotion. [When the heart] is promoted by kidney-fire and kidney-water, [all the parts] connected with the heart will respectively communicate with every Zang-organ and Fu-organ. [Only in such a way] can any obstruction be avoided.

由是而胃既得气之本,乃可下行,以达于足。从气街而下髀关,抵伏兔,下膝膑,循胫下跗,入中指之内庭而终者,皆胃下达之路也。

其支者,从膝之下廉三寸,别入中指之外间,复是旁行之路,正见其多气多血,无往不周也。

其支者,别跗上,入大指间,出足厥阴,交于足太阴,避肝木之克,近脾土之气也。"

雷公曰:"请言三焦之经。"

岐伯曰:"三焦属之手少阳者,以三焦无形,得胆木少阳之气,以生其火,而脉起于手之小指次指之端,故以手少阳名之。

循手腕出臂,贯肘,循臑之外,行手太阳之里,手阳明之外,火气欲通于大小肠也。上肩,循臂臑,交出足少阳之后,正倚附于胆木,以取其木中之火也。

下缺盆,由足阳明之外面交会于膻中。之上焦,散布其气,而络绕于心包络;之中焦,又下膈入络膀胱,以约下焦。若胃若心包络若膀胱,皆三焦之气往来于上中下之际,故不分属于三经而仍专属于三焦也。

然而三焦之气,虽往来于上中下之际,使无根以为主,则气亦时聚时散,不可久矣。讵知三焦虽得胆木之气以生,而非命门之火则不长。三焦有命门以为根,而后布气于胃,则胃始有运用之机;布气于心包络,则心包络始有运行之权;布气于膀胱,则膀胱始有运化之柄也。

Volume 2

In this way, [the heart meridian] communicates with the liver from the left. The liver belongs to wood [when matching with the five elements] and is the mother [that] produces heart [fire]. Although heart-fire originates from innate fire in the life gate, innate fire cannot become effulgent without cultivation of liver-wood. Therefore [the organs] connected with the heart also desire to get Qi for promotion from the liver-wood. [When] liver-Qi is unobstructed, the gallbladder is also unobstructed [because] the gallbladder [is located] beside the liver and is quite easy to be promoted. Besides, the gallbladder is the father of the heart. [In such] a close relationship, certainly there will be no obstruction.

In this way, [the heart meridian] communicates with the spleen. The spleen is the son of the heart. Although spleen-earth does not depend on heart-fire to exist, [stomach-earth has to depend on heart-fire to exist]. Without heart-fire stomach-earth cannot exist [because] the stomach is the son of the heart. Since the heart has formed the stomach, [it] must form the spleen. This is why [the organs that] communicate with the spleen and stomach are connected with each other without any intervals. In this way [the heart] is connected with the lung. Fire tends to flame up and the lobes of the lung prevent it [from flaming up]. [As a result,] the lung is damaged. However, hard metal cannot become soft without fire. [So] there also is a sign of promotion in restriction. If there is no fire in lung-metal, metal [will be] cold and water [will be] chilly, and the transformation source of the stomach and bladder will disappear. How could [it] warm the kidney and transform [it into] the large intestine?

其支者,从膻中而上,出缺盆之外,上项,系耳后,直上出耳上角,至颠,无非随肾之火气而上行也。

其支者,又从耳后入耳中,出耳前,过客主人之穴,交颊,至目锐眦,亦火性上炎,随心包之气上行。然目锐眦实系胆经之穴,仍欲依附木气以生火气耳。"

雷公曰:"请言心主之经。"

岐伯曰:"心主之经即包络之府也,又名膻中。属手厥阴者,以其代君出治,为心君之相臣,臣乃阴象,故属阴。然奉君令以出治,有不敢少安于顷刻,故其性又急,与肝木之性正相同,亦以厥阴名之,因其难顺而易逆也。

夫心之脉出于心之本宫,心包络之脉出于胸中,包络在心之外,正在胸之中,是脉出于胸中者,正其脉属于包络之本宫也。各脏腑脉出于外,心与包络脉出于中,是二经较各脏腑最尊也。

夫肾系交于心包络,实与肾相接,盖心主之气与肾宫命门之气同气相合,故相亲而不相离也。由是下于膈,历络三焦,以三焦之腑气与命门心主之气彼此实未尝异,所以笼络而相合为一,有表里之名,实无表里也。

其支者,循胸中出胁,抵腋,循臑内行于太阴肺脾、少阴心肾之中,取肺肾之气以生心液也。入脉,下臂,入掌内,又循中指以出其端。

其支者,又由掌中循无名指以出其端,与少阳三焦之脉相交会,正显其同气相亲,表里如一也。夫心主与三焦两经也,必统言其相合者,

In such a way, [the heart meridian] will connect with the pericardium [meridian of hand-Jueyin]. The pericardium is Baoluo (elliptic collateral) in Danzhong (CV 17), serving as the prime minister of heart monarch and receiving orders of heart monarch to govern transformation. The meridians [and collaterals that circulate] in and out [from the pericardium] are closer [to heart monarch] than that of the five Zang-organs and six Fu-organs, [in which] there are really manifestations of delight [when] the heart is delightful and anxiety [when] the heart is anxious with correlation between inhalation and exhalation, governing transformation on behalf of heart monarch and enabling Qi from the upper, middle and lower [energizers to flow] freely. [Such] a perforation actually [results from the communication of meridians and collaterals] connected with the heart. "

Leigong asked, "How does the kidney meridian circulate?"

Qibo answered, "The kidney belongs to water and is the image of authentic water of Shaoyin. Sea water is Shaoyin water, exuberance or deficiency [of which] follows [wane and wax of] the moon and [to which water in] the kidney corresponds. [The kidney meridian is] named foot-Shaoyin [because] the meridian starts from the lower [part of] foot-Shaoyin, [running] upwards from the sole, circulating behind the medial ankle, transferring into the heel, rising to the shank and into the popliteal fossa, moving above the knee and penetrating into the spine. [Such a procedure of circulation] is the road of river cart[4], i. e. the road of the conception vessel and governor vessel.

However both [the conception vessel and governor vessel are]

盖三焦无形。借心主之气相通于上中下之间,故离心主无以见三焦之用,所以必合而言之也。

雷公曰:"请言胆经。"

岐伯曰:"胆经属足少阳者,以胆之脉得春木初阳之气,而又下趋于足,故以足少阳名之。

然胆之脉虽趋于足,而实起目之锐眦,接手少阳三焦之经也。由目锐眦上抵头角,下耳循颈,行手少阳之脉前,至肩上,交出手少阳之后,以入缺盆之外,无非助三焦之火气也。

其支者,从耳后入耳中,出走耳前,至目锐眦之后,虽旁出其支,实亦仍顾三焦之脉也。

其支者,别自目外而下大迎,合手少阳三焦,抵于颐下,下颈,复合缺盆,以下胸中,贯膜膈、心包络,以络于肝,盖心包络乃胆之子,而肝乃胆之弟,故相亲而相近也。第胆虽肝之兄,而附于肝,实为肝之表,而属于胆。肝胆兄弟之分,即表里之别也。胆分肝之气,则胆之汁始旺,胆之气始张,而后可以分气于两胁,出气街,统毛际,而横入髀厌之中也。

其直者,从缺盆下腋,循胸过季胁,与前之入髀厌者相合,乃下循髀外,行太阳阳明之间,欲窃水土之气以自养也。出膝外廉,下跗骨,以直抵绝骨之端,下出外踝,循跗上,入小指次指之间,乃其直行之路也。

其支者,又别跗上,入大指歧骨内,出其端,还贯入爪甲,出三毛,以交于足厥阴之脉,亲肝木之气以自旺,盖阳得阴而生也。"

connected with the kidney. [When] there is kidney-water, the river cart is unobstructed; [when] there is no kidney-water, the river cart is obstructed. [When] there is kidney-water, the road [along which] the governor vessel circulates is unobstructed; [when] there is no kidney-water, the road [along which] the governor vessel circulates is obstructed. So the circulation and movement of these two meridians all depend on the kidney. Therefore the road of the river cart and the road of the governor vessel are actually the road of the kidney meridian.

In this way, circulation [of the kidney meridian] into the liver [is just] like a mother entering the room of her son. In this way, circulation [of the kidney meridian] into the spleen [is just] like water running into the earth. Through the liver and spleen meridians, [the kidney meridian is] connected with the bladder [meridian]. The kidney is the internal of the bladder and the bladder is the external of the kidney. The bladder begins to transform [water when it has] received Qi from the kidney. It is just through such a connection that Qi can flow to and fro.

[The kidney meridian is] connected with the bladder, penetrating through the spine to meet the governor [vessel], returning to emerge before the navel and reaching the bladder [when] connected with the conception vessel. Although Qi transformation is possible, [it] in fact [depends on meridian]. [Only when] there is meridian [that is] unobstructed can [Qi flow] freely. [The kidney meridian that] circulates directly [moves] from the liver into the lung, [just like] a son returning to the family of his mother. Circulating from the lung to the throat, [the kidney

雷公曰:"请言膀胱之经。"

岐伯曰:"膀胱之经属足太阳者,盖太阳为巨阳,上应于日,膀胱得日之火气,下走于足,犹太阳火光普照于地也。

其脉起目内眦,交手太阳小肠之经,受其火气也。上额交巅,至耳上角,皆火性之炎上也。其直行者,从巅入络脑,还出别下项,循肩膊内,挟脊两旁下行,抵于腰,入循膂,络肾,盖膀胱为肾之表,故系连于肾,通肾中命门之气,取其气以归膀胱之中,始能气化而出小便也。虽气出于肾经,而其系要不可不属之膀胱也。

其支者,从腰中下挟脊以贯臀,入腘中而止,亦借肾气下达之也。

其支者,从膊内别行,下贯脾膂,下历尻臀,化小便,通阴之器而下出也。过髀枢,循髀外下合腘中,下贯于两踹内,出外踝之后,循京骨,至小指外侧,交于足少阴之肾经,亦取肾之气可由下面升,以上化其水也。"

雷公曰:"请言小肠之经。"

岐伯曰:"小肠之经属手太阳者,以脉起于手之小指,又得心火之气而名之也。夫心火属少阴,得心火之气,宜称阴矣。

然而心火居于内者为阴,发于外者为阳,小肠为心之表也,故称阳而不称阴,且其性原属阳,得太阳之日气,故亦以太阳名之。

其脉上腕出踝,循臂出肘,循臑行手阳明少阳之外,与太阳胆气相通,欲得金气自寒,欲得木气自生也。交肩上,入缺盆,循肩,向腋下行,当膻中而络于心,合君相二火之气也。循咽下膈,以抵于胃,虽火能生胃,而小肠主出不主生,何以抵胃,盖受胃之气,运化精微而生糟粕,犹

meridian finally] reaches the root of tongue and ends [its circulation], indicating the desire to worship the monarch through the throat and tongue.

Although the kidney and the heart restrict each other, in fact [they also] promote each other. That is why the lateral [parts of the kidney meridian] emerge separately around the heart but dare not directly move into the heart monarch. After entering Danzhong (CV 17) and Baoluo (elliptic collateral) in the chest, essential [Qi] from the kidney meridian rises up and transforms into fluid in the heart, indicating that the monarch has received necessity from the subjects and the subjects from remote mountains have paid tributes to the royal court.

Each Zang-organ is just one, but [the Zang-organ of] the kidney is two, [reflecting] the image of two poles[5]. The two poles [refer to] the sun and the moon. The moon represents Yin [while] the sun represents Yang. The kidney seems to be a water Zang-organ and appropriately corresponds to the moon, not to the sun. However [it does not mean that] there is no Qi of Yang in the moon and no Qi of Yin in the sun. [The reason why] the kidney corresponds to [both] the sun and the moon [is that] there are [both] Yin and Yang in it. [In fact,] Yin conceals in Yang and Yang hides in Yin, the interaction [of which] is [mutual] promotion, just like the sun and the moon shine [on the earth]. Actually there are both water and fire in the five Zang-organs and seven Fu-organs. [But] only water and fire in the kidney are invisible because [they are] innate water and fire, not like water and fire in other Zang-organs and Fu-organs [that are] all acquired

之生胃也。故接胃之气,下行任脉之外,以自归于小肠之正宫,非小肠之属而谁属乎。

其支者,从缺盆循颈颊上至目锐眦,入于耳中,此亦火性炎上,欲趋窍而出也。

其支者,别循颊,上颐,抵鼻,至目内眦,斜络于颧,以交足太阳膀胱之经,盖阳以趋阳之应也。"

雷公曰:"请言大肠之经。"

岐伯曰:"大肠之经名为手阳明者,以大肠职司传化,有显明昭著之意,阳之象也。夫大肠属金,宜为阴象,不属阴而属阳者,因其主出而不主藏也。

起于手大指次指之端,故亦以手名之。循指而入于臂,入肘,上臑,上肩,下入缺盆而络于肺,以肺之气能包举大肠,而大肠之系亦上络于肺也。大肠得肺气而易于传化,故其气不能久留于膈中,而系亦下膈,直趋大肠,以安其传化之职。

夫大肠之能开能阖,肾主之,是大肠之气化宜通于肾,何以大肠之系绝不与肾会乎?不知肺金之气即肾中水火之气也,肾之气必来于肺中,而肺中之气既降于大肠之内,则肾之气安有不入于大肠之中者乎?不必更有系通肾,而后得其水火之气,始能传化而开合之也。

其支者,从缺盆上颈贯颊,入下齿缝中,还出夹两口吻,交于唇中之左右,上挟鼻孔,正显其得肺肾之气,随肺肾之脉而上升之征也。"

postnatally.

[The elements in all the Zang-organs and Fu-organs] are all water and fire, [but] only [water and fire] in the kidney are innate, [indicating that] there is actually a governor in between the two kidneys. [Such a] governor [is] the life gate. The life gate is a small heart [which is just] like the image of the supreme pole[6] that produces innate water and fire and [makes it possible for] acquired water and fire to be produced, and therefore [paving the way for] the formation of the five Zang-organs and seven Fu-organs [which are] respectively located in different palaces[7], enjoying happiness provided [by the heart monarch] with everlasting transformation and invigoration."

Leigong asked, "How does the liver meridian circulate?"

Qibo answered, "The liver belongs to foot-Jueyin. [The so-called] Jueyin is reverse Yin. [It] corresponds to thunder and fire in the sky. The meridian starts from the side of big toe [covered with] hair. That is why it is named foot-Jueyin.

Thunder and fire all emerge from the earth, leaping up in the sky, the nature [of which is] impetuous and difficult to control. The liver is also impetuous in nature, the most reverse one among the Yin meridians. [Anything that is] slightly different from it [will] reversely move and never stop. From the tarsus, [it] circulates upwards to the ankle. After communicating behind with the spleen-earth of foot-Taiyin, [it runs] upwards to the medial side of the popliteal fossa, circulating along the abdomen to the pubes, across genitals and into the lower abdomen. Although [it] tends [to circulate] along the path of the liver [meridian], [it] also tends [to

陈远公曰："十二经脉,各说得详尽,不必逐段论之。"

【今译】

雷公请问岐伯:"关于十二经脉,天师巳经详细地解释了,但十二经的往来互通的缘故,还没有详尽地说明,希望天师能说明其中的深奥之义,以便留传给后代,可以吗?"

岐伯说:"可以的。肺属于手太阴经。太阴是月亮之象,月亮属于金,肺也属于金,肺经脉循行于手上,所以称为手太阴肺经。手太阴肺经起始于中焦中的胃脘之上,胃属土,土能生金,所以胃就是肺之母。其向下络属大肠,因为大肠也属于金,是胃的旁系之子。肺则是大肠之兄,而兄是能包容弟的,足以将其予以网罗。所谓络,就是网罗包举的意思。之所以循行于胃口,是因为胃是肺之母,可以接受胃土治气。肺脉又上行于膈位,当胃气充足时,必然会将气分给其子。肺脏得到其母胃腑之气,其气便上行于肺脏,必然由膈膜而上升。肺得到了胃之气的资助,肺脏就会自成一家,其经脉便从中焦发出,横向循行到腋下,因为畏惧心而不敢去触犯心。然而肺之系其实与心是相通的,因为心是肺之君,而肺则是心之臣,臣必然要朝拜君,这是履行其职责之路。向下循行到上臂内侧,然后再循行到手少阴心经和手厥阴心包经之前,这是肺经拜谒相府的门第。心主就是心包络,为心君之相,心包络代替心君行事。心火克肺金,必然要借助心主之气进行刑克。而呼吸与心的相通,全部凭借此处经脉的相互关联。肺禀君主之尊,必然要尊奉

move] along the path of the spleen [meridian].

Since [the liver meridian] tends [to move] to the spleen [meridian], [it] certainly tends [to move] to the stomach [meridian]. Since the laterals of the liver [tend] to communicate with the spleen and stomach, [when] there is any reversal [cold], [it will] inevitably attack the spleen and stomach because the road [along which the spleen and stomach meridians circulate] is familiar [to the liver meridian]. Although the laterals of the liver [meridian] are connected with the spleen and stomach, Qi in the liver must return to the original palace[8]. That is why the laterals [of the liver meridian] circulate again in the lobes of the liver. Beside the lobes of the liver is the gallbladder. The gallbladder is the elder brother of the liver and the liver is the younger brother. [In] the gallbladder, [there are] no collaterals [that connect with] the liver. [But in] the liver, [there are] collaterals [that connect with] the gallbladder, [indicating that] the younger brother is stronger than the elder brother.

Penetrating upwards to the diaphragm, [the liver meridian] tends [to move along] the road of the heart [meridian]. The liver is impetuous [in nature] and should directly move into the palace of the heart[9]. [But it does] not move directly to the heart. [In fact it] moves to the septum, spreading in the hypochondrium and rib-side, [demonstrating] kindness of the mother. The mother loves her son and will try every means [to help] her son increase property. The hypochondrium and rib-side are the warehouses of the heart palace. But [the liver is] impetuous in nature and cannot just stay in the hypochondrium and rib-side. After circulating along

宰相的辅助之令,所以其循行于少阴心经和厥阴心包经之前而不敢有所懈缓。由此而循行向下进入肘中,又循行于前臂内侧,并由前臂循行到寸口和鱼际,这都是肺经相通之道。接着又从鱼际循行到大拇指的末端而出来,这是肺脉循行的末端。经脉循行到末端之后,分支循行,从手腕之后直出次指的内侧,这是从旁边分出的脉络。"

雷公问:"脾经是怎样循行的呢?"

岐伯说:"脾是土脏,本性为湿,以足太阴经命名。太阴之月,夜晚照在土地上,月是阴之象,脾属土,能得到月亮的阴气,因此以太阴命名之。

脾经起始于足大指的末端,所以称为足太阴脾经。脾脉既然起始于足下,必然从下往上循行,由足大指内侧的尺白肉际,经过横骨之后,上行到内踝之前及小腿内侧,循行到胫骨内侧,交互于足厥阴肝经之前,随之进入肝经的循行路线。

肝木克脾,应该为脾土所畏惧,但为什么其经脉的循行反而与肝相通呢?不知道肝木虽然克脾土,然而木也能资助脾土的形成。如果脾土没有得到木气的疏通,脾土就缺少了发生之气。所以脾土既然畏惧肝木的克制,又未尝不喜欢肝木的资助。脾经之所以相交于足厥阴肝经之前,就是为了与肝木之气相合。脾经继续上行到膝盖和大腿内侧之前,然后进入腹部,回归到脾经的本脏。腹脾是脾经的正宫,脾属土,居于中州,中州是天下的腹地。脾是人体的腹地。

the throat, [the liver meridian] moves upwards to Hangsang[10],
connecting with the eyes [and finally] rising to the forehead to meet
the governor vessel at the top of the head. This [is] the road [along
which] wood and fire ascend.

The laterals [of the liver meridian circulate] downwards from
the eyes to the cheeks and around the lips, resolving stagnated fire
of liver-wood through the opening of the mouth and tongue. The
branches [of the liver meridian] stem from the liver, penetrating
through the diaphragm, rising upwards into the lung. [The liver
meridian] fears metal restricting wood, [and therefore its]
connection with [the lung] meridian [through such a branch] is the
way to detect. "

Leigong asked, "I have understood the circulations of [the
meridians of] the five Zang-organs. Please tell [me about the
meridians and collaterals of] the seven Fu-organs."

Qibo answered, "The stomach meridian is also named
Yangming because its meridian is connected with the large intestine
meridian of hand-Yangming, descending downwards from the nose
to the foot. However, the stomach meridian belongs to Yangming,
but is not the same as the large intestine [meridian].

The stomach is a Fu-organ with sufficient Qi and blood,
actually [acting as] an image of the sun and the moon [that are]
shining together. Therefore [the stomach is] a Fu-organ with pure
Yang, functioning to accept [food] and transform [it into essence].
Yang is responsible for rising up, flowing from the forehead to the
teeth, mouth and lips, circulating to the cheeks and before the ears,
and connecting [with other meridians] at the forehead and skull to

脾与胃相为表里,脾在内而胃在外,脾为胃所包,所以脾络属于胃。脾得到胃气,脾气才能开始上升,经脉也因之而随着上行到膈,上行到喉咙后又继续上升到舌根,因为舌根是心之苗,而脾是心之子,子母之气相通贯而不相隔离。

然而舌根为心的外窍,而不是心的内庭,脾脉虽然上升到舌根,单终究没能到达心中,因此分支又继续循行,凭借胃气,从胃的中脘之外上行到膈,使经脉从而贯通到膻中之处,再向上与手少阴心经相交,这是子亲母的表现。"

雷公问:"心经是怎样循行的呢?"

岐伯说:"心是火脏,以手少阴命名之,因为心火为后天之火,后天之火是有形之火,对应于天上的荧惑星。心虽然属于火,但其本性还是属于阴的,且其经脉循行在手上,故而以手少阴经来命名之。

而其他脏腑的经脉都起始于手足,惟独心脉起始于心脏,与其他经脉的起始不同,因为心是君主,总揽权纲,没有将权力给予四肢。心与五脏七腑无不相通,相通最为紧密的是小肠。

小肠是心之表,而心实际上又络属于小肠,向下与任脉通,因此任脉凭借小肠之气上行与心相通,这是臣子朝拜君主的表现。

心经的别支继续上行并与肺相通,沿着咽喉两侧循行到双目之中,以发挥心中文明雅致的光彩。又从心系上行到肺,下行后又从腋下出来,沿着前臂内侧后沿,循行在手厥阴心包经之后,下行到肘,沿着前臂循行到小指的内侧并从其末端出来,这是手少阴心经直行的路径。又经肺部曲折而行至后,并沿着脊椎直接下行,与肾相贯通,到达命门之

demonstrate [the function of] Yang [that can move to] anywhere.

The divergent collaterals [of the stomach meridian] descends from behind the cheeks to Renying (ST 9), circulating along the throat to the supraclavicular fossa, moving at the lateral side of [the kidney meridian of] foot-Shaoyin, running downwards to the diaphragm to connect with Qi in the kidney and pericardium. Since the stomach is the pass of the kidney and functions for the pericardium, [it] gets Qi from two meridians[11], [making it possible for] the stomach to digest water and food and transform into essential nutrients. Since the stomach has received Qi from these two meridians, [it] must return to the stomach and therefore belongs to the stomach.

The divergent [collateral] of the stomach [meridian] connects with the spleen [meridian]. The stomach [serves] as the husband of the spleen and the spleen [serves] as the wife of the stomach. [For this reason,] the spleen obeys the orders of the stomach [to give free rein to] its [function of] transformation. It circulates directly downwards from the supraclavicular fossa to the medial side of the breast, entering Qi street[12] from around the navel. Qi street is an acupoint [named] Qichong (ST 30) [which is] the source of Qi. [Only when] the source [of Qi] is ascertained [can] Qi fill the breast and diffuse to every meridian and collateral. Its branch starts from the opening of the stomach[13], circulating along the abdomen and across the external of [the kidney meridian of] foot-Shaoyin and the internal of the stomach meridian, combining [with the kidney meridian when] moving downwards to Qi street. [Such a circulation, communication and combination is] still to get Qi from

中，这就是心肾既济之路。

心是火脏，畏惧水克，为什么能贯通于肾？难道想让肾水有路径侵犯心火吗？这是因为不知道心脏之火与命门之火原本不可一日不能相互贯通。心脏如果得到命门之火，心火才会有根，心脏如果没有得到肾水之滋润，心火就不会旺盛，因为心火必须得到肾中水火的滋养，以克为生所说的就是这个道理。既然肾火和肾水相生了，心之系就会分别贯通到各个脏腑，从而就不会有阻隔不通之忧了。

由此而向左与肝相通，肝本来属木，是生发心火之母，心火虽然生于命门中的先天之火，但如果没有得到后天肝木的培养，先天之火气也不会旺盛，因此心脉之系与肝相通，也是想得到肝木相生之气。肝气既然贯通了，胆位于肝之旁，贯通了肝脏，就等于贯通了胆腑，这就是对相互贯通这一情势便捷之处的完善。何况胆也是心之父，与原本之亲应该没有任何的阻隔。

心脏由此而与脾脏相贯通，脾也是心之子，虽然脾土不需借助心火而生发，但胃作为心之爱子，离开了心火胃土就不能发生。心既然能生胃，生胃必然就能生脾，这就是脾胃之系彼此可以相连但却从无间断的缘故。由此心脏就与肺脏相贯通。火性炎上，而肺叶予以阻挡，肺金怎么能不受伤？然而顽金得不到火就不会柔软，相克之中也有相生的迹象，如果肺金没有火的温热，就会导致金寒水冷，胃腑与膀胱气化之源就会断绝，这样又怎能温养肾脏并传化到大肠呢？

可见要与心主相通，心主就是膻中的包络，为心君之相臣，尊奉心

the kidney to assist its source of Qi.

In this way, the stomach can get the source of Qi and therefore moves downwards to reach the foot. Downwards from Qi street, [the stomach meridian moves] to Biguan (ST 31), reaching Futu (ST 32), descending to patella in the knee, circulating along the shank to the instep and ending [its circulation when] entering the medial side of the middle toe. This is the path [that] the stomach [meridian] moves downwards.

Its branch [stems from the region] three Cun below the medial side of the knee and enters the lateral side of the middle toe. This is the lateral path for circulation, demonstrating sufficiency of Qi and blood [in the stomach meridian] and perfect circulation all the time.

Its [another] branch stems from instep, entering the big toe, emerging from [the liver meridian of] foot-Jueyin and communicating with [the spleen meridian of] foot-Taiyin to avoid restriction of liver-wood and approach to Qi of spleen-earth."

Leigong asked, "Please tell [me] about the meridian of triple energizer."

Qibo answered, "Triple energizer belongs to hand-Shaoyang and is invisible. [When it has] received Qi from gallbladder-wood of Shaoyang, fire in it is produced. [The triple energizer] meridian starts from the top of the fourth finger, and therefore is named hand-Shaoyang.

Circulating from the wrist to the arm, penetrating through the elbow and moving along the lateral side [of the arm], [the triple energizer meridian then] runs in the internal [of the small intestine

君之令以完成主化之责。其出入之经络,比五脏六腑更加近于心,真有心喜也喜、心忧也忧的表现,呼吸相通,代替君主施管化行,从而使得三焦上中下之气没有不完全通达的,这其实就是通过心之系而相贯相通的。"

雷公问:"肾经是怎样循行的呢?"

岐伯说:"肾属水,是少阴正水之象。海水是少阴水,随着月象而时盈时虚,肾与之相应,因而以足少阴肾经予以命名,因为其经脉起始于足少阴经下的涌泉穴。该经脉由足心开始上行,沿着足踝内侧之后转进入足跟中,再上行到小腿并循行到腘中,然后上行到股部,与脊贯通,这是河车之路,也就是任督二脉的循行之路。

但任、督二脉都属于肾,所以有了肾水河车之路就贯通,如果没有肾水河车之路就会闭塞,有肾水督脉之路就能通行,没有肾水督脉之路就会阻断,所以任、督二脉能否通行,完全取决于肾水,因此河车之路、督脉之路就是肾经循行之路。

由此循行到肝经,正如母入子之室一样。由此而循行到脾,正如水行于地中一样。经过肝脾二经,肾经与膀胱经络属,因为肾是膀胱之里,膀胱为肾之表,膀胱得到肾气才开始气化,正是通过这条相同之路,才使气能得以相互往来。

肾经络属膀胱,贯通于脊而与督脉相会,然后从脐部之前出,贯通任脉并开始到达膀胱,虽然气化可以开始,其实只有内部具备了经络才能贯通。直行的肾经又从肝进入肺,这是子归母室的表现。由肺部而上行到喉咙,然后再循行舌根就终止了,这是因为想去朝拜君主,所

meridian of] hand-Taiyang and the external [of the large intestine meridian of] hand-Yangming, and fire-Qi [in it] tends to connect with the large and small intestines. [Moving] upwards to the shoulder, [the triple energizer meridian] circulates along the lateral side of the arm and meets with [the gallbladder meridian of] foot-Shaoyang behind, just following the gallbladder-wood in order to get fire from wood.

Descending to the supraclavicular fossa, [the triple energizer meridian] meets with Danzhong (CV 17) from the lateral side [of the stomach meridian of] foot-Yangming. Arriving at the upper energizer, [it] diffuses Qi and runs around the pericardium meridian [of hand-Jueyin with its] collateral; arriving at the middle energizer, [it] descends again into the diaphragm and connects with the bladder to control the lower energizer. The stomach, the pericardium and the bladder are all the places [through which] Qi from the triple energizer flows to the upper, middle and lower. In this case [Qi] does not belong to these three meridians, but just belongs to the triple energizer.

Although Qi from the triple energizer flows from the upper, through the middle and to the lower [regions], if there is no root[14] to control, it may now gather and then disperse and cannot maintain for a long time. Although it is well known that the triple energizer can have [fire when] getting Qi from the gallbladder-wood, [it] cannot [have fire] for a long time without [promotion of] fire from the life gate. [Thus in] the triple energizer, the life gate is the root. Later on [the triple energizer] diffuses Qi into the stomach, [making it possible for] the stomach to perform [its] function.

以先通过喉舌而行。

肾与心虽然好像彼此相克,但实际上则是彼此相生,所以其分支又分别出来环绕于心,但又不敢直接去朝拜心君,而是注入胸部的膻中包络,然后肾经之精上奉而转化为心液,这就如君王从民众中获取其所需要的,也如山野之民向国家进贡一样,很有意义。

各脏只有一个,但肾却有两个,这就是两仪的表现。两仪就是日月,月主阴,日主阳。似乎肾脏就是水脏,所以应该与月对应,而不应该与日对应,但月之中并非没有阳气,而日之中也并非没有阴气,肾脏配日月,就是因为其中含有阴和阳,阴藏于阳之中,阳隐于阴之内,相互交叠为用,正如日月照耀人间一样。五脏七腑各有水火,惟独肾之水火无形,因为肾之水火都是先天的,并非如其他各脏腑的水火那样,都属于后天。

同样是水火,惟独肾之水火属于先天,事实上其中有主宰的因素存在于两肾之间。所谓主宰的因素指的就是命门。命门是小心,一如太极之象一样,能生先天之水火,并由此而化生出后天之水火,于是形成了五脏七腑,分别安居在各个宫中,享受所奠定的福分,从而保证了无穷的化生。"

雷公问:"肝经是怎样循行的呢?"

岐伯说:"肝经属于足厥阴,厥阴是逆阴,对应于天上的雷火。足厥阴肝经起始于足大指丛毛之际,因此以足厥阴肝经命名。

雷火都是从地下发起的,升腾于天际之上,其性急躁,不可控制和抑制。肝性也很急躁,是阴经中最为逆行的经脉,这种态势不是很合乎

[When the triple energizer] diffuses Qi into the pericardium, the pericardium begins to have the power to move and transform; [when the triple energizer] diffuses Qi into the bladder, the bladder begins to have the ability to move and transform.

The branch [of the triple energizer meridian circulates] upwards from Danzhong (CV 17), emerging from the lateral side of the supraclavicular fossa, rising to the nape, connecting with [the region] behind the ear, directly moving upwards, emerging from the upper angle of the ear and reaching the infraorbital rim, just ascending together with fire and Qi from the kidney.

The branch [of the triple energizer meridian] enters the ear again from behind the ear, emerging in front of the ear, passing the acupoint [located near] Ke Zhu Ren[15], meeting with the cheek and arriving at the outer canthus. [This is] also [a manifestation of] fire tending to flame up and moving upwards with Qi from the pericardium. However, the outer canthus is actually an acupoint [located on] the gallbladder meridian [of foot-Shaoyang]. [The reason why the triple energizer meridian finally reaches the outer canthus is that it] desires to follow Qi from wood to produce fire-Qi.

Leigong asked, "Please explain the meridian of pericardium."

Qibo answered, "The pericardium meridian is the palace of Baoluo, also known as Danzhong (CV 17). [The reason that the pericardium meridian] belongs to hand-Jueyin [is that it] manages [important affairs] on behalf of the monarch. [So the pericardium] is the minister of heart monarch. Minister is the image of Yin. That is why [the pericardium] belongs to Yin. [As a minister, the

其本意,其循行常常就会厥逆而不可抑止。该经脉从足部的跗骨向上循行,上行到足踝部后,交接并出现于足太阴脾土之后,然后上行到腘部的内侧,再循行到腹部,并进入阴毛中,经过生殖器后抵达小腹部。虽然循行于肝经的运行之路,同时也趋向于循行在脾经的运行之路。

由于趋向于循行在脾经的运行之路,也必然循行于胃经的运行之路。肝经的分支既然能贯通于脾胃,但凡有所逆行,就必然会首先触犯脾胃两经,这也是其循行中所常态化的运行之路。虽然肝经的分支连通于脾胃,但肝气则必然回归于本宫,因此其分支又循行到肝叶之中。肝叶的旁边有附着的胆经,胆是肝之兄,肝是胆之弟,胆不络属于肝,而肝反而络属于胆,这说明弟反而强于兄。

该经脉上行并贯通到膈,这是循行而趋向于心经的路线。肝性急躁,应该直接循行到心宫之中,而不是直行到心包之中,但却反而循行于膜膈,分布在胁肋之间,这种循行的方式体现了母慈之义。既然慈母爱子,必然会以多方曲折的方式资助其子,以增加其收藏之用,而胁肋则正好是心宫的仓库。然而,肝性正处于急躁之时,不能长久安居在胁肋之间,所以循行到喉咙之后就继续上行,进入颃颡,并与双目相连,然后继续上行并出于额间,与督脉交会于头顶,这就是木火上升之路。肝经的分支,从双目之系下行到颊部,环绕口唇,想随着口舌之窍以疏泄肝木中的郁火。

肝经的分支,又从肝脏分出贯通膈膜,向上循行并注入肺中,因其畏惧肺金对木的克制,便通过此经络作为侦探循行路线的途径。"

pericardium] manages [anything by] obeying the orders of the monarch, and therefore never daring to be at ease or lack off [in doing anything]. For this reason, [the pericardium is] impetuous in nature [and is] exactly the same as [that of] the liver-wood. [The pericardium meridian is] also named Jueyin because it is difficult to be normal and easy to be reverse [in circulation].

The heart meridian emerges from the original palace of the heart and the pericardium meridian starts from the chest. The divergent collateral [of the pericardium meridian] stems from the external of the heart and right in the chest. Thus the meridian emerging from the chest actually originates from the original palace of the divergent [collateral of the pericardium meridian]. The meridians of all the other Zang-organs and Fu-organs emerge from the external but the heart and pericardium meridians start from the middle because these two meridians are the most important than [that of the other] Zang-organs and Fu-organs.

The laterals of the kidney [meridians] communicate with the collaterals of the pericardium [meridian], and are also connected with the kidney. In fact Qi from the pericardium [meridian] and Qi from the life gate in the kidney palace are combined with each other, and therefore often getting close to each other but never separating from each other. From here [the pericardium meridian] moves downwards to the diaphragm and is connected with the triple energizer through collaterals. Since Qi in the Fu-organ triple energizer and Qi in the life gate and pericardium are not different, they get together and integrate with each other. [That is why they] have the names of the external and internal, but do not have [the

雷公问："五脏经脉的循行情况我已经知道了,请再详细说明七腑经络的循行吧。"

岐伯说："胃经也称为阳明,因为其经脉与手阳明大肠经相连接,由鼻跟而下行到足部。然而胃经也属于阳明,但却并非与大肠之义相同。

胃是多气多血之腑,其实具有太阳和月亮交相发亮的表现,所以是纯阳之腑,其主要作用是受盛水谷、消化水谷和化生精微物质。阳主上升,由额部循行于牙齿和口唇,又循行到面颊和耳前,并交会于额颅,以显示其中阳气无所不到的运行。

其分支从颐后下行到人迎,并沿着喉咙而进入缺盆,然后循行于足少阴经的外侧,向下循行到隔膜,并与肾和心包之气贯通。因为胃是肾的关口,又行心包的功用,所以只有从少阴肾经和厥阴心包经得气之后,胃才能腐熟水谷,才能化生出精微物质。胃经既然得到了少阴肾经和厥阴心包经之气,必然归属于其本宫胃中,所以仍然属于胃。

胃经的旁支连络与脾经,胃是脾之夫,脾是胃之妇,脾需听从胃的使唤,以便行使好其运化作用。胃经直行时,从缺盆下行到乳房内侧,挟着肚脐而进入气街。气街是气冲的穴位,是生气之源,探明气的渊源之后,气才会充盈于乳房,才能开始散布到各经络之中。胃经的分支,起始于胃口,沿着腹部循行,经过足少阴肾经的外侧和本经的里面,下行到气街并与肾经相合,这仍然是从肾经获取气之本,以资助胃的化气之源。

implications of] the external and internal.

The branch [of the pericardium meridian] circulates in the chest, emerging from the hypochondrium and arriving at the armpit. [Then it] circulates in the medial side of the arm to [the region between] the lung [meridian] of [hand-] Taiyin and the spleen [meridian] of [foot-] Taiyin [as well as] the heart [meridian] of [hand-] Shaoyin and the kidney [meridian] of [foot-] Shaoyin, getting Qi from the lung and kidney [meridians] to produce fluid for the heart. Entering the meridian, [it moves] downwards to the arm, entering the palm, circulating to the middle finger and emerging from the top of the middle finger.

The branch [of the pericardium meridian] circulates again from the palm to the fourth finger and communicates with the triple energizer meridian [of hand-Shaoyang when] emerging from the top of the fourth finger, demonstrating close relationship [between them because they share] the same Qi and integration of the external and internal. As to the pericardium and triple energizer meridians, discussion must focus on their combination because the triple energizer is invisible. [It is only] with the help of Qi from the pericardium [can Qi in the triple energizer] communicate with the upper, middle and lower. Thus without the help of the pericardium [meridian], the triple energizer is useless. Therefore it is necessary to talk about it together [with the pericardium meridian]."

Leigong asked, "Please explain the gallbladder meridian."

Qibo answered, "The gallbladder belongs to foot-Shaoyang because the gallbladder meridian has received Qi from initial Yang of wood in the spring and tends to circulate to the foot. That is why

　　通过这一途径,胃经既然已经获得了气之本,便可由此而下行到腿部和足部,从气街下行到髀关,抵达伏兔穴,然后继续下行到膝盖部的膑骨,沿着胫骨下行到足部的跗骨处,进入足中趾的内庭穴后,其循行便终止了,这都是胃经向下循行的路线。

　　胃经的又一分支,从膝盖下缘下三寸处分出,进入中趾的外间穴,从而成为旁行的路线,这正好显示了胃经多气多血、无往不周的特性。

　　胃经的另一分支,从足背上分出,进入足大趾间,又从足厥阴肝经出来,与足太阴脾经相交,以避免肝木的克制,从而接近了脾土之气。"

　　雷公问:"请说明手少阳三焦经的循行。"

　　岐伯说:"三焦属于手少阳经,因为三焦是无形的,获得了胆木少阳之气才能滋生起三焦中的火,其经脉从手的小指一侧的次指(即无名指)的末端发出,所以就以手少阳来命名。

　　该经沿着手腕循行到手臂,向上贯通肘部,循行于手臂外侧,然后循行在手太阳小肠经之内及手阳明大肠经之外,这是火气欲贯通大小肠的走势。上行到肩部,又沿着手臂并在足少阳胆经之后与其相交,这正是倚附于胆木以便获取木中之火。

　　向下循行到缺盆,又从足阳明胃经的外侧交会于膻中穴并到达上焦,从而散布三焦之气,以络脉环绕于心包络并到达中焦,然后又下行到膈膜并络属于膀胱,以便制约下焦。如胃、心包络和膀胱,都是三焦之气往来于上、中、下之际,所以并不分别属于这三条经脉,而仍然专属于三焦经。

it is named foot-Shaoyang.

Although the gallbladder meridian tends to move to the foot, [it] actually originates from the canthus and connects with the triple energizer of hand-Shaoyang. Rising upwards from the canthus to the angle of head, [it] moves downwards to the ear, circulating along the neck, running before [the triple energizer meridian of] hand-Shaoyang, arriving at the shoulder, communicating with [the triple energizer meridian] behind and entering the external of supraclavicular fossa, [the purpose of which is] just for assisting fire-Qi in the triple energizer.

The branch [of the gallbladder meridian] enters the ear from behind the ear, moving to the front of the ear and arriving at [the region] behind the canthus. Although the branch stems from the side [of the gallbladder meridian], [it is] actually still related to the triple energizer meridian.

Another branch [of the gallbladder meridian] stems from the outer canthus and moves downwards to Daying (ST 5), combining with the triple energizer [meridian of] hand-Shaoyang, moving to [the region] below the eye, descending along the neck, meeting in the supraclavicular fossa, circulating downwards to the chest and penetrating through the diaphragm and the pericardium to connect with the liver. The pericardium is the son of the gallbladder and the liver is the younger brother of the gallbladder. Thus [there is] close relationship between them. Although the gallbladder is the elder brother of the liver and depends on the liver, [it is] actually the external of the liver but belongs to the gallbladder. The difference between the liver and gallbladder as elder brother and younger

　　然而三焦之气虽然往来于上、中、下之际,但如果无根作主,那么气就会时聚时散,不可长久持续了! 虽然三焦获得了胆木之气以便保持生发之用,但是如果没有命门之火则不能生长,三焦实际上以命门为其根,之后才能散布其气于胃,胃才有运作的机制。只有三焦经散布其气于心包络,心包络才有运行的能力。只有三焦经散布其气于膀胱,膀胱才有运化的能力。

　　三焦经的分支,从膻中穴上行,从缺盆穴的外侧出来,然后上行到颈项,连系到耳后,并向上直行,从耳的上角出来,最后到眼眶的下缘,这无非是随着肾脏的火气而上行的结果。

　　三焦经的另一分支,又从耳后进入耳中,绕出耳前,经过客主人这一穴位相交于频部,又到达眼外角,这也是火性的上炎,随着心包之气而上行。然而,眼外角实际上是胆经之穴,依然想依附木气以便能滋生火气。"

　　雷公问:"请说明手厥阴心包经的循行。"

　　岐伯说:"手厥阴心包经是包络所在的府第,又称其为膻中。心包经之所以属于手厥阴,是因为它代替君主治理天下,是心君的相臣,因为臣是阴之象,所以属于阴。由于相臣是奉君主之令治理天下的,所以不敢有丝毫的安逸和懈怠,因此其性情又特别地急躁,与肝木的性情正好相同,也用厥阴予以命名,因为其循行难以平顺而容易上逆。

　　心的经脉从心之本宫发出,心包络的经脉从胸中的包络发出,居于心脏的外面,正好位于胸腔之中,所以其经脉是从胸中发出的,也正好

brother is differentiation of the external and internal. [Only when] the gallbladder has shared Qi from the liver can bile be invigorated and Qi in the gallbladder be exuberant, eventually diffusing Qi to the hypochondria [from which Qi] emerges from Qi street, passing round the pubes and transversely entering the hip joint.

The straight branch [moves] downwards from the supraclavicular fossa to the armpit, circulating along the chest and across the hypochondrium to combine with the one [that has] entered the hip joint before, descending along the lateral side of the hip and moving between the Taiyang and Yangming [meridians] with the desire to grab Qi from water and earth to nourish itself. Emerging from the lateral side of the knee, [it] descends to the tarsus, moving directly to the lower end of the fibula, running downwards to the external ankle and circulating along the instep to [the region] between the small toe and the fourth toe. This is the direct path [that it moves along].

Its another branch stems from the instep, entering into the juncture of bone in the big toe, penetrating through the nail, emerging from [the region covered with] three hairs [in the big toe] and meeting with [the liver] meridian of foot-Jueyin. [It] approaches Qi in the liver-wood [for the purpose of] invigorating itself because Yang depends on Yin to exist.

Leigong asked,"Please explain the bladder meridian."

Qibo answered, " The bladder meridian belongs to foot-Taiyang. Taiyang is great Yang, corresponding to the sun in the sky. [When] receiving fire-Qi from the sun, the bladder [meridian] moves to the foot, just like the sun shining over the earth.

是从包络本宫中发出来的。各个脏腑的经脉都起始于外面,只有心经和心包经是从心脏内发出的,正因为如此,这两条经脉比其他各脏腑的经脉都要尊贵。

肾经的分支与心包络相交,其实更是与肾脏相连接,因为心包经的气与肾宫命门之气属于同气,且相互交合,所以相互亲近而不分离。由此下行到膈膜,通过络脉与三焦连接,因为三焦的腑气与命门、心包之气彼此之间实际上没有什么差异,所以彼此笼络并合而为一,虽然有表里之名,其实却没有表里之义。

心包经的分支,循行到胸中,从胁部出来,抵达腋窝,然后循行于手臂内侧,并到达太阴肺经、太阴脾经以及少阴心经、少阴肾经之间,获取肺和肾之气以滋生心液。然后进入脉中,向下行进到手臂,再进入手掌,又循行到中指,并从中指末端出来。

另外一个分支,又从手掌中央沿着无名指循行到末端,与手少阳三焦经相交会,从而显示出其同气相亲的本性以及表里如一的特性。厥阴心包与少阳三焦两经,必须结合在一起论述其交合的状况,因为三焦是无形的,需要借助心包之气以贯通于上中下之间,因此离开了心包经就无法观察到三焦的功用了,所以必须结合在一起予以说明。”

雷公问:“请说明足少阳胆经的循行情况。”

岐伯说:“胆经属于足少阳,因为胆的经脉获得了春木的初阳之气,而又向下循行到了足部,因此以足少阳经予以命名。然而,胆的经脉虽然循行到足部,其实却起始于眼外角,又连接到手少阳三焦

Volume 2

The [bladder] meridian starts from the inner canthus, meeting the small intestine meridian of hand-Taiyang to receive fire-Qi [from it]. Ascending to the forehead and meeting with the skull, [it] arrives at [the region] above the ear, demonstrating the nature of fire [that tends] to flame up. [The bladder meridian] moves directly from the skull into the brains, emerging separately from below the nape, circulating inside the shoulder and arm, descending along both sides of the spine, arriving at the waist and connecting with the kidney along the spine. The bladder is the external of the kidney, that is why [it] is connected with the kidney. [Only when the bladder has] received Qi from the life gate in the kidney and keeps it in the bladder can [the bladder] transform [water in it] into urine. Although Qi originates from the kidney meridian, its relationship still belongs to the bladder.

The branch [of the bladder meridian] moves downwards from the waist, penetrating through the buttocks along both sides of the spine and ending [circulation when] entering the popliteal fossa. This way of descending depends on kidney-Qi.

Another branch [of the bladder meridian] stems from the medial side of the arm, moving downwards to penetrate through the spleen and hip and across the buttocks and tailbone, transforming urine, connecting with the genitals and continuing to circulate downwards. Across Bishu (GB 30), [it] circulates along the lateral side of the leg to connect [with other meridians] behind the knee, moving downwards to penetrate through the medial side of the shank, emerging from the back of the external ankle and reaching the lateral side of the small toe along Jinggu (BL 64) to connect

经。该经脉由眼外角上行到头角,向下循行到耳部,再沿着颈部循行到手少阳经之前,到达肩上后又在手少阳经之后与之相交,由于进入了缺盆穴之外,就自然地资助了三焦的火气。

胆经的分支,从耳的后面进入耳中,循行到耳部之前,然后又到达眼外角之后,虽然从旁边分出分支,实际上仍然顾及了三焦的经脉。

胆经的另一分支,从两目的外面分出来后向下循行到大迎穴,并与手少阳三焦经相合,抵达眼眶下之后,再向下循行到颈部之后,与缺盆穴会合后继续下行到胸中,并贯通膜膈中的心包络,然后与肝相络连。心包络是胆经之子,而肝是胆之弟,因此彼此之间相亲相近。虽然胆是肝之兄,但却始终依附于肝,实际上是肝之表,肝之表自然属于胆。所以肝胆兄弟的区分就是表里的分别。胆从肝中分出了气,胆汁才开始旺盛,胆气才开始舒张,之后才会将气分布到两胁,从气街出来,绕行于阴毛,然后横行进入髀厌之中。

胆经中所直行的经脉,从缺盆向下循行到腋窝,然后沿着胸部循行,经过季胁而与前面进入髀厌的经脉相结合,再向下循行到股骨之外,行进在太阳经和阳明经之间,想窃取水土之气以实现自养。然后再从膝部外侧的朦骨出来,向下循行到跗骨,以便直接抵达绝骨之端,继续向下到达外踝后出来,再循行于足部的跗骨之上,进入足小趾和次趾之间,这就是其直行之路。

胆经的分支,又从足部的跗骨之上循行,进入足大趾的歧骨,然后又从其里面循行出来,进而贯入爪甲,又从足大趾旁的三毛之际循行出

with the kidney meridian of foot-Shaoyin. [This is] also the way to get Qi from the kidney to rise from the lower in order to transform water [in the bladder when] moving upwards."

Leigong asked, "Please explain the small intestine meridian of hand-Taiyang."

Qibo answered, "The small intestine meridian belongs to hand-Taiyang because this meridian originates from the small finger of hand and also receives Qi from heart-fire. [That is why it is so] named. The heart-fire belongs to Shaoyin. [It has] received Qi from heart-fire and should be named Yin.

But [when] heart-fire is inside, [it] is Yin; [when heart-fire] is outside, [it is] Yang. The small intestine is the external of the heart. That is why [it is] called Yang, not Yin. The nature [of the small intestine meridian] originally belongs to Yang. [Besides, the small intestine meridian also] receives Qi from the sun. That is why [it is] also called Taiyang.

[The small intestine] meridian moves upwards [from the small finger] to the wrist, emerging from the wrist, circulating along the arm upwards to the elbow and at the lateral sides [of the large intestine meridian of] hand-Yangming and [the triple energizer meridian of] hand-Shaoyang, connecting with Qi from the bladder [meridian of foot-] Taiyang. [This is the way it] wants to get metal-Qi to cool itself and to get wood-Qi to promote itself. [Then it] interactes [with other meridians and collaterals] at the shoulder, entering the supraclavicular fossa, moving downwards to the armpit from the shoulder and connecting with the heart [meridian when] reaching Danzhong (CV 17) [in order] to integrate Qi from

来,并与足厥阴经相交合,这样就实现了亲近肝木之气以自旺的目标,这基本上就是阳得阴而生的原因。"

雷公问:"请说明足太阳膀胱经的循行情况。"

岐伯说:"膀胱的经脉属于足太阳,因为太阳是巨阳,相应于天上的太阳,膀胱经得到太阳的火气,就向下循行到足部,犹如太阳的火光普照于大地一样。

足太阳膀胱经起始于眼内角,与手太阳小肠经相交合,受到了小肠经火气的影响。向上循行到额部后,交于头顶,进而循行到耳的上角,这都是火性炎上的表现。足太阳膀胱经直行时,从头顶进入脑并与脑相连络,然后从颈项向下分出,循行到肩膊内,沿着脊柱的两边向下抵达腰部,沿着脊柱两旁的肌肉,与肾脏相连络,因为膀胱是肾之表,所以与肾相连合,并与肾中的命门之气相贯通,以便取得肾气,然后注入膀胱之中,这样才能使膀胱通过气化而排出小便。虽然气出于肾经,但其分支则不能不属于膀胱。

足太阳膀胱经的分支,从腰中向下循行,沿着脊柱而贯入臀部,直到进入膝部之后才终于停止,这也是借助肾气而向下循行。

足太阳膀胱经的另外一个分支,从膊内侧分出,向下循行而到脊部,经过臀部尾椎骨,气化出小便,与阴器相通并从阴器下面继续下行。经过腿部的髀枢穴,又沿着腿骨外侧向下循行,在膝部之后相合,再向下循行而贯通到小腿内侧,然后从外踝之后出来,沿着京骨穴循行到足小趾外侧,并与足少阴肾经相交合,这也是获取肾中之气,因此就能由下而向上升起,以便通过上行来气化膀胱中的

monarch-fire and ministerial fire[16]. Along the throat, [the small intestine meridian] moves downwards to the diaphragm and reaches the stomach. Although [heart] fire can promote the stomach, the small intestine functions to discharge, not to produce. [But] why [does the small intestine meridian] reach the stomach? Because [the small intestine has] received Qi from the stomach to transport and transform essential nutrients and discharge waste, just like invigorating the stomach. That is why [the small intestine meridian] receives Qi from the stomach, moving downwards to the lateral side of the conception vessel and returning to the authentic palace of the small intestine. [It] certainly belongs to the small intestine [meridian], not any other [meridians].

The branch [of the small intestine meridian] circulates from the supraclavicular fossa to the neck and cheek, arriving at the canthus and entering the ear. Such [a circulation] also [indicates the fact that] fire tends to flame up and desires to come out of the upper orifices.

Another branch [of the small intestine meridian] moves upwards to [the region] below the eye along the cheek, arriving at the nose, reaching the inner canthus, obliquely associating with the cheekbone and connecting with the bladder meridian of foot-Taiyang. [Such a way of circulation indicates that] Yang tends [to move to the position of] Yang [in order to] correspond [to it].

Leigong asked,"Please explain the large intestine meridian."

Qibo answered,"The large intestine meridian is named hand-Yangming because the large intestine functions to discharge and transform [waste], indicating the significance of obvious and clear

水液。"

雷公问:"请说明手太阳小肠经的循行情况。"

岐伯说:"小肠之经属于手太阳,因为该经脉起始于手的小指,又因得到了心火之气,所以就以此命名。心火属于少阴,得到心火之气,应当称其为阴。

然而心火居于内的属于阴,勃发于外的属于阳,小肠为心火之表,所以称其为阳而不称其为阴。况且就性质而言,手太阳小肠经本来属于阳,由于得到太阳之阳气,所以也用太阳予以命名。

手太阳小肠经的经脉上行到手腕,从尺骨小头部出来,沿着手臂循行,从肘部上行而出,循行于手臂中的手阳明经和手少阳经的外侧,与太阳的胆气相通,这一循行的线路是为了得到金气以自寒和得到木气以自生。然后相交于肩上,进入缺盆,接着沿肩胛而向腋下循行,到了膻中穴便与心经相连络,以便能交合君火与相火之气。继而沿着咽喉向下循行到膈部,又抵达胃中。虽然心火能促生胃土,但是小肠主要是传出而不是生发,为什么要抵达胃部呢?这是因为小肠经受纳了胃气,从而能运化精微和排泄糟粕,这种情况正如生发胃土一样。因此,小肠经接钠了胃气后就向下循行到任脉之外,以便能回归到小肠的正宫,这样它不属于小肠又该属于什么呢?

手太阳小肠经的分支,从缺盆分出后向上循行到颈部和颊部,继续向上循行到眼外角,然后进入耳中,这也是火性炎上的表现,其目的是想从上窍而出。

手太阳小肠经的另一分支,沿着颊部出,然后向上循行到眼眶下

manifestation [which is] the image of Yang. The large intestine belongs to metal and should be the image of Yin. [The reason why the large intestine meridian] does not belong to Yin but belongs to Yang [is that] it is in charge of excretion, not in charge of storage.

[The large intestine meridian] originates from the top of the forefinger. That is why it is named after hand. Along the forefinger [it] enters the arm and elbow, moving upwards to the medial side of the upper arm, rising to the shoulder, descending to the supraclavicular fossa to connect with the lung [meridian]. Qi from the lung can contain and support the large intestine, and the divergent collaterals of the large intestine [meridian] also connect with the lung. [When] the large intestine has received Qi from the lung, [it is] easy to transport and transform. That is why Qi [from the large intestine meridian] cannot stay in the diaphragm for a long time and the divergent collaterals [of the large intestine meridian] also circulate downwards to the diaphragm in order to perform [the function of] the large intestine to transport and transform.

The ability of the large intestine to open and close [depends on] the support of the kidney because the transformation of Qi in the large intestine is related to the kidney. [But] why do the divergent collaterals of the large intestine [meridian] never connect with the kidney? [Maybe some people] do not know [that] Qi from lung-metal is actually Qi from water and fire in the kidney. [That is to say that] Qi in the kidney originates from the lung and Qi in the lung flows into the large intestine. [For this reason,] Qi from the kidney certainly enters the large intestine. [Thus,] the divergent collaterals [of the large intestine meridian are] unnecessary to connect with the kidney [in order] to receive Qi from

部,抵达鼻部后又继续循行到眼内角,然后斜行而连络于颧骨,以便与足太阳膀胱经相交合,这基本上就是阳经在循行中趋向于阳位的相应体现。"

雷公问:"请说明手阳明大肠经的循行情况。"

岐伯说:"大肠经命名为手阳明,因为大肠的职能是传化水谷的糟粕,主要是为了彰显其实际意思,也是为了体现阳的形象。大肠属金,应当为阴象,之所以不属于阴而属于阳,是因为大肠经主排泄而不主收藏。手阳明大肠经起始于食指的末端,所以也以手命名。沿着食指向上循行到手臂,进入到肘部,上行到手大臂,在向上循行到肩部,然后向下进入缺盆并连络于肺,因为肺气能够包含大肠,而大肠经的分支也向上循行而连络于肺。大肠得到肺气后就比较容易传化,所以大肠之气不能长久地留于膈中,其分支也向下循行到膈部,并直接向大肠的方向循行,以便发挥大肠传化的功能。大肠之所以能开能合,是因为受到肾气的主宰,所以大肠的气化应该与肾气相通。但为什么大肠经的分支却绝不与肾脏相交会呢?孰不知,肺金的气实际上就是肾中的水火之气,肾气必然来自于肺中,而肺中之气既然下降到大肠之内,那么肾气怎么能不进入大肠之中呢?因而不必再有分支连系贯通于肾,然后才能得到肾中的水火之气,这样才能发挥传化和开合的功能。

手阳明大肠经的分支,从缺盆向上循行到颈部,然后贯通颊部,继而进入下齿的缝中,再环绕上下唇而出来,并交合于唇中的左右,然后沿着鼻孔上行,这正显示其得到了肺肾之气的资助,这也是其随着肺肾

water and fire [for the purpose of] transportation, transformation, opening and closure.

The branch [of the large intestine meridian] moves upwards to the neck and penetrates through the cheek from the supraclavicular fossa, entering the slit between the lower teeth, emerging round the lips, connecting with the left and right in the middle of the lips and rising up along the nostrils. [Such a way of circulation] just indicates [that the large intestine mereidian] receives Qi from the lung and kidney and rises up along with the lung and kidney meridians.

Chen Yuangong's comment, "*The twelve meridians are analyzed in details. [But it is] unnecessary to discuss [them] respectively in passages.*"

Notes

[1] To match with the five elements, the stomach corresponds to earth. That is why it is called stomach-earth.

[2] Taiyin (太阴) here refers to the moon because the moon is the source of Yin.

[3] The life gate (命门) here refers to the kidney. In Chapter 36 in *Nan Jing* (《难经》, *Difficult Issues*), it says: "The two kidneys are not all kidneys. The one located in the left is kidney and the one located in the right is the life gate."

[4] River cart (河车), a term in alchemy, usually means two things, water in the kidneys or circulation of genuine water.

[5] Two poles (两仪) originally refer to the sky and earth.

[6] Supreme pole (太极) is a philosophical concept first used in the book written by Zhuang Zi (庄子) about three thousands of

之经而上升的体现。

　　陈远公评论说："十二经脉，分别解说得非常详尽，就不必分段进行评论了。"

years ago. This concept was defined in different ways, including the source Qi of this universe before the sky and the earth were separated, nothingness, Yin and Yang that were not separated from each other, and the universal law, etc.

[7] Palaces here refer to different cavities in the body.

[8] Original palace here refers to the location of the liver.

[9] Palace of the heart refers to the location of the heart.

[10] Hangsang (颃颡), see [3] in Chapter 13.

[11] These two meridians refer to the kidney meridian of foot-Shaoyin and the pericardium meridian of foot-Jueyin.

[12] Qi street (气街) is a common path where meridian Qi from the head, chest, abdomen and shank gathers and accumulates.

[13] Opening of the stomach refers to pylorus.

[14] Root (根) in this paragraph refers to the basic foundation.

[15] Ke Zhu Ren (客主人) refers to the soft region above the cheekbone.

[16] Monarch-fire (君火) refers to heart-fire and ministerial fire (相火) refers to liver-fire and kidney-fire.

包络配腑篇第十八

【原文】

天老问于岐伯曰："天有六气,化生地之五行,地有五行,化生人之五脏。有五脏之阴,即宜有五腑之阳矣,何以脏止五,腑有七也?"

岐伯曰："心包络,腑也,性属阴,故与脏气相同,所以分配六腑也。"

天老曰："心包络既分配腑矣,是心包络即脏也,何不名脏而必别之为腑耶?"

岐伯曰："心包络,非脏也。"

天老曰："非脏列于脏中,毋乃不可乎?"

岐伯曰："脏称五不称六,是不以脏予包络也。腑称六,不称七,是不以腑名包络也。"

天老曰："心包络,非脏非腑何以与三焦相合乎?"

岐伯曰："包络与三焦为表里,二经皆有名无形,五脏有形与形相合,包络无形,故与无形相合也。"

天老曰："三焦为孤脏,既名为脏,岂合于包络乎?"

岐伯曰："三焦虽亦称脏,然孤而寡合,仍是腑,非脏也,舍包络之气,实无可依,天然配合,非勉强附会也。"

天老曰："善。"

Volume 2

【英译】

Chapter 18
Combination of the Pericardium with Fu-organ

Tianlao[1] asked Qibo, "There are six [kinds of] Qi in the sky [that have] transformed the five elements on the earth. The five elements on the earth have transformed the five Zang-organs in the human body. There is Yin in the five Zang-organs, there should also be Yang in the five Fu-organs. Why are there only five Zang-organs [but] seven Fu-organs?"

Qibo answered, "The pericardium is a Fu-organ but belongs to Yin in nature. That is why [it is] the same as Qi in the Zang-organs. For this reason, [it is] classified [into the Fu-organs and] the Fu-organ [become] six."

Tianlao asked, "Although the pericardium is classified into the Fu-organs, it is still a Zang-organ. Why [is it] not named Zang-organ but must be named Fu-organ?"

Qibo answered, "The pericardium [is in fact] not Zang-organ."

Tianlao asked, "[It is] not Zang-organ but included in the Zang-organs. Is it unnecessary?"

Qibo answered, "The Zang-organs are named five, not six, because the Zang-organs do not include the pericardium. The Fu-organs are named six, not seven, because the Fu-organs do not include the pericardium."

雷公曰："肺合大肠,心合小肠,肝合胆,脾合胃,肾合膀胱,此天合也。三焦与心包络相合,恐非天合矣。"

岐伯曰："包络非脏而与三焦合者,包络里三焦表也。"

雷公曰："三焦腑也,何分表里乎?"

岐伯曰："三焦之气,本与肾亲,亲肾不合肾者,以肾有水气也。故不合肾而合于包络耳。"

雷公曰："包络之火气出于肾,三焦取火于肾,不胜取火于包络乎?"

岐伯曰："膀胱与肾为表里,则肾之火气必亲膀胱而疏三焦矣。包络得肾之火气,自成其腑,代心宣化,虽腑犹脏也。包络无他腑之附,得三焦之依而更亲,是以三焦乐为表,包络亦自安于里,孤者不孤,自合者永合也。"

雷公曰："善。"

应龙问曰："包络,腑也,三焦亦自成腑,何以为包络之使乎?"

岐伯曰："包络即膻中也,为心膜鬲,近于心宫,遮护君主,其位最亲,其权最重,故三焦奉令,不敢后也。"

应龙曰："包络代心宣化,宜各脏腑皆奉令矣,何独使三焦乎?"

岐伯曰："各腑皆有表里,故不听包络之使,惟三焦无脏为表里,故包络可以使之。"

应龙曰："三焦何乐为包络使乎?"

岐伯曰："包络代心出治,腑与脏,同三焦听使于包络,犹听使于心,故包络为里,三焦为表,岂勉强附会哉?"

Volume 2

Tianlao asked, "The pericardium is neither a Zang-organ nor a Fu-organ. [But] why is it combined with the triple energizer?"

Qibo answered, "[Because] the pericardium and triple energizer are externally and internally [related to each other] and these two meridians have names but are all invisible. The five Zang-organs are visible and combined with visibility. The pericardium is invisible and therefore combined with invisibility. "

Tianlao asked, "The triple energizer is an isolated Zang-organ. Now that [it is] named Zang-organ, [but] why [is it] combined with the pericardium?"

Qibo answered, "Although the triple energizer is named Zang-organ, [it is] isolated and not combined [with others]. [Therefore it] is still a Fu-organ, not a Zang-organ. Qi [that has] left the pericardium actually has nothing to depend on. This is a natural combination, not reluctant approach. "

Tianlao said, "Right!"

Leigong asked,"The lung is combined with the large intestine, the heart is combined with the small intestine, the liver is combined with the gallbladder, the spleen is combined with the stomach and the kidney is combined with the bladder. This is a natural combination. The combination of the triple energizer with the pericardium may be not natural. "

Qibo answered, "The pericardium is not a Zang-organ but combined with the triple energizer because the pericardium is the internal and the triple energizer is the external. "

Leigong asked,"The triple energizer is a Fu-organ. Why [is it] divided into the external and internal?"

应龙曰："善。"

陈士铎曰："包络之合三焦,非无因之合也;包络之使三焦,因其合而使之也。然合者,仍合于心耳,非包络之司为合也。"

【今译】

天老请问岐伯曰:"天有六气,化生大地中的五行;地有五行,化生人体中的五脏。有五脏的阴,就应当有五腑的阳,为何脏只有五个,而腑却有七个呢?"

岐伯说:"心包络属于腑,其性则属于阴,所以虽然与脏气相同,但还是分配到了六腑。"

天老问:"心包络既然分配到了腑,但心包络却是脏,为什么将其不命名为脏,而将其另外称为腑呢?"

岐伯说:"因为心包络并不是脏。"

天老问:"不是脏而列入脏中,这不是不可以的吗?"

岐伯说:"脏称为五而不称为六,这就是不以脏的名称命名包络;腑称为六而不称为七,这也是不以腑的名称命名包络。"

天老问:"心包络不是脏也不是腑,为什么能与三焦相结合呢?"

岐伯说:"包络与三焦相为表里,这两条经脉都是有名而无形。五脏是有形的,所以与有形者相合;包络是无形的,因此只能与无形者相合。"

天老问:"三焦是孤脏,既然命名其为脏,又为什么能与包络相

Volume 2

Qibo answered, "Qi from the triple energizer is closely related to the kidney. [The reason that it is] close to the kidney but not combined with the kidney [is that] there is water-Qi in the kidney. That is why [the triple energizer is] not combined with the kidney but combined with the pericardium."

Leigong asked, "Fire-Qi from the pericardium originates from the kidney. The triple energizer gets fire from the kidney, [perhaps] not from the pericardium."

Qibo answered, "The bladder and the kidney are externally and internally [related to each other]. So fire-Qi in the kidney must be close to the bladder and far away from the triple energizer. [When] the pericardium has received fire-Qi from the kidney, [it] certainly becomes a Fu-organ, diffusing and transforming on behalf of the heart. Although [the pericardium is] a Fu-organ, [it] actually serves as a Zang-organ. The pericardium is not combined with other organs and appears closer [when] combined with the triple energizer because the triple energizer likes to be in the external and the pericardium likes to be in the internal. [In this way,] the isolated [organ] is not isolated and mutual combination is always in harmony."

Leigong said, "Excellent!"

Yinglong[2] asked, "The pericardium is a Fu-organ and the triple energizer is also a Fu-organ autonomously. [But] why [does the triple energizer] become the follower of the pericardium?"

Qibo answered, "The pericardium is Danzhong (CV 17) and is the membrane of the heart. [It is located] close to the heart palace to protect [heart] monarch. [Thus] its position is the closest [one

合呢?"

岐伯说:"三焦虽然也被称为脏,但它却是孤脏,没能与其他脏器相合,因此它依然是腑,而不是脏。如果离开了包络之气,实际上就没有可以依靠的了。这是天然的配合,而不是勉强的附会。"

天老说:"好!"

雷公问:"肺与大肠相合,心与小肠相合,肝与胆相合,脾与胃相合,肾与膀胱相合,这就是天然的配合。三焦也与心包络相合,这恐怕不是天然地配合吧?"

岐伯说:"包络不是脏,其之所以能与三焦相合,是因为包络为里,三焦为表。"

雷公问:"三焦是腑,怎么会分为表里呢?"

岐伯说:"三焦之气本来与肾脏亲近,虽然与肾脏亲近但却不与肾脏相合,因为肾中有水气,这就是为什么三焦不与肾脏合而与包络相合。"

雷公问:"包络的火气出自于肾脏,三焦从肾脏中获取了火气,这不是更优于从包络中获取火气吗?"

岐伯说:"膀胱与肾相为表里,肾脏的火气必然亲近膀胱而疏远三焦。包络获得了肾脏中的火气,自然就成为腑了,并且代替心脏进行宣化,包络虽然是腑,其功能却像脏一样。包络没有其他腑的依附,当得到三焦的依附时就显得更为亲近,这就是为什么三焦喜欢成为其表,而包络也自然乐于安居其里,由此可见孤腑其实并不孤立,所以自相配合的脏腑也就会永久地相合了。"

to the heart⌉ and its power is the greatest ⌈one⌉. That is why the triple energizer ⌈must⌉ obey the orders ⌈of the pericardium⌉ and dare not be sluggish."

Yinglong asked, "The pericardium diffuse and transform on behalf of the heart and all the Zang-organs and Fu-organs should obey the orders ⌈of the pericardium⌉. ⌈But⌉ why the triple energizer is independent?"

Qibo answered, "There are the external and internal ⌈relationships in⌉ all Fu-organs. That is why ⌈there is⌉ no ⌈need for them to be⌉ the followers of the pericardium. Only the triple energizer has no external and internal ⌈relationship with other organs⌉ and that is why the pericardium orders it."

Yinglong asked, "Why does the triple energizer like to be the follower of the pericardium?"

Qibo answered, "The pericardium governs on behalf of the heart. The Fu-organs and Zang-organs together with the triple energizer obey the orders of the pericardium, just like taking orders from the heart. That is why the pericardium is the internal and the triple energizer is the external. How can it be a reluctant approach?"

Yinglong said, "Good!"

Chen Shiduo's comment, "There must be reasons ⌈why⌉ the pericardium is combined with the triple energizer. The pericardium instructs the triple energizer because ⌈it is⌉ combined ⌈with the triple energizer⌉. However the combination ⌈with the pericardium⌉ is actually a combination with the heart, not just a combination

雷公说："好！"

应龙问："包络既然是腑，三焦也自然成为腑，为何三焦居然成为包络的使者了呢？"

岐伯说："包络就是膻中，是心脏的膜膈，位于心宫的附近，遮护着君主，其位置最近于心脏，其权势也最为重大，所以当三焦奉行包络之令时，就不敢有任何形式的怠慢。"

应龙说："包络代替心脏宣化，各脏腑都应当奉行其令，为什么只有三焦才是其使者呢？"

岐伯说："各脏腑都有表里，所以不一定听从包络之使，只有三焦没有任何脏与其有表里关系，所以包络就可以使唤它。"

应龙说："三焦为何乐意成为包络的使者呢？"

岐伯说："包络代替心脏进行治理，腑与脏同三焦一起听使于包络，正如听从心脏之令一样，正因为如此，包络就为里，三焦则为表，这怎么能是勉强的附会呢？"

应龙说："好！"

陈士铎评论说："包络与三焦相合，并不是没有因由的相合。包络之所以使唤三焦，是因为两者相合。然而就其相合而言，其实依然是与心相合，并不是与包络这一代心行令者相合。"

Volume 2

with the pericardium [that] governs [on behalf of the heart]."

Notes

[1] Tianlao (天老) was a minister of Yellow Emperor. It was said that he wrote a book entitled *Za Zi Yin Dao* (《杂子阴道》) composed of fifteen volumes.

[2] Yinglong (应龙) was a god mentioned in the book entitled *Shan Hai Jing* (《山海经》, *The Classic of Mountains and Rivers*) written before the Qin Dynasty (221 B.C.–207 B.C.).

卷三

胆腑命名篇第十九

【原文】

胡孔甲问于岐伯曰："大肠者,白肠也,小肠者,赤肠也,胆非肠,何谓青肠乎?"

岐伯曰："胆贮青汁,有入无出,然非肠何能通而贮之乎? 故亦以肠名之。青者,木之色,胆属木,其色青,故又名青肠也。"

胡孔甲曰："十一脏取决于胆,是腑亦有脏名矣,何脏分五而腑分七也?"

岐伯曰："十一脏取决于胆,乃省文耳,非腑可名脏也。"

孔甲曰："胆既名为脏,而十一脏取决之,固何所取之乎?"

岐伯天师曰："胆司渗,凡十一脏之气,得胆气渗之,则分清化浊,有奇功焉。"

孔甲曰："胆有入无出,是渗主入而不主出也,何能化浊乎?"

岐伯曰："清渗入则浊自化,浊自化而清亦化矣。"

孔甲曰："清渗入而能化,是渗入而仍渗出矣。"

岐伯曰："胆为清净之府。渗入者,清气也,遇清气之脏腑亦以清气应之,应即渗之机矣,然终非渗也。"

孔甲曰："脏腑皆取决于胆,何脏腑受胆之渗乎?"

岐伯曰："大小肠膀胱皆受之,而膀胱独多焉,虽然膀胱分胆之渗,

Volume 3

【英译】

Chapter 19
Nomenclature of the Gallbladder

Hu Kongjia[1] asked Qibo, "The large intestine is a white intestine [while] the small intestine is a red intestine. The gallbladder is not an intestine. [But] why is it called a blue intestine?"

Qibo answered, "The gallbladder contains blue bile [which just] comes into [the gallbladder and] never comes out [of the gallbladder]. [If it is] not an intestine, how can [it] connect with and store bile? That is why [it is] also named intestine. Blue is the color of wood and the gallbladder belongs to wood and its color is blue. That is why [it is] also known as blue intestine."

Hu Kongjia asked, "The eleven Zang-organs depend on the gallbladder, therefore [the gallbladder] is a Fu-organ [but] also named Zang-organ. [But] why [are] the Zang-organs divided into five and the Fu-organs [are] divided into seven?"

Qibo answered, "The eleven Zang-organs depend on the gallbladder. [This is] just a simplified description. [It does] not [mean that] the Fu-organs can be named Zang-organs."

Kongjia asked, "Now that the gallbladder is named Zang-organ and the eleven Zang-organs depend on it. [But] why must [the eleven Zang-organs] depend on it?"

而胆之气虚矣。胆虚则胆得渗之祸矣,故胆旺则渗益,胆虚则渗损。"

孔甲曰:"胆渗何气则受损乎?"

岐伯曰:"酒热之气,胆之所畏也,过多则渗失所司,胆受损矣,非毒结于脑,则涕流于鼻也。"

孔甲曰:"何以治之?"

岐伯曰:"刺胆络之穴,则病可已也。"

孔甲曰:"善。"

陈士铎曰:"胆主渗,十二脏皆取决于胆者,正决于渗也。胆不能渗,又何取决乎?"

【今译】

胡孔甲请问岐伯:"大肠是白肠,小肠是赤肠。胆不是肠,但为什么将其称为青肠呢?"

岐伯说:"胆囊储藏有青色的胆汁,有入而无出,如果不是肠,为什么能够连通并储藏有胆汁呢? 所以也用肠命名之。青色是木的颜色,而胆也属木,它的颜色也是青色,所以又将其称为青肠。"

胡孔甲问:"十一脏取决于胆,是因为腑也有脏之名,但为何脏有五个而腑却有七个呢?"

岐伯说:"十一脏取决于胆,这是简单的说法,并不是说腑可以命名为脏的。"

胡孔甲问:"胆既然称为脏,而十一脏取决于它,为何脏一定要取决于胆呢?"

Celestial Master Qibo answered, "The gallbladder governs penetration [of bile]. [Only when] Qi from the gallbladder has penetrated through the eleven Zang-organs can Qi [in the eleven Zang-organs] clarify the lucid and transform the turbid. This is a unique function."

Hu Kongjia asked, "[In] the gallbladder, there is [only] penetration and no discharge [of bile]. That means to pour [bile into the gallbladder], not to discharge [bile out of the gallbladder]. [But] how can [it] transform the turbid?"

Qibo answered, "The lucid penetrates into [the gallbladder] while the turbid transforms spontaneously. [When] the turbid transforms spontaneously, the lucid also transforms spontaneously."

Hu Kongjia asked, "The lucid penetrates into [the gallbladder], and also can transform [spontaneously]. Is this penetration and also effusion?"

Qibo answered, "The gallbladder is a clear and pure organ. [The element that] penetrates into [the gallbladder is] lucid Qi. [When] a Zang-organ or a Fu-organ has met lucid Qi, [it will] correspond to it with lucid Qi. [Such] a correspondence indicates the principle of penetration, and certainly not effusion."

Hu Kongjia asked, "[Both] the Zang-organs and Fu-organs depend on the gallbladder. [But] why do the Zang-organs and Fu-organs receive [bile] penetrated [into them from] the gallbladder?"

Qibo answered, "The large intestine, small intestine and bladder all receive [bile from the gallbladder], [among which] the bladder receives most. Since the bladder receives bile from the gallbladder, Qi in the gallbladder becomes deficient. [When Qi in]

岐伯说："胆主渗入，十一脏的气只有得到了胆气才能渗入，才能分清化浊，有奇特的功效。"

胡孔甲问："胆汁有入无出，这是因为渗入，是注入胆汁而不是排出胆汁，为什么能够化浊气呢？"

岐伯说："清气渗入了，浊气就能自化，浊气自化了，清气也能自化。"

胡孔甲问："清气渗入而能化浊气，那么应该是既能渗入又能渗出了。"

岐伯说："胆是清净之府。渗入的是清气，遇到有清气的脏腑，也就以清气与之相应。相应就是渗入的机制，但终究还不是渗出。"

胡孔甲问："脏腑都取决于胆，为何脏腑会都受纳于胆汁的渗入呢？"

岐伯说："大肠、小肠、膀胱都会受纳胆汁，但膀胱惟独所受纳的胆汁比其他的多。膀胱分解了胆所渗出的胆汁，胆气也就因此而虚弱了。胆气虚弱，说明是因胆汁出现渗漏而导致的祸害。因此，胆气旺盛时渗入的胆汁多，胆气虚弱时渗入的胆汁少。"

胡孔甲问："胆汁渗入了，为什么气会受损呢？"

岐伯说："酒热之气是胆所畏惧的。饮酒过多，就会影响其分泌胆汁的功用，胆也就会因之而遭受损害。这与毒气结于脑而鼻涕从鼻孔流出不同。"

胡孔甲问："可以用什么方法来治疗呢？"

岐伯说："可以针刺胆络之穴，这样病就可以痊愈。"

胡孔甲说："好！"

陈士铎评论说："胆主胆汁的分泌，十二脏之所以都取决于胆，实际上就是取决于胆汁的渗入。如果胆汁不能渗入，十二脏又怎么能够取决于胆呢？"

the gallbladder is deficient, the gallbladder will suffer from leakage. So [when Qi in] the gallbladder is exuberant, more [bile will be] penetrated [into the gallbladder]; [when Qi in] the gallbladder is deficient, [bile] penetrated [into the gallbladder will be] reduced."

Hu Kongjia asked, "What will reduce [Qi when bile] penetrates into the gallbladder?"

Qibo answered, "Heat-Qi from wine [is what] the gallbladder fears. [Drinking] too much [wine] will affect the function [of the gallbladder] and harm the gallbladder. [It is] different from toxin [that] binds in the brains and outflows from the nose."

Hu Kongjia asked, "How to treat it?"

Qibo answered, "To needle the acupoints [located on] the collateral of the gallbladder [meridian] can treat such a disease."

Kongjia said, "Good!"

Chen Shiduo's comment , " The gallbladder governs secretion [of bile] and the twelve Zang-organs all depend on the gallbladder . [If bile] cannot penetrate into the gallbladder, how can [the twelve Zang-organs] depend on [it]?"

Notes

[1] Hu Kongjia (胡孔甲) was a historian of Yellow Emperor.

任督死生篇第二十

【原文】

雷公问曰:"十二经脉之外,有任督二脉,何略而不言也?"

岐伯曰:"二经之脉不可略也。以二经散见于各经,故言十二经脉而二经已统会于中矣。"

雷公曰:"试分言之。"

岐伯曰:"任脉行胸之前,督脉行背之后也。任脉起于中极之下,以上毛际,循腹里,上关元,至咽咙上颐,循面入目内眦,此任脉之经络也。

督脉起于少腹,以下骨中央,女子入系廷孔,在溺孔之际,其络循阴器合纂间,统纂后,即前后二阴之间也,别绕臀,至少阴与巨阳中络者,合少阴,上股内后廉,贯脊属肾,与太阳起于目内眦,上额交巅上,入络脑,至鼻柱,还出别下项,循肩膊,挟脊,抵腰中,入循膂,络肾。其男子循茎下至纂,与女子等,其少腹直上者,贯脐中央,上贯心,入喉上颐环唇,上系两目之下中央,此督脉之经络也。

虽督脉止于龈交,任脉止于承浆,其实二脉同起于会阴。止于龈交者未尝不过承浆,止于承浆者未尝不过龈交,行于前者亦行于后,行于后者亦行于前,循环周流彼此无间,故任督分之为二,合之仍一也。

夫会阴者,至阴之所也。任脉由阳行于阴,故脉名阴海。督脉由阴

Volume 3

【英译】

Chapter 20
Life and Death Related to the
Conception Vessel and Governor Vessel

Leigong asked, "Beside the twelve meridians, there are conception vessel and governor vessel. Why do people ignore [these two meridians] and avoid talking [about them]?"

Qibo answered, "These two meridians cannot be ignored. [In fact,] these two meridians are involved in other meridians. Thus [when] talking about the twelve meridians, these two meridians are already involved."

Leigong asked, "Please explain [them] in addition."

Qibo answered, "The conception vessel circulates in front of the chest and the governor vessel circulates in the back. The conception vessel starts from below Zhongji (CV 3), rising up to the pubes, moving in the abdomen, reaching Guanyuan (CV 4), arriving at the throat, ascending to the chin and entering the inner canthus along the cheek. This is the collateral of the conception vessel.

The governor vessel starts from the lower abdomen, moving downwards to the center of pelvis. [In] women, [this meridian here is] connected with the vaginal orifice. Around the urethral meatus, its collateral circulates in the genitals, meeting behind the perineal region [which is the place] between the genitals and anus. Its

行于阳,故脉名阳海。非龈交穴为阳海,承浆穴为阴海也。阴交阳而阴气生,阳交阴而阳气生,任督交而阴阳自长,不如海之难量乎,故以海名之。"

雷公曰:"二经之脉络,予已知之矣。请问其受病何如?"

岐伯曰:"二经气行则十二经之气通,二经气闭则十二经之气塞,男则成疝,女则成瘕,非遗溺即脊强也。"

雷公曰:"病止此乎?"

岐伯曰:"肾之气必假道于任督二经,气闭则肾气塞矣。女不受妊,男不射精,人道绝矣。然则任督二经之脉络,即人死生之道路也。"

雷公曰:"神哉论也。请载《外经》,以补《内经》未备。"

陈士铎曰:"任督之路,实人生死之途,说得精妙入神。"

【今译】

雷公问道:"十二正经之外,还有任脉和督脉这两条经脉,为什么将其忽略而不谈呢?"

岐伯说:"这两条经脉其实是不能忽略的。因为这两条经脉散见于其他各条经脉中,所以当谈到十二经脉时,这两条经脉都已经包含在里面了。"

雷公问道:"请分别予以解说吧。"

岐伯说:"任脉循行在胸部之前,督脉循行在背部之后。任脉起始于中极穴之下,向上循行到毛际,沿着腹部的里面上行到关元穴,然后

branch surrounds the buttocks and circulates to the collateral between Shaoyin [meridian] and Taiyang [meridian], combining with Shaoyin [meridian]. Ascending to [the region] behind the lateral side of the thigh, penetrating through the spine and connecting with the kidney, moving upwards to the forehead with Taiyang [meridian] starting from the inner canthus, meeting at the skull, entering into and communicating with the brains and reaching the nasal bridge. Its branch moves downwards along the neck, circulating to the shoulder, descending along both sides of the spine to the waist, entering the buttocks and connecting with the kidney. [In] men, [the governor vessel] circulates along the penis to the pubes in the same way [as that of] women. [The branch] ascends directly from the lower abdomen, penetrating through the center of the navel upwards to the heart, entering the throat, ascending to the chin, surrounding the lips, and rising up to meet the center behind the middle of the two eyes. This is the meridian and collateral of the governor vessel.

Although the governor vessel ends at Yinjiao (GV 28) and the conception vessel ends at Chengjiang (CV 24), these two meridians actually all start from Huiyin (CV 1). [The governor vessel that] ends at Yinjiao (GV 28) also passes by Chengjiang (CV 24), [the conception vessel that] ends at Chengjiang (CV 24) also passes by Yinjiao (GV 28), [the meridian that] moves in front [of the body] also moves at the back [of the body], [the meridian that] moves at the back [of the body] also moves in front [of the body], [all of which] move in circles and never disconnect from each other. That is why the governor vessel and the conception vessel are two

向上循行到咽喉,再向上循行到下颌部,并沿着面部而进入眼内角,这是任脉的经络。

督脉起始于少腹,向下循行到骨中央,女子与里面的阴道口相连,在尿道开口的附近,其络脉循行至阴部,在会阴部会合后再合并到会阴之后,也就是会合到前后二阴之间。然后其分支环绕臀部,循行到少阴与太阳中的络脉,与少阴经相合,继续向上循行到大腿内侧之后,贯通脊部并连接到肾,与起于眼内角的太阳经一起向上循行到额部,相交于头顶,然后进入脑内,与脑络相连,继而向下循行到鼻柱。其分支环绕颈项后向下循行,沿着肩膊和脊部两侧下行到腰中部,然后从臀部联系到肾。男子的经脉,沿着阴茎向下循行到会阴部,与女子经脉的循行相同。从少腹直接向上的分支,贯通到脐部中央,向上循行并贯通心脏,进入喉咙,继续向上循行到下颌部,环绕嘴唇,向上循行并联系到两目之下的中央,这是督脉的经络循行的路径。

虽然督脉的循行止于龈交穴,任脉的循行止于承浆穴,实际上这两条经脉都同时起始于会阴部。循行中止在龈交穴的督脉,未尝不经过承浆穴;循行中止在承浆穴的任脉,未尝不经过龈交穴。循行于人体之前的经脉,也循行于人体之后;循行在人体之后的经脉,也循行于人体之前。所以其循环往复周流,彼此之间没有任何间断。因此任脉与督脉可以分为两条经脉,但合并起来依然是一条经脉。

会阴穴是极阴之处。任脉由阳循行到阴,所以任脉也可以称为阴海;督脉由阴循行到阳,所以督脉也可以称为阳海。但并不是龈交穴可以称为阳海,也不是承浆穴可以称为阴海。阴与阳相交则阴气生,阳与

meridians but are actually integrated into one.

Huiyin (CV 1) is the location of Zhiyin (BL 67). The conception vessel circulates from Yang to Yin, and therefore [it is] named Yin sea. The governor vessel circulates from Yin to Yang, and therefore [it is] named Yang sea. Yinjiao (GV 28) is not Yang sea, [but] Chengjiang (CV 24) is Yin sea. [When] Yin is combined with Yang, Yin Qi [will be] produced; [when] Yang is combined with Yin, Yang Qi [will be] produced; [when] the conception vessel and the governor vessel are combined with each other, Yin and Yang will grow spontaneously. [Is it] not like the sea [that is] difficult to measure? That is why [it is] named after sea.

Leigong asked, "I have understood the circulation of these two meridians. How about the diseases occurring in them?"

Qibo answered, "[Only when] Qi in these two meridians flow [smoothly can] Qi in the twelve meridians circulate normally [without any hindrance]. [If] Qi in these two meridians is blocked, Qi in the twelve meridians [will be] stagnated. [If such a problem has happened, it will cause] hernia in men and abdominal mass in women, either enuresis or stiffness of spine."

Leigong asked, "Just such a disease?"

Qibo answered, "Qi in the kidney must depend on the conception [vessel] and governor [vessel to flow]. [When] Qi [in these two meridians are] blocked, Qi in the kidney [will be] stagnated. [If such a problem has happened,] women are unable to be pregnant and men are unable to ejaculate, the way [to conceive a baby is] lost. So the conception vessel, governor vessel and collaterals are the roads of human life."

阴相交则阳气生,任脉和督脉相交则阴阳自然生发,这不正如大海一样,难以测量吗? 所以就用海来命名之。"

雷公问:"任脉和督脉的循行,我已经知道了,请问其所引发的疾病会怎么样的呢?"

岐伯说:"任督二脉之气通行,十二经之气则通畅无阻;任督二脉之气闭塞,十二经之气则闭塞不通。在这种情况下,男子则会得疝病,女子则会得瘕症,不是遗尿,就是脊柱强直。"

雷公问:"任督二脉所引发的疾病只有这些吗?"

岐伯说:"肾气之运行必须凭借任、督二脉的循行路线,当任督二脉之气闭塞了,肾气也将随之而闭塞不通。在这种情况下,女人不能受孕,男子不能射精,生育的功能就断绝了。所以任督两经的脉络,实际上就是人的死生道路啊!"

雷公说:"真神妙论述啊! 请将其载录于《外经》,以补充《内经》的不足。"

陈士铎评论说:"任督二脉的循行路线,就是人的生死途径,说得精妙如神啊!"

Volume 3

Leigong said, "What a marvelous explanation! Please record [it] in [Yellow Emperor's] External Canon of Medicine to supplement what [Yellow Emperor's] Internal Canon [of Medicine] lacks."

Chen Shiduo's comment, "The paths of the conception [vessel] and governor [vessel] are the ways of life and death for human beings. The explanation is marvelous."

阴阳二跷篇第二十一

【原文】

司马问曰:"奇经八脉中有阴跷阳跷之脉,可得闻乎?"

岐伯曰:"《内经》言之矣。"

司马曰:"《内经》言之,治病未验或有未全欤?"

岐伯曰:"《内经》约言之,实未全也。阴跷脉足少阴肾经之别脉也,起于然骨之照海穴,出内踝上,又直上之,循阴股以入于阴,上循胸里,入于缺盆,上出人迎之前,入于目下鸠,属于目眦之睛明穴,合足太阳膀胱之阳跷而上行,此阴跷之脉也。

阳跷脉足太阳膀胱之别脉也,亦起于然骨之下申脉穴,出外踝下,循仆参,郗于附阳,与足少阳会于居髎,又与手阳明会于肩髃及巨骨,又与手太阳阳维会于臑俞,与手足阳明会于地仓及巨髎,与任脉足阳明会于承泣,合足少阴肾经之阴跷下行,此阳跷之脉也。

然而跷脉之起止,阳始于膀胱而止于肾,阴始于肾而止于膀胱,此男子同然也,若女子微有异。男之阴跷起于然骨,女之阴跷起于阴股;男之阳跷起于申脉,女之阳跷起于仆参。知同而治同,知异而疗异,则阳跷之病不至阴缓阳急,阴跷之病不至阳缓阴急,何不验乎?"

司马公曰:"今而后,阴阳二跷之脉昭然矣。"

Volume 3

【英译】

Chapter 21
Yin Heel Vessel and Yang Heel Vessel

Si Ma asked, "Eight extra meridians include Yin heel vessel and Yang heel vessel. Can I listen [to your explanation]?"

Qibo answered, "[It is already] explained in [*Yellow Emperor's*] *Internal Canon* [*of Medicine*]."

Si Ma asked, "[Although it is already] explained in [*Yellow Emperor's*] *Internal Canon* [*of Medicine*], [some of the therapeutic methods used] to treat disease are not confirmed. Is it not completely explained?"

Qibo answered, "The explanation in [*Yellow Emperor's*] *Internal Canon* [*of Medicine*] is brief, not complete. Yin heel vessel is the divergent meridian of the kidney meridian of foot-Shaoyin, starting from Zhaohai (KI 6) located in Rangu[1], emerging from the medial ankle, rising up directly, circulating along the medial side of the thigh into the pubes, moving upwards to the chest, entering the supraclavicular fossa, emerging [from the area] before Renying (ST 9), entering the cheekbone, connecting with Jingming (BL 1), combining with the bladder meridian of foot-Taiyang and moving upwards with Yang heel vessel. This is Yin heel vessel.

Yang heel vessel is the divergent meridian of the bladder meridian of foot-Taiyang, also starting from Shenmai (BL 62)

陈士铎曰："二跷之脉,分诸男女,《内经》微别,人宜知之,不可草草看过。"

【今译】

司马问道："奇经八脉之中,有阴跷之脉和阳跷之脉,可否听听您的解释吗?"

岐伯说："《内经》已经讲过了。"

司马问："《内经》虽然已经讲过了,但用来治病时还没有得到应验,是否有些讲得不够全面呢?"

岐伯说："《内经》只是简约地作了论述,确实没有全面地予以说明。阴跷之脉,实际上是从足少阴肾经分出的别脉。该别脉起始于足然骨下的照海穴,从足内踝上出来后又直接向上循行,沿着大腿内侧上行而进入阴部。然后继续向上循行到胸内,并进入缺盆,再向上循行,从人迎穴之前出来,进入眼睛下面的颧部,这就是眼内角的睛明穴,与足太阳膀胱经的阳跷合并后一起上行,这就是阴跷之脉。阳跷脉是足太阳膀胱经的别脉,也起始于然骨之下的申脉穴,从足外踝下出来,循行到仆参穴之中,即以附阳为穴,与足少阳胆经会于居髎穴,又与手阳明大肠经会于肩髃穴和巨骨穴,又与手太阳小肠经的阳维穴会于臑俞穴,又与足阳明胃经会于地仓穴和巨髎穴,又与任脉、足阳明胃经会于承泣穴,又与足少阴肾经的阴跷脉合并后向下循行,这就是阳跷脉。

然而,就跷脉的起始和终止而言,阳跷脉起始于膀胱而终止于肾,阴跷脉则起始于肾而终止于膀胱。该经脉在男子体内的循行都是这

located below Rangu, emerging from below the external ankle, circulating to Pucan (BL 61) and Fuyang[2], meeting with [the bladder meridian of] foot-Shaoyang in Juliao (GB 29), meeting with [the large intestine meridian of] hand-Yangming in Jianyu (LI 15) and Jugu (LI 16), meeting with [the small intestine meridian of] hand-Taiyang and Yang link vessel in Naoshu (SI 10), meeting with [the stomach meridian of] foot-Yangming in Dicang (ST 4) and Juliao (ST 3), meeting with the conception vessel and [the stomach meridian of] foot-Yangming in Chengqi (ST 1), and combining with Yin heel vessel of the kidney meridian of foot-Shaoyin. This is Yang heel vessel.

However in terms of the beginning and ending of the heel vessels, Yang [heel vessel] starts from the bladder and ends at the kidney, Yin [heel vessel] starts from the kidney and ends at the bladder, [the circulation of which is] the same in men and slightly different in women. The Yin heel vessel starts from Rangu in men and from the medial side of the thigh in women, the Yang heel vessel starts from Shenmai (BL 62) in men and from Pucan (BL 61) in women. [If the meridians in men and women are] the same, treatment [of diseases is] also the same; [if the meridians in men and women are] different, treatment [of disease is] also different. [To deal with disease in this way,] disease [related to] Yang heel vessel will not lead to slowness of Yin and contracture of Yang, and disease [related to] Yin heel vessel will not result in slowness of Yang and contracture of Yin. How could it not be well confirmed?"

Si Ma said, "From now on, the [knowledge about] Yin heel vessel and Yang heel vessel is very clear."

样,但在女子体内的循行则稍有差异。男子的阴跷脉起始于然骨,而女子的阴跷脉则起始于阴股;男子的阳跷脉起始于申脉穴,而女子的阳跷脉则起始于仆参穴。男女经脉的起始和终止相同,疾病的治疗也相同;男女经脉的起始和终止有差异,疾病的治疗也有差异。这样的话,阳跷脉所引起的疾病就不至于发展到阴缓阳急的状况,阴跷脉所引起的疾病也不至于发展到阳缓阴急的状况,哪有不能应验疾病的呢?"

司马说:"从今以后,阴跷脉和阳跷脉的情况就非常明确了!"

陈士铎评论说:"阴跷和阳跷之脉,男女中都是有所区别的,对此《内经》略微作了一些分析说明,大家应当了解,阅读时不能草草看过了事。"

Volume 3

Chen Shiduo's comment，" These two heel vessels differ from men and women. In ［Yellow Emperor's］ Internal Canon ［of Medicine］，there are some brief explanations which should be well understood，not just read hastily."

Notes

［1］Rangu（然骨）refers to the area before the medial ankle and in the depression below the big bone.

［2］Fuyang（附阳）is an acupoint located three *Cun* above the area behind the external ankle.

奇恒篇第二十二

【原文】

奢龙问于岐伯曰："奇恒之腑，与五脏并主藏精，皆可名脏乎？"

岐伯曰："然。"

奢龙曰："脑、髓、骨、脉、胆、女子胞，既谓奇恒之腑，不宜又名脏矣？"

岐伯曰："腑谓脏者，以其能藏阴也。阴者，即肾中之真水也。真水者，肾精也。精中有气，而脑髓骨脉胆女子胞皆能藏之，故可名腑，亦可名脏也。"

奢龙曰；"修真之士，何必留心于此乎？"

岐伯曰："人欲长生，必知斯六义，而后可以养精气，结圣胎者也。"

奢龙曰："女子有胞以结胎，男子无胞，何以结之？"

岐伯曰："女孕男不妊，故胞属之女子，而男子未尝无胞也，男子有胞而后可以养胎息，故修真之士，必知斯六者。至要者，则胞与脑也。脑为泥丸，即上丹田也；胞为神室，即下丹田也。骨藏髓，脉藏血，髓藏气，脑藏精，气血精髓尽升泥丸，下降于舌，由舌下华池，由华池下廉泉、玉英，通于胆，下贯神室。世人多欲，故血耗气散，髓竭精亡也。苟知藏而不泻，即返还之道也。"

奢龙曰："六者宜藏，何道而使之藏乎？"

Volume 3

【英译】

Chapter 22
Extraordinary Fu-organs

Shelong[1] asked Qibo, "The extraordinary Fu-organs and the five Zang-organs all store essence. Can 〔the extraordinary Fu-organs be〕 named Zang-organs?"

Qibo answered, "Yes."

Shelong asked, "The brains, marrow, bones, vessels, bladder and uterus are called extraordinary Fu-organs. Are they unnecessary to be named Zang-organs?"

Qibo answered, "〔The reason that〕 the Fu-organs are called Zang-organs 〔is that〕 they can store Yin 〔essence〕. Yin 〔essence〕 refers to genuine water in the kidney. Genuine water is essence in the kidney. There is Qi in essence 〔which〕 can be stored in the brains, marrow, bones, vessels, bladder and uterus. That is why 〔they〕 can be named Fu-organs and can also be named Zang-organs."

Shelong asked, "Why do those cultivating genuineness[2] care about such positions?"

Qibo answered, "Those 〔who〕 want to live a long life must know the meaning of this six 〔extraordinary Fu-organs〕. 〔Only with such a knowledge can they〕 cultivate essential Qi and conceive a baby."

Shelong asked, "Women can conceive a baby because 〔they〕

岐伯曰："广成子有言,毋摇精,毋劳形,毋思虑营营,非不泻之谓乎?"

奢龙曰;"命之矣。"

陈士铎曰:"脑、髓、骨、脉、胆、女子胞,非脏也,非脏而以脏名之,以其能藏也,能藏故以脏名之,人可失诸藏乎?"

【今译】

奢龙请问岐伯:"奇恒之腑与五脏并主藏精,可以用'脏'来对其予以命名吗?"

岐伯说:"可以的。"

奢龙问:"脑、髓、骨、脉、胆和女子胞,既然称为奇恒之腑,难道就不宜又命名为脏了吗?"

岐伯说:"之所以将腑称为脏,是因为其能够藏阴。所谓阴,指的就是肾脏中的真水。肾脏中的真水就是肾精。肾精中存在着气,而脑、髓、骨、脉、胆与女子胞都能对此加以贮藏,所以既可以将其命名为腑,也可以将其命名为脏。"

奢龙问:"修身养性、保持真精的人士,为何特别留心于这些情况呢?"

岐伯说:"人想长生,就必须知道这六种奇恒之腑的意义,这样才能滋养精气,才能孕育成圣胎。"

奢龙问:"女子有胞宫就能孕育出胎儿,男子没有胞胎,为何也能

have uterus. Men do not have uterus. How can they conceive a baby?"

Qibo answered, "Women can conceive a baby and men cannot. That is why uterus is in women. However [it does not mean that] men do not have uterus. [Only when] men have uterus [can they] cultivate fetus. So those cultivating genuineness must know [these six extraordinary Fu-organs]. Among these six [extraordinary Fu-organs,] the most important are the uterus and brains. The brains is Ni Wan (muddy pill)[3], also known as upper Dantian (the upper elixir field)[4]; the uterus is the root of spirit, also known as lower Dantian (the lower elixir field). The bones store marrow, the vessels store blood, the marrow stores Qi and the brains store essence. Qi, blood, essence and marrow all ascend to Ni Wan, descending to the tongue, moving downwards from the tongue to Huachi[5] and from Huachi to Lianquan (CV 23) and Yuying[6], penetrating through the gallbladder and entering the root of spirit. Human beings have a lot of desires. That is why blood is often consumed, Qi is always dispersed, marrow is frequently exhausted and essence is inevitably lost. If [one] knows [the principle of] storage without excretion, [he or she will certainly] return to the [right] way [of living]."

Shelong asked, "[Essence in] the six [extraordinary Fu-organs] should be stored. How to store it?"

Qibo answered, "Guang Chengzi has said, never shake essence, never overstrain the body, never contemplate too much. [Isn't it the right way] not to excrete?"

Shelong said, "[I will] follow this way."

孕育胎儿呢?"

岐伯说:"女子能怀孕,男子却不能怀孕,所以胞宫就属于女子的器官,然而男子却并不是没有胞宫。男子只有具备了胞宫之后,才能养育胎息。所以修身养性、保持真精的人士必须要了解这六种奇恒之腑。这六种奇恒之腑中最重要的,是脑与胞。脑为泥丸宫,也就是上丹田;胞为神室,也就是下丹田。骨藏髓,脉藏血,髓藏气,脑藏精,气血髓精,这些都上升到了泥丸宫,然后下降到舌,并由舌而下降到华池,再由华池下降到廉泉、玉英,然后与胆相通,接着继续向下循行,贯通神室。世人多有性欲,因而导致了血耗气散、髓竭精亡的后果。如果懂得了藏而不泄的重要性,那就懂得了返还之道的真谛。"

奢龙问:"这六种奇恒之腑都应当藏,但用什么方法才能使其藏而不泻呢?"

岐伯说:"广成子说过,不要摇动精气,不要劳累形体,不要有思虑繁杂,所强调的不就是藏而不泄吗?"

奢龙说:"我当谨遵此命!"

陈士铎评论说:"脑、髓、骨、脉、胆、女子胞,并非脏。不是脏却以脏命名之,就是因为它们能藏精,所以凡是能够藏精的都可用脏予以命名,人怎么能够失去这些贮藏呢?"

Volume 3

Chen Shiduo's comment, " *The brains*, *marrow*, *bones*, *vessels*, *gallbladder and uterus are not Zang-organs*. [*They are*] *not Zang-organs but named Zang-organs because they can store* [*essence*]. *That is why* [*they are*] *named Zang-organs. How can human beings lose* [*what is*] *stored* [*in these six extraordinary Fu-organs*]?"

Notes

[1] Shelong (奢龙) was the minister of Yellow Emperor.

[2] To cultivate genuineness means to cultivate life and health.

[3] Ni Wan (泥丸), literally muddy pill, refers to the brains used in Daoism. Daoism believes that human being is a small universe composed of small sky and earth. In the human body, the brains represent the earth because it is yellow in color and the earth is also yellow in color.

[4] Dantian (丹田), usually translated as the upper elixir field, originally referred to the place where Daoist practiced alchemy. Later on it was adopted in medicine and refers to three important regions in the human body, i. e. the region between the eye brows known as the upper Dantian (upper elixir field), the region below the heart known as the middle Dantian (middle elixir field) and the region below the navel known as the lower Dantian (lower elixir field).

[5] Huachi (华池) is an extra acupoint where Yin fluid is produced.

[6] Yuying (玉英) is an acupoint located below the tongue.

小络篇第二十三

【原文】

应龙问于岐伯曰："膜原与肌腠有分乎？"

岐伯曰："二者不同也。"

应龙曰："请问不同？"

岐伯曰："肌腠在膜原之外也。"

应龙曰："肌腠有脉乎？"

岐伯曰："肌腠膜原皆有脉也，其所以分者，正分于其脉耳。肌腠之脉，外连于膜原，膜原之脉，内连于肌腠。"

应龙曰："二脉乃表里也，有病何以分之？"

岐伯曰："外引小络痛者，邪在肌腠也。内引小络痛者，邪在膜原也。"

应龙曰："小络又在何所？"

岐伯曰："小络在膜原之间也。"

陈士铎曰："小络一篇，本无深文，备载诸此，以小络异于膜原耳。知膜原之异，即知肌膜之异也。"

Volume 3

【英译】

Chapter 23
Small Collaterals

Yinglong asked Qibo, "Is there any difference between Mo Yuan (interpleuro-diaphragmatic space) and Ji Cou (muscular striae)?"

Qibo answered, "They are different."

Yinglong asked, "What is the difference?"

Qibo answered, "Ji Cou (muscular striae) is located outside of Mo Yuan (interpleuro-diaphragmatic space)."

Yinglong asked, "Is there any meridian in Ji Cou (muscular striae)?"

Qibo answered, "Ji Cou (muscular striae) and Mo Yuan (interpleuro-diaphragmatic space) all have meridians. The reason [why they are] different [is that] the meridians in them are different. The meridian of Ji Cou (muscular striae) is externally connected with Mo Yuan (interpleuro-diaphragmatic space) and the meridian of Mo Yuan (interpleuro-diaphragmatic space) is internally connected with Ji Cou (muscular striae)."

Yinglong asked, "These two meridians are externally and internally [related to each other]. How to differ [when] there is disease?"

Qibo answered, "[If there is] disease caused externally in the small collateral, evil is in Ji Cou (muscular striae); [if there is]

【今译】

应龙请问岐伯："膜原与肌腠有区分吗?"

岐伯说："两者并不相同。"

应龙问："请问有何不同?"

岐伯说："肌腠在于膜原之外。"

应龙问："肌腠有经脉吗?"

岐伯说："肌腠、膜原都是有经脉的,它们之所以被分开,正是因为它们的经脉是有区别的,肌腠的经脉在外连接着膜原,膜原的经脉在里连接着肌腠。"

应龙问："这两个经脉互为表里,其引发疾病后又该如何区别呢?"

岐伯说："如果在外引起小络疼痛的,病邪则隐藏在肌腠中;如果在里而引起小络疼痛的,病邪则隐藏在膜原中。"

应龙问："小络又在什么地方呢?"

岐伯说："小络处在膜原之间的位置上。"

陈士铎评论说："小络这一篇,本来没有什么深奥的文字,之所以记载于此,主要因为小络与膜原有差异。懂得了膜原的差异,也就懂得了肌腠的差异了。"

disease caused internally in the small collateral, evil is in Mo Yuan (interpleuro-diaphragmatic space)."

Yinglong asked, "Where is the small collateral located?"

Qibo answered, "The small collateral is [located in the region] between Mo Yuan (interpleuro-diaphragmatic space)."

Chen Shiduo's comment , "This chapter about small collateral is simple. To record such [information in] this [chapter] is to show the difference between small collateral and Mo Yuan (interpleuro-diaphragmatic space). [If one] knows the difference of Mo Yuan (interpleuro-diaphragmatic space), [he or she will] certainly know the difference of Ji Cou (muscular striae)."

肺金篇第二十四

【原文】

少师问曰："肺金也，脾胃土也，土宜生金，有时不能生金者谓何？"

岐伯曰："脾胃土旺而肺金强，脾胃土衰而肺金弱，又何疑乎？然而脾胃之气太旺，反非肺金所喜者，由于土中火气之过盛也。土为肺金之母，火为肺金之贼，生变为克，乌乎宜乎？"

少师曰："金畏火克，宜避火矣，何又亲火乎？"

岐伯曰："肺近火，则金气之柔者必销矣。然肺离火，则金气之顽者必折矣。所贵微火以通薰肺也。故土中无火，不能生肺金之气。而土中多火，亦不能生肺金之气也。所以烈火为肺之所畏，微火为肺之所喜。"

少师公曰："善。请问金木之生克？"

岐伯曰："肺金制肝木之旺，理也。而肝中火盛，则金受火炎，肺失清肃之令矣。避火不暇，敢制肝木乎？即木气空虚，已不畏肺金之刑，况金受火制，则肺金之气必衰，肝木之火愈旺，势必横行无忌，侵伐脾胃之土，所谓欺子弱而凌母强也。肺之母家受敌，御木贼之强横，奚能顾金子之困穷，肺失化源，益加弱矣。肺弱欲其下生肾水难矣，水无金生则水不能制火，毋论上焦之火焚烧，而中焦之火亦随之更炽甚，且下焦之火亦挟水沸腾矣。"

Volume 3

【英译】

Chapter 24
Lung-Metal

Shaoshi asked, "The lung [belongs to] metal, the spleen and stomach [belong to] earth, and earth produces metal[1]. [But] why [earth] cannot produce metal sometimes?"

Qibo answered, "[When] earth [-Qi] in the spleen and stomach is exuberant, lung-metal is strong; [when] earth [-Qi] is debilitated, lung-metal is weak. Why is there doubt? However, [if] Qi in the spleen and stomach is very effulgent, lung-metal actually dislikes because fire-Qi in earth is too exuberant. Earth is the mother of lung-metal and fire is the thief[2] of lung-metal. [In this case,] mutual promotion becomes mutual restriction. How could it be appropriate to produce metal?"

Shaoshi asked, "Metal fears restriction of fire and fire should be avoided. [But] why [does it] like fire?"

Qibo answered, "[When] the lung is close to fire, weakness of metal Qi will certainly be resolved. But [if] the lung leaves fire, obstinateness of metal-Qi must be broken. The important [thing is that] moderate fire can unobstruct and fumigate the lung. Thus [if] there is no fire in earth, [it] cannot produce metal-Qi in the lung. But [if] there is excessive fire in earth, [it] cannot also produce metal-Qi in the lung. For this reason, raging fire is [what] the lung fears and moderate fire is [what] the lung likes."

少师曰："何肺金之召火也?"

岐伯曰："肺金,娇脏也,位居各脏腑之上,火性上炎,不发则已,发则诸火应之。此肺金之所以独受厥害也。"

少师曰："肺为娇脏,曷禁诸火之威逼乎? 金破不鸣,断难免矣。何以自免于祸乎?"

岐伯曰："仍赖肾子之水以救之。是以肺肾相亲更倍于土金之相爱。以土生金,而金难生土。肺生肾,而肾能生肺,昼夜之间,肺肾之气实彼此往来两相通,而两相益也。"

少师曰："金得水以解火,敬闻命矣。然金有时而不畏火者,何谓乎?"

岐伯曰："此论其变也。"

少师曰："请尽言之。"

岐伯曰："火烁金者,烈火也。火气自微何以烁。金非惟不畏火,且侮火矣。火难制金,则金气日旺。肺成顽金,过刚而不可犯,于是肃杀之气必来伐木。肝受金刑力难生火,火势转衰,变为寒火,奚足畏乎? 然而火过寒无温气以生土,土又何以生金。久之火寒而金亦寒矣。"

少师曰："善。请问金化为水,而水不生木者,又何谓乎?"

岐伯曰："水不生木,岂金反生木乎? 水不生木者,金受火融之水也。真水生木而融化之水克木矣。"

少师曰："善。"

陈士铎曰："肺不燥不成顽金,肺过湿不成柔金,以肺中有火也。

Volume 3

Shaoshi said: "Good! Please explain the promotion and restriction of metal and wood."

Qibo answered, "Lung-metal controls effulgence of liver-wood. [This is] a principle. [If] fire in the liver is exuberant, metal [will be] restricted [by] flaming fire and the lung [will] lose its function of clarification and depuration. [If lung-metal] just tries to avoid fire, how can it control liver-wood? If wood-Qi is empty and deficient, [it] will not fear restriction of lung-metal. Now that metal is controlled by fire, metal-Qi in the lung must be weakened. The more effulgent fire in liver-wood is, the more wildly [it] acts [in] invading and striking earth [Qi in] the spleen and stomach, known as "bullying weak son and insulting strong mother". [When] the lung's mother family[3] is invaded, [it just tries] to resist wood-thief's[4] violence [and is] impossible to care about predicament of metal's son[5]. [When] the lung has lost [its] source of transformation, [it will become] weaker and weaker. [When] the lung is weak, [it is] difficult to produce kidney-water in the lower. [If] water cannot be produced by metal, it is unable to control fire. [As a result,] fire in the upper energizer will be burning, fire in the middle energizer will be more blazing accordingly, and fire in the lower energizer will leap up with water".

Shaoshi asked, "Why is lung-metal restricted by fire?"

Qibo answered, "Lung-metal is a delicate Zang-organ located above all the Zang-organs and Fu-organs. Fire tends to flame up. [If] it does not flame up, nothing [will happen]. [If it] flames up, all fire will correspond to it. That is why only lung-metal is restricted and damaged."

肺得火则金益,肺失火则金损。故金中不可无火,亦不可多火也。水火不旺,金反得其宜也。总不可使金之过旺耳。"

【今译】

少师问道:"肺属于金,脾胃属于土,土应该生金,但有时却不能生金,这是什么原因呢?"

岐伯说:"脾胃之土旺盛,肺金则强大;脾胃之土衰弱,肺金则衰弱。这还有什么疑问吗?但是,如果脾胃之气太旺,反而不是肺金所喜欢的,这是土中的火气过于旺盛的缘故。土为肺金之母,火为肺金在贼,这样相生就会变为相克,这又怎么会适宜其生金呢?"

少师问:"金畏惧火克,应当避火,但为什么金又亲近火呢?"

岐伯说:"如果肺亲近火,金气的柔软部分就会销溶。然而,如果肺离开了火,金气的顽固部分必然被折断,重要的是微火能贯通燎薰肺金。所以如果土中没有火,就不能生肺金之气;而如果土中火多,也不能生肺金之气。所以,烈火是肺金所畏惧的,微火是肺金所喜爱的。"

少师说:"好!请问金木的生克是怎样的呢?"

岐伯说:"肺金克制肝木的旺盛,这是正常的。然而如果肝中火气旺盛,金就会受到炎火的克制,从而就使肺金失去清肃之令。肺金避火可谓惟恐不及,哪还敢克制肝木呢?即使木气空虚,也不会畏惧肺金的刑伐,况且金受到火的克制,则肺金之气就必然会衰弱,肝木之火也就会越来越旺,这样就势必会横行无忌,从而侵袭和克伐脾胃之土,这就是所谓欺负衰弱之子以凌侮强母的意思。肺之母的家室遭受到敌对方

Volume 3

Shaoshi asked, "The lung is a delicate Zang-organ. Could [it] control threat of all fire? [When] metal is broken, [there will be] no sound. [Such a result] cannot be avoided. How to avoid such a disaster?"

Qibo answered, "[It] still depends on water from the kidney to save. Thus the close relationship between the lung and the kidney is more important than that between earth and metal because earth can produce metal but metal cannot produce earth. [However,] the lung can promote the kidney and the kidney can also promote the lung. [Therefore] in the daytime and at night, Qi from the lung and the kidney communicates with each other and promotes each other."

Shaoshi asked, "[I have well understood the fact that] metal gets water to resolve fire under [your] guidance. [But] why does metal not fear fire sometimes?"

Qibo answered, "This is a discussion about its changes."

Shaoshi asked, "Please explain it."

Qibo answered, "Fire [that] burns metal is blazing fire. [If] fire-Qi is moderate, how [can it] burn [metal]? Metal not only fears fire, but also insults fire. [If] fire is difficult to control metal, [it indicates that] metal-Qi is increasingly effulgent. [If] the lung becomes obstinate, [it will be] too strong to be invaded. [In this case,] sough-Qi [is formidable and] certainly strikes wood. [When] striken by metal, the liver is difficult to produce fire. [As a result,] fire tends to decline and changes into cold fire. What else to fear then? If fire is too cold, there is no warm Qi to produce earth. [If this happens,] how can earth produce metal? [If] fire is cold for a

的攻击,就会连忙抵御木贼的强行横暴,又怎么能够顾及金之子的困难和穷境呢?肺金失去了化生之源,就会日益虚弱。肺金虚弱,想再往下继续生出肾水,就很难了。水如果没有金生,水就不能制火,更不要说上焦之火的焚烧了,但中焦的火也会随之更加炽热,而下焦的火也同样会随着水气而沸腾了。"

少师问:"为什么肺金会召火呢?"

岐伯说:"肺金是颇为娇嫩的脏器,而且位于各个脏腑之上。火性上炎,不发作就无所谓了,一旦发作所有的火就会随之相应。这就是肺金独自遭受到火的攻击和克制的主要原因。"

少师问:"肺为娇嫩的脏器,怎么还能够遏制各种火势的威逼呢?可见金破不鸣的情况,的确是绝对难以避免的了。但为什么还可以自免于火力的祸害呢?"

岐伯说:"这仍然需要依靠肾子之水予以挽救。这就是为什么肺肾两脏相互如此亲近,比土金之间的相亲相爱更加亲密亲近。因为土能生金,而金却难以生土。不同的是,肺能生肾,而肾也能生肺。白昼和黑夜之间,肺肾之气实际上一直彼此往来,两相贯通,所以互相都能受益。"

少师问:"金得到水的资助就能解火,我已经非常幸运地得到了指教。但金有时却不畏惧火,这又是为什么呢?"

岐伯说:"这是涉及其中的变化。"

少师说:"请予以详细说明吧。"

岐伯说:"火如果能烁金,此火就是烈火。如果火气自身衰微,又

long time, metal [will] also becomes cold. "

Shaoshi asked, "Good! Please explain why metal transforms water but water cannot produce wood. "

Qibo answered, "[If] water does not produce wood, how can metal produce wood? [The reason why] water does not produce wood [is that such a kind of] water is produced [by] fire melting metal. Genuine water produces wood. But water [produced by fire melting metal] can only restrict wood. "

Shaoshi said, "Good!"

Chen Shiduo's comment, "[If] the lung is dry, [it] cannot become obstinate metal; [if] the lung is too damp, [it] cannot become soft metal because there is fire in the lung. [When] the lung acquires fire, metal will be promoted; [when] the lung has lost fire, metal will be damaged. Thus there must be fire in metal and fire [in metal] must not be excessive. [If] water and fire are not vigorous, [it will be] beneficial to metal. Anyway metal itself should not be too vigorous. "

Notes

[1] Combination of the spleen and stomach with earth and connection of the lung with metal are related to coordination of the five elements [which are composed of wood, fire, earth, metal and water] with the five Zang-organs [which include the heart, liver, spleen, lung and kidney]. Traditionally the heart matches with fire, known as heart-fire; the liver matches with wood, known as liver-wood; the spleen matches with earth, known as spleen-earth;

怎么能够烁金呢？这种情况下，金不仅不畏惧火，而且还会欺侮火。火难以克制金，金气就会日益旺盛。肺就会变成顽金，由于过于刚硬就不会得到侵犯了，于是肺金的肃杀之气就必然会来克伐肝木。肝受到金的刑伐，就难以生火，火势就会因之而转衰，从而变为寒火，这又怎么可能令金畏惧呢？然而，如果火过于寒冷，就没有温暖之气以生土，这样土又怎么可能生金的呢？久而久之，由于火寒，金也随之而变寒了！"

少师说："好！请问金化为水，而水却不能生木，这又是为什么原因呢？"

岐伯说："水不能生木，金又怎么可能生木呢？水不能生木，是因为此水属于金被火克伐之后而融化的水。真水生木，而金受火克伐而融化的水，不但不会生木，反而会克木。"

少师说："好！"

陈士铎评论说："如果肺不干燥就不会成为顽金，如果肺过湿就不能成为柔金，因为肺中是有火的。肺得到了火，金就会受益，肺失去了火，金就会受损，所以金中不可以没有火，也不可以有太多的火。只有水火不旺的时候，金反而才能得到其适宜发展的条件。总而言之，不能使金气太过旺盛。"

the lung matches with metal, known as lung-metal; and the kidney matches with water, known as kidney-water.

[2] Thief here refers to pathogenic factors.

[3] The lung's mother family here refers to the spleen. According to the five elements, earth produces metal. That is to say earth is the mother of metal. When matching with the five elements, the lung belongs to metal and the spleen belongs to earth.

[4] Wood-thief here refers to the pathogenic factors related to the liver which matches with wood in the five elements.

[5] Metal's son here refers to the kidney which matches with water in the five elements.

肝木篇第二十五

【原文】

少师曰："肝属木，木非水不养，故肾为肝之母也。肾衰则木不旺矣，是肝木之虚，皆肾水之涸也。然而肝木之虚，不全责肾水之衰者何故？"

岐伯曰："此肝木自郁也。木喜疏泄，遇风寒之邪，拂抑之事，肝辄气郁不舒。肝郁必下克脾胃，制土有力，则木气自伤。势必求济肾水，水生木而郁气未解，反助克土之横。土怒水助转来克水。

肝不受肾之益，肾且得土之损，未有不受病者也。肾既病矣，自难滋肝木之枯，肝无水养，其郁更甚。郁甚而克土愈力。脾胃受伤气难转输，必求救于心火，心火因肝木之郁全不顾心，心失化源，何能生脾胃之土乎？

于是怜土予之受伤，不敢咎肝母之过逆，反嗔肺金不制肝木，乃出其火而克肺，肺无土气之生，复有心火之克则肺金难以自存。听肝木之逆，无能相制矣。"

少师曰："木无金制，宜木气之舒矣，何以仍郁也？"

岐伯曰："木性曲直，必得金制有成。今金弱木强，则肝寡于畏，任郁之性以自肆，土无可克，水无可养，火无可助，于是木空受焚矣，此木无金制而愈郁也。

【英译】

Chapter 25
Liver-Wood

Shaoshi asked, "The liver belongs to wood and wood cannot be cultivated [if there is] no water. Therefore the kidney is the mother of the liver. [When] the kidney is debilitated, wood becomes weakened. [When] liver-wood is weakened, water in the kidney is completely dry. However, deficiency of liver-wood is not only caused by decline of kidney-water. What is the reason?"

Qibo answered, "This is [due to] spontaneous depression of liver-wood. Wood likes free coursing. [When] meeting with evil wind and cold and encountering depression, the liver [will] suddenly become stagnated and uncomfortable. [When] the liver [becomes] stagnated, [it will] inevitably restrict the spleen and stomach below. [When] earth[1] is strongly controlled, wood-Qi[2] will be damaged spontaneously. [In this case, it] tends to get aid from kidney-water. [Although] water promotes wood, stagnated Qi is not resolved. Instead, [it has] promoted [wood] to restrict earth transversely. [As a result,] earth [-Qi becomes] furious and turns to restrict water [when] assisted by water.

[When] the liver fails to benefit from the kidney and the kidney is damaged by earth, disease is inevitable. [When] the kidney is in disorder, [it is] difficult to mosten liver-wood [that is] dry. [If] the liver has no water to nourish, its stagnation will be

所以治肝必解郁为先，郁解而肝气自平。何至克土？土无木克则脾胃之气自易升腾，自必忘克，肾水转生肺金矣。肺金得脾胃二土之气，则金气自旺，令行清肃。肾水无匮乏之忧，且金强制木，木无过旺肝气平矣。少师曰：肝气不平可以直折之乎？”

岐伯曰：“肝气最恶者郁也。其次则恶不平，不平之极即郁之极也。故平肝尤尚解郁。”

少师曰：“其故何也？”

岐伯曰：“肝气不平，肝中之火过旺也。肝火过旺，由肝木之塞也。外闭内焚，非烁土之气即耗心之血矣。夫火旺宜为心之所喜，然温火生心，烈火逼心，所以火盛之极，可暂用寒凉以泻。肝火郁之极，宜兼用舒泄以平肝也。”

少师曰：“善。”

陈士铎曰：“木不郁则不损，肝木之郁，即逆之之谓也。人能解郁，则木得其平矣。何郁之有？”

【今译】

少师说：“肝属木，木如果没有水就不能滋养，所以肾水是肝木之母，肾衰木就不会旺盛。所以肝木的虚衰，都是因为肾水干涸的缘故。但是，肝木的虚衰，又不能完全责怪肾水的衰竭，这是什么原因呢？”

岐伯说：“这是肝木自郁的原因。木喜欢疏泄，遇到风寒之邪及抑郁之事，肝木动辄就会气郁，因而感觉很不舒畅。如果肝木抑郁，就必

more serious. [If the liver is] more stagnated, earth will be more seriously restricted. [When] the spleen and stomach are damaged, Qi is difficult to transfer and [it is quite] necessary to get help from fire-Qi. [When] heart-fire [is affected by] stagnation of liver-wood, [it is] unable to promote the heart. [When] the heart has lost [its] source of transformation, how can [it] produce earth for the spleen and stomach?

Thus [it is] pitiful [that] earth is damaged, [but] the liver, [as] the mother [of fire], should not be blamed for reverse [activity]. On the contrary, lung-metal should be blamed for failing to control liver-wood. [For this reason,] fire should be stimulated to restrict the lung. [When] there is no production of earth-Qi in the lung but there is heart-fire to restrict, lung-metal is difficult to exist. [Under such a condition, it] has to allow reverse [activity of] liver-wood and is unable to control [it]."

Shaoshi asked, "[If] wood is not controlled by metal, wood-Qi will be diastolic. [But] why [it is] still stagnated?"

Qibo answered, "Wood tends to bend in nature. [Only when] cut by metal [can wood be] made into utensil. Now metal is weak and wood is strong. [But] the liver is powerless and depression is more serious. [In this case,] earth is unable to restrict [anything], water is unable to nourish [anything] nor to resist [anything]. [As a result,] wood [-Qi] is empty and is burnt [by fire]. This [is the reason why] wood is not restricted by metal but is stagnated more seriously.

So to treat the liver, stagnation should be resolved first. [Only when] stagnation is resolved [can] liver-Qi is harmonized

然会向下克制脾胃。如果脾土被有力地克制了,木气就会自行受伤,势必要向肾水求助。虽然水生木,但木的郁气却并没有被解除,反而资助木气横克脾土。土气会因此而怒发,得到水的资助后就转而克制水了。

肝如果不能接受肾所给予的益处,肾水反而会受到脾土的损害,在这种情况下肾水没有不引发疾病的。肾既然有病了,肾水自然就难以滋养干枯了的肝木,如果肝没有得到水的滋养,抑郁就更加严重了。抑郁严重了,其克制脾土之力就会更加强大。脾胃受伤之后,其气就难以转输,就必然要求救心火的资助,因为肝木的抑郁,心火已经完全不能顾及心了,心火失去其化生之源,又怎么能资助脾胃之土的生发呢?

于是,怜惜的脾土之子就要遭受伤害,又不敢归咎于肝母过于逆克的失职,反而要嗔怒肺金不能克制肝木,于是就激发其火去克制肺金,肺由于没有土气的生发,又再次遭受心火的克制,肺金就难以自存了,只能听任肝木的上逆,根本没有办法去克制了。”

少师问:“如果木没有金的克制,木气就应当舒张了,但为什么仍然郁闭呢?”

岐伯说:“木性曲直,只有得到金的克制才能成形。如今金虚弱而木强盛,肝木独自强盛而不畏惧任何东西,其郁闭之性就会更加放肆。土不能克制,水不能滋养,火没有资助,于是虚空的木气就遭受了火的焚烧,这就是木没有金的克制但却更加郁闭的缘故。所以治疗肝病,必然以解郁为先,只有将抑郁解除了,肝气才会自然平和,又何至于仅仅克制脾土呢? 土如果没有木的克制,那么脾胃之气就会很自然地容易升腾,自然就会忘记克制,肾水因此便转而生发肺金。肺金得到脾胃二

spontaneously. Why [is it] only necessary to restrict earth? [If] earth is not restricted by wood, Qi in the spleen and stomach will spontaneously leap up and certainly forget to restrict [kidney-water]. Kidney-water then transfers to promote lung-metal. [When] lung-metal has received Qi from spleen-earth and stomach-earth, metal-Qi will spontaneously become vigorous and begin to clarify and depurate. [In this case,] kidney-water will have no problem of shortage. Moreover, metal [becomes] strong and controls wood. [Since] wood is not quite vigorous, liver-Qi is harmonized."

Shaoshi asked, "[If] liver-Qi is not harmonized, can [it] be directly pacified?"

Qibo answered, "Liver-Qi mostly dislikes stagnation and also hates disharmony. Extreme disharmony means extreme stagnation. Thus to harmonize the liver is [the right way] to resolve stagnation."

Shaoshi asked, "What is the reason?"

Qibo answered, "Disharmony of liver-Qi [means that] fire in the liver is blazing. [If] fire in the liver is blazing, liver-wood will be obstructed. External blockage and internal burning indicate [that] Qi in earth is burnt or blood in the heart is consumed. Blazing fire [originally] is [what] the heart likes. However, moderate fire promotes the heart and blazing fire threatens the heart. So [if] fire increasingly blazes, [it] can temporarily be purged [with medicinals] cold and cool [in property]. [If] fire in the liver is extremely stagnated, [it is] appropriate to harmonize the liver by relaxation and purgation."

土之气,金气自然就会旺盛,并受令而行施清肃之职,这样肾水就没有匮乏之忧了,并且金强壮而克制木气,这样木气就不会过于旺盛,肝气就会因此而平和了。"

少师问:"如果肝气不平和,可以直接予以平折吗?"

岐伯说:"肝气最厌恶的是抑郁,其次厌恶的是不平。不平的极点,就是抑郁的极点,所以平肝就是解郁之法。"

少师说:"其原因是什么呢?"

岐伯说:"如果肝气不平,肝中的火气就会过于旺盛。肝火过于旺盛,则是由于肝木闭塞所致。如果外部郁闭了,里边就会遭遇焚烧,如果这不是烁烧脾胃之土,就是耗散心中之血。火旺盛本来应该是心所喜欢的,但是只有温火才能生心,而烈火则只能逼心。所以如果火盛到了极点,可以暂用寒凉的药物予以泻之。如果肝火郁闭到了极点,就应该采用舒散和泄泻的治疗方法予以处理,从而使肝木之气得以平和。"

少师说:"好!"

陈士铎评论说:"木不抑郁就不会造成损毁。肝木的抑郁,就是木气逆行的意思。如果人能解除抑郁,肝就会平和了。能做到这一点,还会有什么抑郁呢?"

Shaoshi said, "Good!"

Chen Shiduo's comment, "No stagnation of wood, no damage [of earth]. Thus stagnation of liver-wood actually means reverse [circulation of Qi in wood]. [When] stagnation is resolved, wood will be pacified. What stagnation will there be?"

Notes

[1] Earth in this chapter refers to the spleen and stomach.

[2] Wood-Qi here refers to liver-Qi.

[3] Liver-mother means that the liver is the mother of the heart. According to traditional Chinese medicine, the liver belongs to wood and the heart belongs to fire. Since wood produces fire, wood is likened to mother of fire.

肾水篇第二十六

少师曰："请问肾水之义。"

岐伯曰："肾属水,先天真水也。水生于金,故肺金为肾母。然而肺不能竟生肾水也,必得脾土之气薰蒸,肺始有生化之源。"

少师曰："土克水者也,何以生水?"

岐伯曰："土贪生金,全忘克水矣。"

少师曰："金生水而水养于金,何也?"

岐伯曰："肾水非肺金不生,肺金非肾水不润。盖肺居上焦,诸脏腑之火,咸来相逼,苟非肾水灌注,则肺金立化矣。所以二经子母最为关切。无时不交相生,亦无时不交相养也。是以补肾者必须益肺,补肺者必须润肾,始既济而成功也。"

少师曰："肾得肺之生即得肺之损,又何以养各脏腑乎?"

岐伯曰："肾交肺而肺益生肾,则肾有生化之源。山下出泉涓涓,正不竭也。肾既优渥,乃分其水以生肝。肝木之中本自藏火,有水则木且生心,无水则火且焚木,木得水之济,则木能自养矣。木养于水,木有和平之气,自不克土。而脾胃得遂其升发之性,则心火何至躁动乎? 自然水不畏火之炎,乃上润而济心矣。"

少师曰："水润心固是水火之既济,但恐火炎而水不来济也。"

岐伯曰："水不润心,故木无水养也。木无水养肝必干燥,火发木

Volume 3

【英译】

Chapter 26
Kidney-Water

Shaoshi asked, "Please explain the meaning of kidney-water."

Qibo answered, "The kidney belongs to water [which is] innate genuine water. Water produces metal. That is why lung-metal is the mother of the kidney. However, the lung cannot produce kidney-water alone and must depend on fumigation and steaming of Qi from earth. [Only in this way can] the lung have the source of production and transformation."

Shaoshi asked, "Earth restricts water. [But] why [can it] produce water?"

Qibo answered, "[Because] earth just wants to produce metal and forgets to restrict water."

Shaoshi asked, "Why does metal produce water and water nourish metal?"

Qibo answered, "Without lung-metal, kidney-water cannot be produced; without kidney-water, lung-metal cannot be moistened. Because the lung is located above the upper energizer, fire from each Zang-organ and Fu-organ all threatens [it]. If there is no kidney-water to pour [into it], lung-metal will be immediately dissolved. So the mother-child [relationship between these] two meridians[1] is the closest, [which is characterized by] constant

焚,烁尽脾胃之液,肺金救土之不能,何暇生肾中之水。水涸而肝益加燥,肾无沥以养肝,安得余波以灌心乎!肝木愈横,心火愈炎,肾水畏焚,因不上济于心,此肾衰之故,非所谓肾旺之时也。"

少师曰:"肾衰不能济心,独心受其损乎?"

岐伯曰:"心无水养,则心君不安,乃迁其怒于肺金,遂移其火以逼肺矣。肺金最畏火炎,随移其热于肾,而肾因水竭,水中之火正无所依,得心火之相会,翕然升木,变出龙雷,由下焦而腾中焦,由中焦而腾上焦,有不可止遏之机矣。是五脏七腑均受其害,宁独心受损乎!"

少师曰:"何火祸之酷乎?"

岐伯曰:"非火多为害,乃水少为炎也。五脏有脏火,七腑有腑火,火到之所,同气相亲,故其势易旺,所异者,水以济之也。而水止肾脏之独有,且水中又有火也。水之不足,安敌火之有余。此肾脏所以有补无泻也。"

少师曰:"各脏腑皆取资于水,宜爱水而畏火矣。何以多助火以增焰乎?"

岐伯曰:"水少火多,一见火发,惟恐火之耗水,竟来顾水,谁知反害水乎? 此祸生于爱,非恶水而爱火也。"

少师曰:"火多水少,泻南方之火,非即补北方之水乎?"

岐伯曰:"水火又相根也。无水则火烈,无火则水寒,火烈则阴亏也,水寒则阳消也。阴阳两平,必水火既济矣。"

少师曰:"火水既济独不畏土之侵犯乎?"

岐伯曰:"土能克水,而土亦能生水也。水得土以相生,则土中出

mutual communication and constant mutual cultivation. Thus to tonify the kidney is certainly beneficial to the lung and to tonify the lung is surely to moisten the kidney. [Only in such a way can] the function of mutual assistance and mutual achievement be performed."

Shaoshi asked, "The kidney is promoted by the lung, but also damaged by the lung. How [can it] nourish all the Zang-organs and Fu-organs?"

Qibo answered, "[When] the kidney communicates with the lung, the lung can produce kidney [-water] and the kidney will have the source of production and transformation. [It is just like] water that trickles constantly and inexhaustibly from the spring below the mountain. Since kidney [-water] is abundant, [it will] separate some water to promote the liver. [In] liver-wood, fire is originally stored. [When] there is water [to nourish], wood will produce heart [-fire]; [when] there is no water [to nourish], fire will burn wood; [when] wood is nourished by water, wood will nourish itself. [Only when] wood is nourished by water [can] it bear Qi of peace and will not restrict earth. [Under such a condition,] the spleen and stomach will naturally ascend. How can heart-fire move restlessly? Naturally water will not fear flaming fire and move upwards to moisten and nourish the heart."

Shaoshi asked, "[Kidney-] water moistens heart [fire]. [This is] certainly mutual promotion between water and fire. However, mutual promotion may fail if fire flames up?"

Qibo answered, "[If kidney-] water does not moisten the

水,始足以养肝木而润各脏腑也。第不宜过于生之,则水势汪洋亦能冲决堤岸,水无土制,变成洪水之逆流,故水不畏土之克也。"

少师曰:"善。"

陈士铎曰:"五行得水则润,失水则损。况取资多而分散少乎。故水为五行之所窃,不可不多也。说得水之有益,有此刻悟水矣。"

【今译】

少师问道:"请问肾水是什么意思?"

岐伯说:"肾属水,是先天的真水。水由金所生,所以肺金是肾水之母。然而,肺却不能独自地生出肾水,还必须得到脾土之气的薰蒸,这样肺才能有生化之源。"

少师问:"土是克水的,为什么还能生水呢?"

岐伯说:"土热衷于生金,全然忘了对水的克制。"

少师问:"金是生水的,但为什么水反而能滋养金呢?"

岐伯说:"肾水如果没有肺金就不能生发,肺金如果没有了肾水不能滋润。因为肺居于上焦,各脏腑之火都想对其加以逼迫,如果不是肾水的灌注,肺金顷刻之间就会被火熔化了。所以,肺与肾这两经的子母关系最为密切,无时无刻不互相交合和相互滋生,同时也无时无刻不互相滋养。所以补肾时就必须要补益肺,补肺时也必须要滋润肾,这样才能实现相互既济、相互而成的目标。"

少师问:"肾得到肺的资助才能生发,既然受到了肺的损害,又怎

heart, wood will certainly have no water to nourish. [If] wood has no water to nourish, the liver will become dry. [When] fire flames up and wood is burnt, fluid in the spleen and stomach will be boiled away. [If] lung-metal is unable to save earth, how can [it] produce water for the kidney? [When] water dries up, the liver will increasingly become dry. [If] the kidney has no water to nourish the liver, how can [it] have extra water to irrigate the heart? [As a result,] liver-wood [acts] more transversely[2] and heart-fire flames more seriously. Kidney-water fears to be burnt and therefore does not flow up to nourish the heart. This is the cause of kidney debilitation, not the time [when] the kidney becomes vigorously."

Shaoshi asked, "Debilitated kidney cannot nourish heart [-fire]. Does it only damage heart [-fire]?"

Qibo answered, "[If] the heart has no water to nourish, the heart monarch [feels] unease, blaming lung-metal and transferring heart-fire to threaten lung [-metal]. [In fact,] lung-metal mostly fears flaming fire and transports heat [-Qi in heart-fire] to the kidney, consequently leading to exhaustion of water in the kidney. [In this case,] fire [-Qi] in [kidney-] water has nothing to depend on. [When] meeting with heart-fire, [fire-Qi] immediately rises up to [liver-] wood and changes into Loong[3] thunder, soaring from the lower energizer to the middle energizer, from the middle energizer to the upper energizer, continuously and uncreasingly. [Actually] the five Zang-organs and seven Fu-organs are all damaged by [fire-Qi], not only the heart is damaged."

Shaoshi asked, "Why is damage [caused by] fire so serious?"

么能够滋养各个脏腑呢?"

岐伯说:"肾与肺相交,肺就会因此而受益,因此就有利于生肾,这样肾就有了生化之源,正如山下泉水涓涓而流,正好取之不尽,用之不竭。肾中之水既然充盈了,于是就会分水来生肝。肝木之中本来就自行藏火,一旦有了水,木就会生心。如果没有水的滋生,火就会焚烧肝木。木一旦得到水的资助,就能自行养育了。木得到水的养育,木就有了和平之气,自然就不会克制土了,脾胃因此就能发挥好其升发之性了,这样心火又怎么会躁动呢? 水自然就不会不畏惧火的上炎,于是便向上滋润并对心加以济助。"

少师说:"水润心,这固然是水火之间的相互既济,但是恐怕火上炎后水就不能相互既济了。"

岐伯说:"如果水不润心,木就失去了水的滋养。如果木失去了水的滋养,肝就必然会干燥,从而导致火生发而木焚烧,同时也烁尽了脾胃中的津液,这样肺金就无力救援土了,哪有可能资助肾中之水的生发呢? 水干涸后肝就日益干燥,肾也没有多少水去滋养肝了,又怎么可能有多余的水去灌心呢? 其结果是肝木更加横逆,心火更加上炎,肾水畏惧焚烧,所以就不能向上既济于心了,这就是造成肾衰的主要原因,不是所谓的肾旺时节所导致的。"

少师问:"肾衰不能济心,是否只有心才会遭受损害吗?"

岐伯说:"心没有水的滋养,心君不能安宁,因此就会迁怒于肺金,于是便转移其火以逼迫肺金。实际上肺金最畏惧烈火,于是便将其热气转移到肾脏,肾水便因此而枯竭。此时的水中之火正好无所依靠,一

Qibo answered, "[This] damage is not caused by fire, actually caused by shortage of water [that leads to] blazing [of fire]. [In] the five Zang-organs, [there is] Zang-organ fire; [in] the seven Fu-organs, [there is] Fu-organ fire. [No matter where] fire reaches, [it will] meet closely with Qi. That is why it tends to blaze. The difference is [that] water can support [fire]. [Among the Zang-organs and Fu-organs,] only in the kidney there is water and in the water there is fire. [If] water is insufficient, how can [it] resist excessive fire? That is why the kidney only needs tonification, not purgation."

Shaoshi asked, "Every Zang-organ and Fu-organ gets [necessary nutrient] from water and certainly loves water and fears fire. [But] why most [Zang-organs and Fu-organs] assist fire to increase [its] flaming?"

Qibo answered, "[In the body] there is less water and more fire. When seeing fire, there is fear [that it might] consume water [and measures will be taken] immediately to defend water. Who knows [that this actually] damages water? This is harm caused by love, not aversion to water and love of fire."

Shaoshi asked, "[If there is] more fire and less water, is purgation of fire in the south not supplementation of water in the north?"

Qibo answered, "Water and fire are the roots of each other. [If] there is no water, fire will blaze; [if] there is no fire, water will be cold. [When] fire is blazing, Yin will be deficient; [when] water is cold, Yang [Qi] will disperse. [Only when] Yin and Yang

旦得到心火的交会,肝木就会勃然升发,变化得像龙雷一样,由下焦而升腾到中焦,由中焦而升腾到上焦,其升腾之势几乎不可遏止。所以五脏七腑均遭受其危害,怎么可能只有心才会遭受损害的呢?"

少师问:"为什么火的危害如此严酷呢?"

岐伯说:"这并不是火多而造成的危害,而是由于水少而导致火不断炎上。五脏有脏火,七腑有腑火,火到之处,同气相亲,因此火势就容易旺盛。所不同的是,水可以与火相济。但只有肾中才独自有水,而且水中又有火。水的不足,又怎么敌过火之有余呢? 这就是肾脏有补无泻的缘故。"

少师问:"各脏腑都取资于水,应当爱水而畏火,但为什么多数情况下会助长火势以增强其焰力呢?"

岐伯说:"如果人体水少火多,一旦火开始生发,惟恐水就会遭遇消耗。在这种情况下,如果一味地顾水,谁会知道这样反而会损害水呢? 这一祸害源自于彼此之间的恩爱,并非因为恶水而爱火的缘故。"

少师问:"火多水少,泻去南方的火,难道不正好补了北方的水吗?"

岐伯说:"水火相互为根。如果没有水,火势就会猛烈;如果没有火,水就会变寒。如果火势猛烈,就会导致阴的亏损;如果水变寒了,就会导致阳的消散。只有阴阳相互平衡,才必然会实现水火的既济。"

少师问:"火水既济,惟独不畏惧土的侵犯吗?"

岐伯说:"土能克水,但土也能生水。水得到土而相生,土中就能生出水来,才能开始滋养肝木,并滋润各个脏腑。但生水也不宜太过,

are balanced can water and fire promote each other. "

Shaoshi asked, "Fire and water promote each other. [What about] invasion of earth? No one fears [about it]?"

Qibo answered, "Earth can restrict water and produce water. Water depends on earth to exist. [When] earth has produced water, liver-wood will be nourished, every Zang-organ and Fu-organ will be moistened. However, [it is] inappropriate to produce too much [water]. [If too much water is produced, it] floods tempestuously and bursts the bank. Without the control of earth, water becomes flood and adverse current. That is why water does not fear the restriction of earth. "

Shaoshi said, "Good!"

Chen Shiduo's comment, "[When] getting water, the five elements will be moistened; [when] losing water, [the five elements will be] damaged, let alone more acquirement and less dispersion. Thus water is what the five elements [try] to steal. [For this reason, water] must be acquired more. [This chapter] discusses the benefit of water, [enabling people] to understand [the significance of] water."

Notes

[1] These two meridians refer to the lung meridian and the kidney meridian.

[2] The word "transversely" here means reverse activity.

[3] Loong (龙) is the legendary ancestor of the Chinese nation.

生水太过就会导致水势汪洋,从而导致凶猛之水冲决堤岸。在这种情况下水就无法得到土的克制,最终变成逆流的洪水,水也就因此而不畏惧土的克制了。"

少师说:"好!"

陈士铎评论说:"五行得到水会就能滋润,失去水就会遭受损害。更何况获取多而分散少呢?所以水为五行所窃取,不可不多得一些。所论述的得水之益处颇有意义,据此就可以领悟到水的重要性了。"

Volume 3

Now in the whole world，the Chinese Loong（龙）is wrongly translated as "dragon". Every Westerner knows that "dragon" in the West is a monster，absolutely not equilent to Loong（龙）.

心火篇第二十七

【原文】

少师曰："心火，君火也。何故宜静不宜动？"

岐伯曰："君主无为，心为君火，安可有为乎！君主有为，非生民之福也。所以心静则火息，心动则火炎。息则脾胃之土受其益，炎则脾胃之土受其灾。"

少师曰："何谓也？"

岐伯曰："脾胃之土喜温火之养，恶烈火之逼也。温火养则土有生气而成活土，烈火逼则土有死气而成焦土矣。焦火何以生金，肺金干燥，必求济于肾水，而水不足以济之也。"

少师曰："肾水本济心火者也，何以救之无裨乎？"

岐伯曰："人身之肾水原非有余。况见心火之太旺，虽济火甚切，独不畏火气之烁乎？故避火之炎，不敢上升于心中也。心无水济则心火更烈，其克肺益甚。肺畏火刑，必求援于肾子，而肾子欲救援而无水，又不忍肺母之凌烁，不得不出其肾中所有，倾国以相助。于是水火两腾，升于上焦，而与心相战。心因无水以克肺，今见水不济心火来助肺，欲取其水而转与火，相合则火势更旺。于是肺不受肾水之益，反得肾火之虐矣。斯时肝经之木见肺金太弱，亦出火以焚心，明助肾母以称，于实报肺仇而加刃也。"

Volume 3

【英译】

Chapter 27
Heart-Fire

Shaoshi asked, "Heart-fire [is] monarch-fire. Why [is it] appropriate to be calm, not to be active?"

Qibo answered, "The monarch does nothing [for interference]. The heart is monarch-fire, how can [it] do anything [against nature]? [If] the monarch does something, [it is] not to bring benefits to the people. Thus [only when] the heart is calm, fire [can] be quenched. [If] the heart is startled, fire [will] flame up. [When fire is] quenched, earth[1] in the spleen and stomach [will be] invigorated; [when fire] flames up, earth in the spleen and stomach [will be] damaged."

Shaoshi asked, "What is the reason?"

Qibo answered, "Earth in the spleen and stomach likes to be nourished by moderate fire and dislikes to be threatened by blazing fire. [When] nourished by moderate fire, there is vital Qi in earth and earth is active. [When] threatened by blazing fire, there is dead Qi in earth and earth is scorched. How can scorched earth produce metal? [When] lung-metal is dry, [it] certainly needs help from kidney-water. But [kidney-] water is insufficient and unable to help it."

Shaoshi asked, "Kidney-water originally helps heart-fire. [But]

少师曰："何以解氛乎?"

岐伯曰："心火动极矣,安其心而火可息也。"

少师曰："可用寒凉直折其火乎?"

岐伯曰："寒凉可暂用,不可久用也。暂用则火化为水,久用则水变为火也。"

少师曰："斯又何故欤?"

岐伯曰："心火必得肾水以济之也。滋肾安心则心火永静,舍肾安心则心火仍动矣。"

少师曰："凡水火未有不相克也,而心肾水火何相交而相济乎?"

岐伯曰："水不同耳。肾中邪水最克心火,肾中真水最养心火,心中之液即肾内真水也。肾之真水旺,而心火安。肾之真水衰,而心火沸。是以心肾交而水火既济,心肾开而水火未济也。"

少师曰："心在上,肾在下,地位悬殊,何彼此乐交无间乎?"

岐伯曰："心肾之交,虽胞胎导之,实肝木介之也。肝木气通,肾无阻隔,肝木气郁,心肾即闭塞也。"

少师曰："然则肝木又何以养之?"

岐伯曰："肾水为肝木之母,补肾即所以通肝。木非水不旺,火非木不生,欲心液之不枯,必肝血之常足。欲肝血之不乏,必肾水之常盈,补肝木,要不外补肾水也。"

少师曰："善。"

陈士铎曰："心火者,君火也。君心为有形之火,可以水折。不若

why can [it] not help?"

Qibo answered, "Originally kidney-water in the human body is not sufficient, let alone excessive blazing of heart-fire. Although [it is] quite urgent to help [heart-] fire, [it is also] quite fearful of fire-Qi [that is] blazing. Thus [it tries] to avoid flaming fire and dares not to rise up to the heart. Without help of water, heart-fire [will become] more blazing and restrict the lung more seriously. The lung fears restriction of fire and certainly tries to get help from its son kidney[2]. [As] the son [of the lung], the kidney certainly desires to save [the lung], but there is no water [in the kidney]. Nevertheless, [it] cannot bear [that] mother lung is burnt [by fire] and has to take all [water] from the kidney, just like [to make use of] the whole country to help [it]. As a result, [both] water and fire rise up to the upper energizer to fight with the heart. [Since] the heart has no water to restrict the lung,[kidney-] water fails to enable heart-fire to assist the lung. In order to get water, [it] transfers to combine with fire. Combination [with fire makes] fire blaze more seriously. As a result, the lung not only fails to get benefit from kidney-water, but also is damaged by kidney-fire. At that time, wood in the liver meridian finds [that] lung-metal is too weak and wants to produce fire to burn the heart. [Superficially, such an activity seems] to help mother kidney, [In fact it is] to avenge lung-metal with a knife."

Shaoshi asked, "How to resolve such a crisis?"

Qibo answered, "Heart-fire [now is] active to the extreme. [Only when] the heart is calm [can heart-] fire be pacified."

肾中之火，为无形之火也。无形之火，可以水养。知火之有形、无形，而虚火、实火可明矣。"

【今译】

少师问："所谓心火，就是君火，为什么心火宜静而不宜动呢？"

岐伯说："君主无为，心为君火，怎么能有所为呢？君主有为，并不是万民的幸福。所以，只有心安静了，火才能安息了，如果心躁动，火就会上炎。如果火安息了，脾胃之土能受益匪浅；如果火上炎了，脾胃之土遭受火的灭顶之灾。"

少师问："这是什么道理呢？"

岐伯说："脾胃之土喜欢获得温火的养育，厌恶烈火的威逼。获得温火的养育，土就有生气，从而成为活土；遭遇烈火的威逼，土就会成为死气，从而变成焦土。焦土怎么能生金呢？肺金干燥了，必然要求助于肾水的滋养，然而肾水由于不足，就无法既济肺金。"

少师问："肾水本来是既济心火的，为什么救济而没有获益呢？"

岐伯说："人身的肾水，原本就没有多余。何况由于心火太旺，虽然济火甚为紧迫，难道就不怕火气的灼烧吗？所以要避免火的上炎，不敢让其上升到心中。如果心火没有得到水的既济，就会变得更加猛烈，对肺金的克制就会更加严厉。肺本来就畏惧火的刑伐，必然要向肾子求助。尽管肾子想要救助，但却因为没有水，又不忍心看到肺母遭受凌烁，就不得不拿出肾中所有的水予以倾国式的相助。结果就导致了水与火的同时升腾，当升腾到上焦的时候，就开始与心相搏斗。心因为没

Volume 3

Shaoshi asked, "Can fire be broken by cold and chill?"

Qibo answered, "Cold and chill can be used temporarily, but not for a long time. Temporary use will transform fire into water [while] long-term use will transform water into fire."

Shaoshi asked, "What is the reason?"

Qibo answered, "Heart-fire can only be helped by kidney-water. [Only when] the kidney is nourished and the heart is pacified, heart-fire can be calmed forever. [However,] to neglect the kidney and only to pacify the heart will make heart-fire move [wantonly]."

Shaoshi asked, "Water and fire never stop restricting each other. [But] why do water and fire in the kidney and heart help each other instead of interacting with each other?"

Qibo answered, "[Because] water [in it] is different. [In] the kidney, evil water is especially able to restrict heart-fire and genuine water in the kidney is especially able to nourish heart-fire. Fluid in the heart is the genuine water from the kidney. [When] genuine water in the kidney is rich, heart-fire is calm; [when] genuine water in the kidney declines, heart-fire is burning. Therefore mutual communication between the heart and the kidney [enables] water and fire to help each other, separation of the heart and kidney [prevents] water and fire from helping each other."

Shaoshi asked, "The heart [is located] in the upper and the kidney [is located] in the lower, [their] positions are different. [But] why [can they] communicate with each other without any intervals?"

有得到水去克制肺,如看到水不能济助于心,火就来资助肺,想要取得水,然后转而与火相合,火势因此而变得更加旺盛。于是,肺就无法得到肾水的益处,反而遭受肾火的虐待。此时,肝经之木看到肺金太弱,也生出火来焚烧心,表面上似乎是资助肾母一起战斗,其实是报复肺金之仇而对其加以刑罚。"

少师问:"如何解除危机状况呢?"

岐伯说:"心火动到了极点的时候,只要心安静了,火就能安息。"

少师问:"是否可用寒凉法斩断火势呢?"

岐伯说:"寒凉可以暂时使用,但不可长期使用。暂时使用,火就会化而为水;长期使用,水就会变而为火了。"

少师问:"这又是什么原因呢?"

岐伯说:"心火必须得到肾水才能相济。如果滋养肾而安静心,心火就会永远安静;如果舍弃肾而安静心,心火就会依然妄动不止。"

少师问:"凡是水火没有不相克的,然而心肾中的水火为什么相交而又相济呢?"

岐伯说:"水是不同的。肾中的邪水,最易于克制心火;肾中的真水,最善于滋养心火。心中的液体,就是肾内的真水。肾中的真水旺盛,心火就因此而安息;肾中的真水衰弱,心火就会转而沸腾。所以心肾相交,水火就能既济;心肾相离,水火就无法既济。"

少师问:"心在上,肾在下,地位悬殊,为什么彼此相交而无间呢?"

岐伯说:"心肾相交,虽然有胞胎的导引,但更重要的是肝木的介入。肝木的气通了,肾就没有任何阻隔了;肝木的气郁了,心肾就会因

Volume 3

Qibo answered, "[In terms of] communication between the heart and kidney, the uterus is the guidance while liver-wood is the media. [When] Qi in liver-wood is uninhibited, the kidney is unobstructed; [when] Qi in liver-wood is stagnated, the heart and kidney are obstructed."

Shaoshi asked, "But how can liver-wood be nourished?"

Qibo answered, "Kidney-water is the mother of liver-wood [and therefore] to tonify the kidney is to unobstruct liver-wood. Without water, fire cannot be effulgent; without wood, [fire] cannot be produced. To avoid dryness of heart fluid, liver blood must be sufficient. To keep liver blood enough, kidney-water must be always sufficient. [Thus the key point for] tonifying liver-wood is to tonify kidney-water."

Shaoshi said, "Excellent [explanation]!"

Chen Shiduo's comment, "Heart-fire is monarch-fire. Monarch heart is visible fire and can be broken by water. [It is] unlike fire in the kidney [which] is invisible fire. Invisible fire can be nourished by water. [If one] knows visible fire and invisible fire, [he or she will certainly be] clear about deficiency-fire and excess-fire."

Notes

[1] Earth in this chapter mainly refers to the nature of the spleen and stomach which belong to earth when matching with the five elements.

[2] When matching with the five elements, the lung belongs to

此而闭塞了。"

少师问："但肝木又依靠什么来滋养呢？"

岐伯说："肾水为肝木之母，所以补肾就可以通肝。没有了水，木不能旺盛；没有了木，火不能生发。要想心液不枯，肝血就必须要经常充足；要想肝血不乏，肾水就必须要经常充盈。所以补肝木的要点，就是对肾水的补充。"

少师曰："好！"

陈士铎评论说："心火是君火。心君是有形之火，可以用水折伐。不像肾中之火，为无形之火。无形之火，可以用水滋养。知道火的有形和无形，就可以明白什么是虚火，什么是实火了。"

metal and the kidney belongs to water. According to the principle of the five elements, metal produces water and therefore water is the son of metal. That is why the kidney is taken as the son of the lung.

卷四

脾土篇第二十八

【原文】

少师问曰："脾为湿土，土生于火，是火为脾土之父母乎？"

岐伯曰："脾土之父母，不止一火也。心经之君火，包络、三焦、命门之相火皆生之。然而君火之生，脾土甚疏；相火之生，脾土甚切，而相火之中命门之火，尤为最亲。"

少师曰："其故何欤？"

岐伯曰："命门盛衰，即脾土盛衰。命门生绝即脾土生绝也。盖命门为脾土之父母，实关死生。非若他火之可旺、可微、可有、可无也。"

少师曰："命门火过旺，多非脾土之宜，又何故乎？"

岐伯曰："火少则土湿，无发生之机；火多则土干，有燥裂之害。盖脾为湿土，土中有水。命门者，水中之火也。火藏水中，则火为既济之火，自无亢焚之祸，与脾土相宜，故火盛亦盛，火衰亦衰，火生则生，火绝则绝也。若火过于旺，是火胜于水矣。水不足以济火，乃未济之火也。火似旺而实衰，假旺而非真旺也。与脾土不相宜耳。非惟不能生脾，转能耗土之生气，脾土无生气，则赤地干枯，欲化精微以润各脏腑难矣。且火气上炎，与三焦、包络之火直冲而上，与心火相合。火愈旺而土愈耗，不成为焦土得乎？"

Volume 4

【英译】

Chapter 28
Spleen-Earth

Shaoshi asked, "The spleen is damp earth and earth is produced by fire. Is fire the parent of spleen-earth?"

Qibo answered, "The parent of spleen-earth is not just one kind of fire. Monarch-fire in the heart meridian and ministerial fire in the uterus, triple energizer and the life gate[1] all produce [earth]. However, [it is] difficult for monarch-fire to produce spleen-earth, [but it is] easy for ministerial fire to produce [spleen-earth]. And [among all kinds of] ministerial fire, fire from the life gate is the closest [one in producing spleen-earth]."

Shaoshi asked, "What is the reason?"

Qibo answered, "The prosperity and debilitation of the life gate are also the prosperity and debilitation of spleen-earth. [So] the existence and annihilation of the life gate also [demonstrate] the existence and annihilation of spleen-earth because the life gate is the parent of spleen-earth, quite related to life and death. [Thus it is] not like other [kinds of] fire [that can be] effulgent or moderate and exist or disappear."

Shaoshi asked, "Why is fire in the life gate too effulgent and inappropriate to spleen-earth?"

Qibo answered, "[If] fire is too little, earth will be damp and

少师曰："焦土能生肺金乎？"

岐伯曰："肺金非土不生。今土成焦土，中鲜润泽之气，何以生金哉？且不特不生金也，更且嫁祸于肺矣，盖肺乏土气之生，又多火气之逼，金弱木强，必至之势也。木强凌土而土败更难生金，肺金绝而肾水亦绝也，水绝则木无以养，木枯自焚，益添火焰，土愈加燥矣。"

少师曰："治何经以救之？"

岐伯曰："火之有余水之不足也，补水则火自息。然而徒补水则水不易生，补肺金火气，则水有化源，不患乎无本也。肾得水以制火，则水火相济，火无偏旺之害。此治法之必先补水也。"

少师曰："善。"

陈士铎曰："脾土与胃土不同。生脾土与生胃土不同，虽生土在于火也，然火各异。生脾土必须于心，生胃土必须于心包。心为君火，包络为相火也。二火断须补肾，以水能生火耳。"

【今译】

少师问道："脾为湿土，土生于火，火是脾土之父母吗？"

岐伯说："脾土之父母，不仅仅是一种火。心经的君火，包络、三焦、命门的相火，都能生脾土。但君火生脾土则比较疏远，相火生脾土则比较切近。在相火之中，命门之火尤其亲近。"

少师问："其原因是什么呢？"

岐伯说："命门旺盛了或衰微了，脾土也随之旺盛火衰微；命门生

cannot be produced [by fire]; [if] fire is too much, earth will be dry and broken. Because the spleen is damp earth and there is water in earth. The life gate is fire in water. [When] fire stays in water, it is helpful [to earth] and will certainly not burn [earth]. [Under such a condition,] there is co-adaptation between [fire] and spleen-earth. That is why [when] fire is effulgent, [earth is] also effulgent; [when] fire is debilitated, [earth is] also debilitated; [when] fire is exhausted, [earth is] also exhausted. [But] if fire is too effulgent, it will outstrip water. [As a result,] water is insufficient [and unable] to nourish fire and therefore [fire becomes] unhelpful fire. [In this case,] fire appears effulgent but actually debilitated, [that is] falsely effulgent and not truly effulgent, inappropriate to spleen-earth. [In fact such a seemingly effulgent fire is] not only unable to promote the spleen, but also consumes vital Qi in earth. [When] there is no vital Qi in spleen-earth, [it appears like] completely dry earth and is difficult to transform nutrients [from water and food] to moisten all Zang-organs and Fu-organs. Besides, [when] fire Qi flames up, [it] runs straight upwards together with fire from the triple energizer and uterus to connect with heart-fire. The more effulgent fire [is], the more damage earth [suffers]. [It will] inevitably become scorched earth!"

Shaoshi asked, "Could scorched earth produce lung-metal?"

Qibo answered, "Without earth, lung-metal could not be produced. Now earth becomes scorched, [in which] there is no moist Qi. How could [it] produce metal? [It is] not only unable to produce metal, but also transfers harm [caused by fire] to the lung.

发了或断绝了，脾土也随之生发了或断绝了。因为命门是脾土之父母，实际上关乎到脾土的生死，所以并不像其他各类的火，可以旺盛也可以衰微，可以存在可以消亡。"

少师问："命门之火过旺，但大多情况下却不适宜于脾土，这又是什么原因呢？"

岐伯说："如果火少了，土就会变湿，就没有了生发的机会；如果火多了，土就会变干，其干燥破裂就会造成危害。因为脾是湿土，而土中是有水的。命门是水中之火，而火也藏于水中，这样火就成为既济之火，自然就不会导致亢焚式的祸害，并且与脾土相适宜。因此当火旺盛的时候，土也会随之而旺盛；当火衰弱的时候，土也会随之而衰弱；当火生长的时候，土也会随之而生长；当火灭绝的时候，土也会随之灭绝。如果火过于旺盛，这是因为火比水更强胜；如果水不足以济火，这就是未能既济之火。火似乎是旺盛的，但实际上却是衰弱的。如果是假旺的而不是真旺的，就与脾土不相适应了。在这种情况下，火不仅无法生发脾土，还会转而消耗脾土的生气。如果脾土没有生气，赤地就会变得干枯，要想转化水谷的精微以滋润各个脏腑，那就很难了。而且由于火气上炎，便与三焦、包络之火直冲而上，与心火相合，从而使火气更加旺盛，而土气则更加耗散，这怎么可能不成为焦土吗？"

少师问："焦土能生肺金吗？"

岐伯说："肺金没有了土就不能生发，如今土变成了焦土，其中缺乏润泽之气，怎么能够生金呢？不仅不能生金，而且还会将祸转嫁于肺。因为肺缺乏土气的资助，又遭遇更多火气的威逼，结果就导致了金

[As a result,] the lung lacks assistance of earth-Qi and is frequently threatened by fire-Qi. [Since] metal is weak and wood is strong, this is certainly the inevitable tendency. [When] wood is strong, [it will] damage earth; [when] earth is damaged, [it is] very difficult to produce metal; [when] lung-metal is exhausted, kidney-water is also exhausted; [when] water is exhausted, wood [is] unable to be nourished; [when] wood is dry, [it will] burn itself and increase flaming of fire; [when wood is burnt and flaming fire is increased,] earth [will be] scorched more."

Shaoshi asked, "Which meridian can be treated to save [earth]?"

Qibo answered, "[When] there is excessive fire, water [will be] insufficient. [When] water is enriched, fire [will] harmonize spontaneously. However, just to supplement water is not easy to produce water. [Only when] lung-metal and fire-Qi are supplemented can water have a source of transformation and avoid any damage of the root[2]. [When] the kidney has got water to control fire, water and fire will coordinate with each other and fire will not be increasingly effulgent and damage [water]. Thus in terms of treatment, [measures should be taken] first to supplement water."

Shaoshi said, "Excellent [explanation]!"

Chen Shiduo's comment, "Spleen-earth and stomach-earth are different. To produce spleen-earth and to produce stomach-earth are also different. Although to produce earth depends on fire, fire differs one from another. To produce spleen-earth depends on the

的衰弱和木的强盛,这是不可避免的态势。木强盛就会欺凌土,而土的衰败更难以生金了。如果肺金绝灭了,肾水也会随之而绝灭。如果水绝灭了,木就无法得到滋养了。如果木干枯而自焚,就会增加火焰的沸腾之势,土就会更加干燥了。"

少师问:"治疗哪一条经脉才能获得救助呢?"

岐伯说:"火的有余,是水气的不足所致。只有补益了水,火才会自然安息。然而,如果仅仅是一味地补水,水也不易生发。只有补益肺金和火气,水才会有化生之源,这样才不用担心没有本源了。肾得到水才能制火,这样水火就会相济,火就不会引发偏旺之害。所以在治疗方法上,就必须先行补水。"

少师说:"好!"

陈士铎评论说:"脾土与胃土不同。生脾土与生胃土也不同,虽然生土取决于火,但各种火中也存在着各种差异。生脾土必须依赖于心,生胃土必须依靠包络。心为君火,包络为相火。这两种火就必须要补肾,因为水是能生火的。"

heart while to produce stomach-earth depends on the pericardium. The heart is monarch-fire while the pericardium is ministerial fire. All [these two kinds of] fire need to tonify the kidney because only water can produce fire."

Notes

[1] See [3] in Chapter 17.

[2] Root here refers to the source for producing water.

胃土篇第二十九

【原文】

少师问曰："脾胃皆土也,有所分乎?"

岐伯曰："脾,阴土也;胃,阳土也。阴土逢火则生,阳土必生于君火。君火者,心火也。"

少师曰："土生于火,火来生土,两相亲也,岂胃土遇三焦命门之相火,辞之不受乎?"

岐伯曰："相火与胃不相合也,故相火得之而燔,不若君火得之而乐也。"

少师曰："心包亦是相火,何与胃亲乎?"

岐伯曰："心包络代君火以司令者也,故心包相火即与君火无异,此胃土之所以相亲也。"

少师曰："心包代心之职,胃土取资心包,无异取资心火矣。但二火生胃土则受益;二火助胃火则受祸者,何也?"

岐伯曰："胃土衰则喜火之生,胃火盛则恶火之助也。"

少师曰："此又何故欤?"

岐伯曰："胃阳土宜弱不宜强。"

少师曰："何以不宜强也?"

岐伯曰："胃多气多血之府,其火易动,动则燎原而不可制,不特烁

Volume 4

【英译】

Chapter 29
Stomach-Earth

Shaoshi asked, "Both the spleen and stomach are earth[1]. What is the difference [between them]?"

Qibo answered, "The spleen [belongs to] Yin-earth [while] the stomach [belongs to] Yang-earth. [When] meeting with fire, Yin-earth begins to grow. [However,] Yang-earth must depend on monarch-fire to grow. [The so-called] monarch-fire [refers to] heart-fire."

Shaoshi asked, "Earth originates from fire and fire produces earth, [there is a] close relationship between them. But why does stomach-fire refuse to accept fire from the triple energizer and the life gate[2] [when] meeting [with it]?"

Qibo answered, "Ministeral fire and the stomach are not coordinated with each other. That is why [the stomach becomes] red-hot [when] meeting ministerial fire, quite different from meeting monarch-fire with happiness."

Shaoshi asked, "Pericardium is also ministerial fire. [But] why [is it] close to the stomach?"

Qibo answered, "The pericardium, on behalf of monarch-fire, is responsible for administration. That is why there is no difference between ministerial fire from the pericardium and monarch-fire. This [is the reason] why stomach-earth and [ministerial fire from

肺以杀子,且焚心以害母矣,且火之盛者,水之涸也。火沸上腾必至有焚林竭泽之虞,烁肾水,烧肝木,其能免乎?"

少师曰:"治之奈何?"

岐伯曰:"火盛必济之水,然水非外水也,外水可暂救以止炎,非常治之法也。必大滋其内水之匮。内水者,肾水也。然而火盛之时,滋肾之水不能泻胃之火,以火旺不易灭,水衰难骤生也。"

少师曰:"又将奈何?"

岐伯曰:"救焚之法,先泻胃火,后以水济之。"

少师曰:"五脏六腑皆借胃气为生,泻胃火不损各脏腑乎?吾恐水未生,肾先绝矣。"

岐伯曰:"火不熄则土不安,先熄火后济水,则甘霖优渥,土气升腾,自易发生万物。此泻胃正所以救胃,是泻火非泻土也。胃土有生机,各脏腑岂有死法乎?此救胃又所以救肾并救各脏腑也。"

少师曰:"胃气安宁,肝木来克奈何?"

岐伯曰:"肝来克胃,亦因肝木之燥也,木燥则肝气不平矣,不平则木郁不伸,上克胃土,土气自无生发之机,故调胃之法以平肝为重。肝气平矣又以补水为急,水旺而木不再郁也,惟是水不易旺仍须补肺金,旺则生水,水可养木,金旺则制木,木不克土,胃有不得其生发之性者乎?"

少师曰:"善。"

陈士铎曰:"胃土以养水为主,养水者助胃也。胃中有水则胃火不

the pericardium are] close to each other. "

Shaoshi asked, "The pericardium fulfils the responsibility on behalf of the heart. [So when] stomach-earth takes resource from the pericardium, [it is] the same as taking it from heart-fire. But [when these] two [kinds of] fire produce stomach-earth, it is beneficial; [when these] two [kinds of] fire assist stomach-fire, it is harmful. Why?"

Qibo answered, "[When] stomach-earth is debilitated, [it] likes to be promoted by fire; [when] stomach-fire is exuberant, [it] dislikes assistance of harmful fire. "

Shaoshi asked, "What is the reason?"

Qibo answered, "[Because] Yang-earth in the stomach should be weak, not strong. "

Shaoshi asked, "Why should [it] not be strong?"

Qibo answered, "The stomach [is a] Fu-organ with excessive Qi and blood. [That is why] its fire tends to scurry. [When stomach fire] scurries, [it begins] to burst and cannot be controlled. [In this case, it] not only burns the lung, but also kills the son[3] and burns the heart to harm the mother[4]. The more blazing fire is, the more withered water becomes. [When] fire flames up, [it] must burn trees [in the forest] and exhaust [water in] the pools, [actually] scorching kidney-water and burning liver-wood. How can it be avoided?"

Shaoshi asked, "How to treat it?"

Qibo answered, "[When] fire is exuberant, [it] must be improved by water. However water [mentioned here] is not external water. External water can prevent [fire from] blazing for

沸。故补肾正所以益胃也。可见胃火之盛由于肾水之衰,补肾水正补胃土也。故胃火可杀,胃土宜培,不可紊也。"

【今译】

少师问道:"脾胃都是土,它们有什么区别吗?"

岐伯说:"脾属于阴土,胃属于阳土。阴土遇到火就会生发,而阳土则必须遇到君火才能生发。君火就是心火。"

少师问:"土生于火,火来生土,所以两者极为亲近,但为什么胃土遇到命门、三焦的相火反而会不予接受呢?"

岐伯说:"因为相火与胃不相配合,所以胃遇到相火就会炽热起来,不像遇到了心火而乐于获益。"

少师问:"心包络也是相火,但为什么与胃亲近呢?"

岐伯说:"因为心包络替代君火实施其政。所以心包络的相火与君火是没有什么差异的,这就是胃土与心包络的火相彼此亲近的缘故。"

少师问:"心包代替君火行施其职,胃土从心包获取资助,这与取资于心火没有什么差异。但心包络的相火与心君之火资生,胃土就会受益,而资助胃火时则会造成祸害,这是什么原因呢?"

岐伯说:"胃土衰弱,则喜欢得到火的资生;胃火炽盛,则厌恶火的资助。"

少师问:"这又是什么原因呢?"

岐伯说:"胃属阳土,适宜虚弱而不适宜强壮。"

the time being. [But this is] not the commonly [used] method to deal with [it]. [What] must [be done is] to enrich internal water. Internal water is kidney-water. However [when] fire is exuberant, to enrich water in the kidney cannot purge fire in the stomach because blazing fire is not easy to extinguish and declined water is difficult to enrich immediately."

Shaoshi asked, "What else can be done then?"

Qibo answered, "The method for stopping blazing [fire is] to purge stomach-fire first and then improve water."

Shaoshi asked, "The five Zang-organs and six Fu-organs all depend on stomach-Qi to exist. Can purgation of stomach-fire damage the Zang-organs and Fu-organs? I am afraid [that] kidney [-Qi] will be exhausted before water is produced."

Qibo answered, "[If] fire is not harmonized, earth cannot be pacified. [What should be done is] to extinguish fire first and then improve water. [Only in this way can there be] sufficient timely rainfall, [can] earth-Qi rise up [and can] all things spontaneously and easily arise. [In this case,] to purge the stomach is actually to assist the stomach and to purge fire is actually to purge earth. [When] there is vitality in stomach-earth, how can the Zang-organs and Fu-organs collapse? Such [a way of treatment indicates that] to rescue the stomach is to rescue the kidney and also to rescue all the Zang-organs and Fu-organs."

Shaoshi asked, "Stomach-Qi is harmonized. [But] what will happen [if] liver-wood restricts [it]?"

Qibo answered, "The liver restricts the stomach because of dryness of liver-wood. [When] wood is dry, liver-Qi is in

少师问:"为什么不适宜强壮呢?"

岐伯说:"因为胃是多气多血之腑,所以胃火易动,胃火动了之后就会开始燎原,而且不可遏制。结果不仅烁伤了肺,而且还会扼杀其子,并且会焚烧心,从而危害了土之母。当火旺盛的时候,水就会变得干涸。当火开始向上沸腾的时候,必然会造成焚烧山林和干涸水泽的后果。在这种情况下,烁肾水而烧肝木的危害又怎么能避免呢?"

少师问:"如何治疗呢?"

岐伯说:"如果火炽盛,就必须用水既济。然而水可不是外水,外水可暂时用以救助,以便抑止火的上炎,但这却不是常用的治疗方法。应该做的是要加大对内水匮乏的滋润。所谓内水,指的就是肾水。然而当火盛的时候,只能滋养肾中之水,而不能泻胃中之火,因为火旺盛了就不容易灭掉,而水衰弱了就难以生发。"

少师问:"这又将怎么办呢?"

岐伯说:"救助火焚之法,首先要泻胃火,然后再以水相济。"

少师问:"五脏六腑都借助胃气来生发,难道泻胃火不会损害各脏腑吗?我担心水还没有生发但肾可能就已经绝断了。"

岐伯说:"如果火不平熄,土就难以平安。所以要先熄火,然后再济水。这样甘霖就会充沛,土气就会升腾,自然就易于促使万物的发生,所以此时的泻胃正是为了救胃,因为这是泻火而不是泻土。胃土有了生机,各脏腑又怎么会有死法呢?所以这样做既是救胃,也是救肾,同时救助了其他各个脏腑。"

少师问:"胃气安宁了,肝木来克制,其结果又会是怎样的呢?"

disharmony. [When liver-Qi is in] disharmony, wood [-Qi] will be stagnated and unable to prevail, [eventually moving] upwards to restrict stomach-earth and preventing earth-Qi from arising. Hence the method for regulating the stomach [should] focus on harmonizing the liver. [When] liver-Qi is harmonized, [measures must be taken] immediately to supplement water. [When] water is enriched, wood will not be stagnated. However water is uneasy to enrich, [efforts] should [be made] to supplement lung-metal. [When metal is] effulgent, water will be produced and will nourish wood; [when] metal is effulgent, wood will be controlled and will not restrict earth. How could the stomach not bear the property of development?"

Shaoshi said, "Excellent [explanation]!"

Chen Shiduo's comment, "Stomach-earth is mainly responsible for nourishing water. Nourishing water indicates assistance of the stomach. [When] there is water in the stomach, fire in the stomach will not blaze. That is why to supplement the kidney is just to benefit the stomach. [It shows that] exuberance of stomach-fire is due to debilitation of kidney-water [and that] to supplement kidney-water is to supplement stomach-earth. Hence stomach-fire can be extinguished and stomach-earth should be cultivated. [Such a procedure] cannot be deranged."

Notes

[1] Both the spleen and stomach belong to earth when matching with the five elements.

岐伯说:"肝之所以来克胃,也是因为肝木枯燥的缘故,木枯燥了肝气就不能平静。如果肝气不平,木气就会抑郁不堪,于是便克制胃土,这样土气自然就不会有生发的机遇了。所以调胃的方法,主要是以平肝为主。当肝气平和了,又必须紧急补水,只有水旺了,木才不再抑郁。当水不易旺盛的时候,仍然必须补肺。金旺了就会生水,水旺了就能养木。金旺了就会克制木,而木就因此而不克土。这样胃怎么能不恢复其生发之性呢?"

少师说:"好!"

陈士铎评论说:"胃土以养水为主,养水就是助胃。只有胃中有了水,胃火才不再沸腾。这就是为什么补肾而有益于胃。可见胃火之盛是由于肾水之衰所致,所以补益肾水也正是为了补胃土。因此胃火可以消除,而胃土则应该培养,不能造成混乱。"

Volume 4

[2] See [3] in Chapter 17.

[3] The son refers to metal (lung) that is produced by earth (spleen).

[4] The mother refers to fire (heart) that produces earth (spleen).

包络火篇第三十

【原文】

少师曰："心包之火无异心火，其生克同乎？"

岐伯曰："言同则同，言异则异。心火生胃，心包之火不止生胃也。心火克肺，心包之火不止克肺也。"

少师曰："何谓也？"

岐伯曰："心包之火生胃，亦能死胃。胃土衰，得心包之火而土生，胃火盛，得心包之火而土败。土母既败，肺金之子何能生乎？"

少师曰："同一火也，何生克之异？"

岐伯曰："心火阳火也，其势急而可避；心包之火阴火也，其势缓而可亲。故心火之克肺，一时之刑，心包之克肺，实久远之害。害生于刑者，势急而患未大；害生于恩者，势缓而患渐深也。"

少师曰："可救乎？"

岐伯曰："亦在制火之有余而已。"

少师曰："制之奈何？"

岐伯曰："心包阴火，窃心之阳气以自养之，亦必得肾之阴气以自存。心欲温肾，肾欲润心，皆先交心包以通之。使肾水少衰，心又分其水气，肾且供心火之不足，安能分余惠以慰心包。心包干涸，毋怪其害胃土也。补肾水之枯，则水足灌心而化液，即足注心包而化津，此不救

Volume 4

【英译】

Chapter 30
Pericardium-Fire

Shaoshi asked, "Pericardium fire and heart-fire are not different. Are [their] production[1] and restriction the same?"

Qibo answered, "To say [that they are] the same, [they are] certainly the same; to say [that they are] different, [they are] certainly different. Heart-fire produces the stomach, [but] pericardium-fire does not only produce the stomach. Heart-fire restricts the lung, [but] pericardium-fire does not only restrict the lung."

Shaoshi asked, "What does it mean?"

Qibo answered, "Fire in the pericardium produces the stomach, but also kills the stomach. [When] stomach-earth is debilitated, earth [can be] produced [after] getting fire from the pericardium; [when] stomach-fire is exuberant, earth [will be] damaged [after] getting fire from the pericardium. When the mother of earth[2] is damaged, how can the son of lung-metal[3] be produced?"

Shaoshi asked, "[They are] the same [kind of] fire. Why are [their] production and restriction different?"

Qibo answered, "Heart-fire [is] Yang-fire. Its tendency is urgent but avoidable; pericardium-fire is Yin-fire. Its tendency is moderate and kind. Thus [when] heart-fire restricts the lung, [it is just] temporary punishment; [when] pericardium [-fire] restricts

胃,正所以救胃也。"

少师曰:"包络之火可泻乎?"

岐伯曰:"胃土过旺,必泻心包之火。然心包之火,可暂泻而不可久泻也。心包逼近于心,泻包络则心火不宁矣。"

少师曰:"然则奈何?"

岐伯曰:"肝经之木,包络之母也。泻肝则心包络之火必衰矣。"

少师曰:"肝亦心之母也,泻肝而心火不寒乎?"

岐伯曰:"暂泻肝则包络损其焰,而不至于害心。即久泻肝则心君减其炎,亦不至于害包络,犹胜于直泻包络也。"

少师曰:"诚若师言,泻肝经之木,可救急而不可图缓,请问善后之法?"

岐伯曰:"水旺则火衰,既济之道也。安能舍补肾水别求泻火哉。"

少师曰:"善。"

陈士铎曰:"包络之火为相火,相火宜补不宜泻也。宜补而用泻,必害心包矣。"

【今译】

少师问:"心包之火与心火没有差异,其生克是相同的吗?"

岐伯说:"说是相同就是相同,说是不同就是不同。心火能生胃,但心包之火不仅仅是生胃。心火能克肺,但心包之火不仅仅是克肺。"

少师问:"这是什么意思呢?"

the lung, [it is] long-term damage. Damage caused by punishment is immediate but not great; [damage] caused by kindness is moderate but more and more serious."

Shaoshi asked, "Can [it be] saved?"

Qibo answered, "[It] depends on controlling excessive fire."

Shaoshi asked, "How to control?"

Qibo answered, "Yin-fire in the pericardium steals Yang Qi from the heart to nourish itself and must get Yin Qi from the kidney to ensure its existence. [When] the heart desires to warm the kidney and the kidney desires to moisten the heart, [they] both have to connect with the pericardium first to unobstruct [their communication]. If kidney-water is less and debilitated, [if] the heart disperses water [from the kidney] and [if] the kidney cannot provide heart-fire with enough [Qi], how can [it] share [its] extra resource[4] with the pericardium? [When water in] the pericardium is dry, [it] certainly damages stomach-earth. [When] dried kidney-water is supplemented, [kidney-] water [will be] sufficient, irrigating[5] the heart to transform into humor[6] and pouring into the pericardium to transform into fluid[7]. Such [an activity] seems not to save the stomach, [but] in fact [it] certainly saves the stomach."

Shaoshi asked, "Can fire in the pericardium be purged?"

Qibo answered, "[If] stomach-earth is too prosperous, [it] must purge fire in the pericardium. But fire in the pericardium can only be purged temporarily, not for a long time. The pericardium is quite close to the heart, [and therefore] purgation [of fire in] the pericardium will disturb heart-fire."

岐伯说："心包之火既能生胃，也能亡胃。胃土衰弱的时候，得到心包之火，土就能生；胃火旺盛的时候，得到心包之火，土就会败。土之母既然都败了，肺金之子又怎么能生发呢？"

少师问："同样是火，为什么其生克会有差异呢？"

岐伯说："心火是阳火，其势急迫是不可避开的。心包之火是阴火，其势虽然缓慢，但却显得比较亲切。因此心火之所以克肺，是因为一时的刑伐；心包之火之所以克肺，其实体现的是长久的危害。由刑伐而造成的危害，其势虽然急迫，但隐患还不太大。由恩爱而造成的祸害，其势虽然缓慢，但隐患却不断加深！"

少师问："有办法治疗吗？"

岐伯说："该治法也是在遏制有余之火。"

少师问："如何遏制有余之火呢？"

岐伯说："心包属于阴火，通过窃取心中之阳气就可以自养，同时也必须得到肾的阴气才能得以自存。心想温暖肾，肾想滋润心，这都需要首先与心包相交，这样才能保证彼此贯通。假如肾水衰少，心就会分散肾中的水气，而肾供给心火的水气就不足了，这又怎么能分出多余的水气以慰心包呢？如果心包之水干涸了，自然就会危害胃土，没有什么奇怪的。如果补助了肾水的枯竭，肾水就会充足，就能灌溉心而化为液，就足以灌注心包而化为津液，这就是没有救胃却反而救了胃的缘故。"

少师问："包络之火可以泻吗？"

岐伯说："如果胃土过于旺盛，必然要泻心包之火。虽然心包之火

Volume 4

Shaoshi asked, "How to solve it?"

Master Qibo answered, "Wood in the liver meridian [is] the mother of the pericardium. [Thus] to purge the liver will certainly debilitate fire in the pericardium."

Shaoshi asked, "The liver is also the mother of the heart. Does heart-fire [become] cold [when] the liver is purged?"

Qibo answered, "To temporarily purge the liver will damage flaming [fire in] the pericardium, but will not harm the heart. Even the liver [is] purged for a long time, [it will] reduce the flame [of fire in] heart monarch, but will not harm the pericardium. [Such a way of purgation is] even better than direct purgation [of fire] in the pericardium."

Shaoshi asked, "[It is] just as what the Master have said, purgation of wood in the liver meridian can resolve urgency but cannot be [taken as] an ordinary way. What is the following way [to deal with it]?"

Qibo answered, "[When] water is prosperous, fire will decline. [This is] the right way of mutual support [between water and fire]. How can [one] abandon [the way] to supplement kidney-water and just adopt [the way] to purge fire?"

Shaoshi said, "Excellent [explanation]!"

Chen Shiduo's comment, "Fire in the pericardium is ministerial fire and ministerial fire can be supplemented but cannot be purged. [If it is] in need of supplementation but is purged, [it] certainly damages the pericardium."

可以暂时泻之,但却不可长久泻之。心包接近于心脏,如果持续泻包络之火,心火就不会安宁。"

少师问:"那该怎么办呢?"

岐伯说:"肝经之木,是包络之母。泻肝则必然导致心包络之火的衰微。"

少师问:"肝也是心之母。难道泻肝时心火不会变寒吗?"

岐伯说:"暂时泻肝,包络的火焰就会受到一定的折损,但还不至于危害到心。如果长期泻肝,心君将会减少其火焰,但也不至于危害到包络,这比直接泻包络的效果还要好。"

少师问:"正像天师所说的那样,泻肝经之木,可以救急但却不能救缓,请问该如何善后呢?"

岐伯说:"水旺则会导致火衰,这是水火既济的常规,又怎么能舍弃补肾水之法而借用其他的泻火之法呢?"

少师说:"好!"

陈士铎评论说:"包络之火是相火,相火适宜补不适宜泻。应当补但却反而泻了,则必然会危害心包。"

Volume 4

Notes

[1] Production here means promotion or support.

[2] Mother of spleen-earth refers to heart-fire because in the five elements fire produces earth.

[3] Son of lung-metal refers to kidney-water because in the five elements metal produces water.

[4] Resource here means kidney-water.

[5] Irrigating means to provide water for the heart.

[6] Humor is a special translation of the Chinese concept 液. In traditional Chinese medicine，液 means a sort of thick fluid.

[7] Fluid refers to the Chinese concept 津 which means a sort of fluid that is thinner than 液.

三焦火篇第三十一

【原文】

少师曰："三焦无形，其火安生乎？"

岐伯曰："三焦称腑，虚腑也。无腑而称腑，有随寓为家之义。故逢木则生、逢火则旺。即逢金，逢土亦不相仇而相得。总欲窃各脏腑之气以自旺也。"

少师曰："三焦耗脏腑之气，宜为各脏腑之所绝矣，何以反亲之也？"

岐伯曰："各脏腑之气非三焦不能通达上下，故乐其来亲而益之以气，即有偷窃亦安焉而不问也。"

少师曰："各脏腑乐与三焦相亲，然三焦乐与何脏腑为更亲乎？"

岐伯曰："最亲者，胆木也。胆与肝为表里，是肝胆为三焦之母，即三焦之家也。无家而寄生于母家，不无府而有府乎？然而三焦之性喜动恶静，上下同流，不乐安居于母宅，又不可谓肝胆之宫竟是三焦之府也。"

少师曰："三焦火也，火必畏水，何故与水亲乎？"

岐伯曰："三焦之火最善制水，非亲水而喜入于水也，盖水无火气之温则水成寒水矣。寒水何以化物。故肾中之水，得三焦之火而生；膀胱之水，得三焦之火而化。火与水合，实有既济之欢也。但恐火过于热，制水太甚，水不得益而得损，必有干燥之苦也。"

少师曰："然则何以治之？"

Volume 4

【英译】

Chapter 31
Triple Energizer Fire

Shaoshi asked，"The triple energizer is invisible. How is its fire produced?"

Qibo answered，"The triple energizer is called Fu-organ. [Actually it is a] nominal Fu-organ. [The reason why it is] not a Fu-organ but called Fu-organ [is that] the place [where it is located is taken] as its home. Thus [when] meeting with wood, [it] will grow; [when] meeting with fire, [it] will be prosperous. Even [when] meeting with metal and earth, [it] will not hate [them], but achieve with them. On the whole [it] desires to acquire Qi from every Zang-organ and Fu-organ to develop itself."

Shaoshi asked，"The triple energizer consumes Qi in all the Zang-organs and Fu-organs. Every Zang-organ and Fu-organ should oppose to it. [But] why are [they] close to it?"

Qibo answered，"Without [the help of] the triple energizer, every Zang-organ and Fu-organ is unable to connect with the upper and lower. That is why they like [the triple energizer to be] close [to them and] provide Qi [for them]. Even if [the triple energizer] steals [Qi from them, they are] still quite calm and never blames [it]?"

Shaoshi asked，"Every Zang-organ and Fu-organ likes to be close to the triple energizer. Which Zang-organ or Fu-organ does

岐伯曰："泻火而水自流也。"

少师曰："三焦无腑,泻三焦之火,何从而泻之?"

岐伯曰："视助火之脏腑以泻之,即所以泻三焦也。"

少师曰："善。"

陈士铎曰："三焦之火附于脏腑,脏腑旺而三焦旺,脏腑衰而三焦衰,故助三焦在于助各脏腑也,泻三焦火可置脏腑于不问乎? 然三焦盛衰,全在各脏腑也。"

【今译】

少师问："三焦是无形的,其火又是怎么发生的呢?"

岐伯说："三焦称为腑,实际上是虚腑。不是腑但却反而被称为腑,即将其所在之处作为其家室的意思,因此遇到木就会生发,遇到火就会旺盛。即便使遇到金和土,彼此之间也不会相互仇视,而会相互得益。总而言之,就是想要获取各个脏腑之气以实现自旺的目的。"

少师问："三焦耗散了各个脏腑之气,理应被各个脏腑所根绝,为什么各脏腑反而与之亲密无间呢?"

岐伯说："各脏腑之气如果没有与三焦相合,就不能通达上下,所以都喜欢与三焦亲近,以便能补充其所需之气,即便三焦窃取了其中之气,也自然会安于现状而不过问。"

少师问："各脏腑喜欢与三焦相亲,但三焦则乐于与哪个脏腑更亲呢?"

岐伯说："三焦最亲近的是胆木。胆与肝为表里,所以肝胆是三焦

the triple energizer like best to be close to [it]?"

Qibo answered, "[The triple energizer] likes the best is gallbladder-wood. The gallbladder and the liver are externally and internally [related to each other] and are the mother of the triple energizer and the home of the triple energizer. [The triple energizer] has no home but stays in mother's home, [that is why it is] not a Fu-organ but called a Fu-organ. However the triple energizer likes to move and dislikes to be quiet, [therefore] flowing upwards and downwards and unwilling just to stay at mother's home. So the palace[1] of the liver and gallbladder can be regarded as the palace of the triple energizer."

Shaoshi asked, "The triple energizer [belongs to] fire and fire must fear water. [But] why does [it] like water?"

Qibo answered, "Fire in the triple energizer tends to control water. [It is] not close to water, but likes to enter water because water will become cold [if there is] no fire-Qi in it. Cold water is unable to transform anything. That is why [only when] water in the kidney has acquired fire from the triple energizer can [it be] produced and [only when] water in the bladder has obtained fire from the triple energizer can [it be] transformed. Combination of fire and water actually indicates mutual benefit. But if fire is too hot, [it will] extremely control water. [As a result,] water will not get any benefit. [Instead, water] will be damaged and become withered[2]."

Shaoshi asked, "How to treat it then?"

Qibo answered, "To purge fire [will enable] water to flow spontaneously."

之母,也是三焦的家园。三焦自身无家,所以寄生于其母之家,这不就是既无府第但却又有府第的缘故吗?但三焦的本性则是喜动而恶静,总是与上下进行交流,并不乐于安居在其母之家。所以不能就此认为肝胆之宫居然就是三焦的府第。"

少师问:"三焦属于火,火必然畏惧于水,为什么三焦居然与水亲近呢?"

岐伯说:"三焦之火最善于制水,所以并不是亲近水,而是喜欢进入水中。因为水如果没有火气的温暖,就会变成寒水了,而寒水又怎么能化为人体所需的精微之物?所以肾中之水只有得到三焦之火的资助才能生发,膀胱之水只有得到三焦之火的资助才能气化。而火与水的相合,实际上存在着水火既济的益处。但又担心火过于热,太热之火制水就会太过严厉,这样水不但不会受益,反而会遭受损害,必然造成干燥的后果。"

少师问:"但对此该怎么治疗呢?"

岐伯说:"只要泻下了火气,水就会自然流通了。"

少师问:"三焦没有腑,如果要泻三焦之火,又该从何处泻呢?"

岐伯说:"要根据助长火气的脏腑进行泻火,这样就可以泻三焦了。"

少师说:"好!"

陈士铎评论说:"三焦之火附着于脏腑,脏腑旺盛三焦也会旺盛,脏腑衰弱三焦也会衰弱。所以资助三焦的关键在于资助各个脏腑。由此可见,要泻三焦之火,怎么可能置脏腑于不闻不问呢?所以三焦的盛衰,完全取决于各个脏腑的状况。"

Volume 4

Shaoshi asked, "The triple energizer is not a Fu-organ. How to purge fire from the triple energizer?"

Qibo answered, "To observe [which] Zang-organ or Fu-organ promotes fire and purge it, [fire in] the triple energizer will certainly be purged too."

Shaoshi said, "Excellent [explanation]!"

Chen Shiduo's comment, "Fire in the triple energizer is attached to Zang-organs and Fu-organs. [Therefore, when] the Zang-organs and Fu-organs are prospersous, the triple energizer is also prospersous; [when] the Zang-organs and Fu-organs are debilitated, the triple energizer is also debilitated. Thus to assist the triple energizer depends on the assistance of the Zang-organs and Fu-organs. How [can one] neglect the Zang-organs and Fu-organs [when] purging fire in the triple energizer? So the wax and wane of the triple energizer all depend on that of the Zang-organs and Fu-organs."

[1] Palace here refers to the location of the liver and gallbladder.

[2] Wither here means dryness.

胆木篇第三十二

【原文】

少师曰:"胆寄于肝,而木必生于水。肾水之生肝即是生胆矣,岂另来生胆乎?"

岐伯曰:"肾水生木必先生肝,肝即分其水以生胆。然肝与胆皆肾子也,肾岂有疏于胆者乎?惟胆与肝为表里,实手足相亲,无彼此之分也。故肾水旺而肝胆同旺,肾水衰而肝胆同衰。非仅肝血旺而胆汁盈,肝血衰而胆汁衰也。"

少师曰:"然亦有肾水不衰,胆气自病者何也?"

岐伯曰:"胆之汁主藏,胆之气主泄,故喜通不喜塞也。而胆气又最易塞,一遇外寒,胆气不通矣;一遇内郁,胆气不通矣。单补肾水不舒胆木,则木中之火不能外泄,势必下克脾胃之土,木土交战多致胆气不平,非助火以刑肺,必耗水以亏肝,于是胆郁肝亦郁矣。肝胆交郁,其塞益甚。故必以解郁为先,不可徒补肾水也。"

少师曰:"肝胆同郁,将独鲜胆木之塞乎?"

岐伯曰:"郁同而解郁,乌可异哉?胆郁而肝亦郁,肝舒而胆亦舒。舒胆之后济之补水,则水荫木以敷荣,木得水而调达,既不绝肝之血,有不生心之液者乎?自此三焦得木气以为根,即包络亦得胆气以为助,十二经无不取决于胆也。何忧匮乏哉!"

Volume 4

【英译】

Chapter 32
Gallbladder-Wood

Shaoshi asked, "The gallbladder is attached to the liver and wood must originate from water. [The fact that] kidney-water produces liver [-wood actually] means [that kidney-water] produces gallbladder [-wood]. Does it mean that [kidney-water] produce gallbladder [-wood] in another way?"

Qibo answered, "Kidney-water produces wood and must produce the liver first. And the liver then separates some water to produce the gallbladder. However, both the liver and gallbladder are the sons of the kidney, how can the kidney estrange from the gallbladder? Besides, the gallbladder and the liver are externally and internally [related to each other], [indicating that they are] actually close to each other and not different from each other. Thus [when] kidney-water is prosperous, the liver and gallbladder are also prospersous; [when] kidney-water is debilitated, the liver and gallbladder are also debilitated. [The fact is] not just [when] liver blood is prosperous bile is exuberant and [when] liver blood is debilitated bile is also debilitated."

Shaoshi asked, "However, there are [some people whose] kidney-water is not debilitated but [whose] bile itself is in disorder. Why?"

Qibo answered, "Bile in the gallbladder is responsible for

少师曰:"善。"

陈士铎曰:"肝胆同为表里,肝盛则胆盛,肝衰则胆衰,所以治胆以治肝为先。肝易于郁,而胆之易郁,又宁与肝胆殊乎,故治胆必治肝也。"

【今译】

少师问:"胆寄于肝的位置,而木则必然生于水中,肾水对肝的滋生,也就是对胆的滋生,怎么能另行生胆呢?"

岐伯说:"肾水滋生木,但也必然先滋生肝,而肝也就是从中分出一部分水去滋生胆。然而,肝与胆都是肾之子,肾怎么能疏远其子胆呢?只是胆与肝互为表里,也就像手足一样颇为亲近,彼此之间没有任何分别的。所以肾水旺盛时,肝胆也会同时旺盛;肾水衰弱时,肝胆也同时会衰弱。这不仅仅是肝血旺盛了胆汁才会充盈,肝血衰弱了胆汁也会衰弱。"

少师问:"但是有时肾水并不衰弱,但胆气却自行发病了,这是为什么呢?"

岐伯说:"因为胆汁主藏,胆气主泄,所以胆喜疏通而不喜闭塞。但是胆气又最易于闭塞,一旦遇到外寒胆气就不通了,一旦遇到内郁胆气也不通了。如果只是单一地补肾水,而没有舒张胆木,那么木中之火不能外泄,势必向下克制脾胃之土。木与土发生交战,多数情况下会导致胆气的不平,这不仅是助长心火而刑伐肺金,而且也必然消耗水而亏

storage [while] Qi in the gallbladder is responsible for purgation. That is why [it] likes unobstruction and dislikes obstruction. But gallbladder-Qi is easy to be obstructed. Thus [when] meeting external cold, gallbladder-Qi is obstructed; [when] meeting internal stagnation, gallbladder-Qi is also obstructed. [If] only kidney-water is supplemented but gallbladder-wood is not relaxed, fire in wood cannot be purged. [Instead, it] must restrict earth in the spleen and stomach in the lower [position]. [When] wood and earth fight against each other, [it will] often cause imbalance of gallbladder-Qi, not only assisting fire to damage the lung, but also consuming water to weaken the liver. [As a result,] the gallbladder is stagnated and the liver is also stagnated. [When both] the liver and gallbladder are stagnated, obstruction is more serious. Thus [in terms of treatment, what should do] first is to resolve stagnation, not just to supplement kidney-water."

Shaoshi asked, "If the liver and gallbladder are both stagnated, would the gallbladder-wood be obstructed alone?"

Qibo answered, "Stagnation is the same. How could the way to resolve stagnation is different? [When] the gallbladder is stagnated, the liver is also stagnated; [when] the liver is relaxed, the gallbladder is also relaxed. [When] the gallbladder is relaxed, [it can be] promoted by supplementing water. [In this way,] water [in the kidney] will [nourish gallbladder-] wood [which will become] prosperous and wood [will be well] regulated and promoted [when] getting water. Since blood in the liver is not exhausted, how could [it] not produce fluid in the heart? From then on, the triple energizer gets wood-Qi as its root, just like the pericardium [that]

损肝,不仅导致胆郁,而且也导致肝郁。如果肝胆都抑郁了,其闭塞就会更加严重。所以治疗时必须首先解郁,而不是单一地补肾。"

少师问:"如果肝胆同时抑郁了,胆木是否会有独自的闭塞呢?"

岐伯说:"既然肝胆同时抑郁了,解郁之法又有何异呢?如果胆抑郁了,肝自然也会抑郁;如果肝舒张了,胆也会舒张。舒张了胆之后,再用补水之法予以调济,那么水就会荫育胆木,木也会因之而茁壮成长,而且木得到了水也随之而发达。既然并没有断绝肝中之血,怎么能不生发心中之液呢?从此以来,三焦得到木气就有了自身的根基,同时包络也得到了胆气的资助,所以十二经没有不取决于胆的,怎么还担忧匮乏的出现呢?"

少师说:"好!"

陈士铎评论说:"肝胆同为表里,肝旺盛则胆也旺盛,肝衰弱则胆也衰弱,所以要治疗胆病,就必须先治疗肝病。肝容易抑郁,胆也容易抑郁,肝胆又会有什么特殊的差异呢?所以治疗胆病时,就必须先治疗肝病。"

gets gallbladder-Qi as its assistance. [In fact] all the twelve meridians depend on the gallbladder. There is no need to worry about any shortage."

Shaoshi said, "Excellent [explanation]!"

Chen Shiduo's comment, "The liver and the gallbladder are externally and internally [related to each other]. [When] the liver is exuberant, the gallbladder is also exuberant; [when] the liver is debilitated, the gallbladder is also debilitated. So for treating the gallbladder, the liver [should be] treated first. The liver is easy to be stagnated and the gallbladder is also easy to be stagnated. [There is] no special difference between the liver and gallbladder. Therefore to treat the gallbladder, the liver [should be] treated first."

膀胱水篇第三十三

【原文】

少师曰："水属阴,膀胱之水谓之阳水,何也?"

岐伯曰："膀胱之水,水中藏火也。膀胱无火,水不化,故以阳水名之。膀胱腑中本无火也。恃心肾二脏之火相通化水,水始可藏而亦可泄。夫火属阳,膀胱既通火气,则阴变为阳矣。"

少师曰："膀胱通心肾之火,然亲于肾而疏于心也。心火属阳,膀胱亦属阳,阳不与阳亲,何也?"

岐伯曰："膀胱与肾为表里,最为关切,故肾亲于膀胱。而膀胱亦不能疏于肾也。心不与膀胱相合,毋怪膀胱之疏心矣。然心虽不合于膀胱,而心实与小肠为表里,小肠与膀胱正相通也。心合小肠,不得不合膀胱矣。是心与膀胱其迹若远而实近也。"

少师曰："然则膀胱亲于心而疏于肾乎?"

岐伯曰："膀胱阳水也,喜通阴火而不喜通阳火,似心火来亲未必得之化水。然而肾火不通心火,则阴阳不交,膀胱之阳火正难化也。"

少师曰："此又何故欤?"

岐伯曰："心火下交于肾,则心包三焦之火齐来相济,助胃以化膀胱之水。倘心不交肾,心包三焦之火各奉心火以上炎,何敢下降以私通于肾。既不下降,敢代君以化水乎?"

Chapter 33
Bladder-Water

Shaoshi asked, "Water belongs to Yin. [But] why is water in the bladder known as Yang water?"

Qibo answered, "[In] water of bladder [there is] fire stored in it. [If] there is no fire in the bladder, water [in it] cannot be transformed. That is why [water in the bladder is] called Yang water. [In] the bladder, [which is a] Fu-organ, originally there is no fire. [It] depends on fire from the heart and kidney to unobstruct and transform water, [enabling] water to store and drain. Fire belongs to Yang. Since the bladder can unobstruct fire-Qi, Yin [in it can] transform into Yang."

Shaoshi asked, "The bladder interacts with fire from the heart and kidney. But [it is] close to the kidney and estranges from the heart. Heart-fire belongs to Yang and the bladder also belongs to Yang. Why is Yang not close to Yang?"

Qibo answered, "The bladder and the kidney are externally and internally [related to each other]. [This is] more important. That is why the kidney is close to the bladder. In fact the bladder cannot estrange from the kidney. The heart is unable to coordinate with the bladder, [but] the bladder cannot be blamed of estranging from the heart. Although the heart is unable to coordinate with the bladder, the heart and the small intestine are externally and internally [related to each other], the small intestine and the bladder

少师曰："君火无为，相火有为，君火不下降，包络相火正可代君出治。何以心火不交，相火亦不降乎？"

岐伯曰："君臣一德而天下治。君火交而相火降，则膀胱得火而水化。君火离而相火降，则膀胱得火而水干。虽君火恃相火而行，亦相火必藉君火而治。肾得心火之交，又得包络之降，阴阳合为一性，竟不能分肾为阴、心为阳矣。"

少师曰："心肾之离合，膀胱之得失如此乎？"

岐伯曰："膀胱，可寒而不可过寒，可热而不可过热。过寒则遗，过热则闭，皆心肾不交之故也。此水火所以重既济耳。"

少师曰："善。"

陈士铎曰："膀胱本为水腑。然水中藏火，无水不交，无火亦不交也。故心肾二脏皆通于膀胱之腑。膀胱不通，又何交乎？交心肾，正藏水火也。"

【今译】

少师问："水属于阴，为什么膀胱之水则被称为阳水呢？"

岐伯说："膀胱的水，其中藏有火。如果膀胱没有火水，就不能气化，所以便用阳水予以命名。膀胱腑中本来是没有火的，所以只有依靠心肾二脏的火的相通才能化水，这样水才能开始贮藏，而且也才能开始排泄。火属于阳，膀胱既然与火气相通，阴自然就变为阳了。"

少师问："膀胱与心肾火气相通，但却亲近于肾而疏远于心。心火

coordinate with each other. [Since] the heart coordinates with the small intestine, [it] certainly coordinates with the bladder. Thus the heart and the bladder seem to separate [from each other] but actually are close [to each other]."

Shaoshi asked, "Is the bladder close to the heart or estranging from the kidney?"

Qibo answered, "The bladder [is] Yang water, liking to communicate with Yin fire but disliking to interact with Yang fire. Although heart-fire is close [to the kidney], [but] is uncertain to transform water [when getting it]. However, [if] kidney-fire does not interact with heart-fire, Yin and Yang are unable to communicate [with each other] and Yang fire in the bladder is difficult to transform."

Shaoshi asked, "What is the reason?"

Qibo answered, "[When] heart-fire interacts with the kidney in the lower, fire from the pericardium and triple energizer will work together to support [it], assisting the stomach to transform water in the bladder. If the heart does not interact with the kidney, fire from the pericardium and triple energizer flames up together with heart-fire. How can it descend to communicate privately with the kidney? Since it cannot descend, how dares it to transform water on behalf of the monarch?"

Shaoshi asked, "Monarch-fire does not need to act [but] ministerial fire must act. Monarch-fire does not descend, [but] pericardium fire [must be responsible for] managing [necessary business] on behalf of the monarch. Why does heart-fire not interact [with others] and ministerial fire also never descend?"

属于阳,膀胱也属于阳,为什么阳反而不与阳相亲近呢?"

岐伯说:"膀胱与肾脏相为表里,彼此关系最为密切,所以肾亲近于膀胱,而膀胱也就不能疏远肾了。心如果不与膀胱相合,膀胱疏远于心也就不奇怪了。然而,心虽然不与膀胱相合,但却与小肠相为表里,而小肠与膀胱也正好相通。心既然与小肠相合,那就不能不与膀胱相合了。所以表面上看心与膀胱相疏远,其实彼此之间还是颇为亲近的。"

少师问:"但是膀胱为什么亲近于心而疏远于肾呢?"

岐伯说:"膀胱属于阳水,喜欢与阴火相通而不喜欢与阳火相通,这就像心火的亲近一样,未必因为得到了就能化水。然而,如果肾火不能与心火想通,那么阴阳就不能相交,而膀胱的阳火也就更难以气化了。"

少师问:"这又是什么原因呢?"

岐伯说:"当心火向下与肾相交时,心包和三焦之火都会相互既济,资助胃来化膀胱之水。如果心不与肾相交,那么心包和三焦的火就会各自随着心火而上炎,怎么敢私自下降与肾相通呢?既然不能下降,又怎么敢代替君火来化水呢?"

少师问:"君火是无为的,相火是有为的,君火不下降,但包络之相火正好可以代替君火出来治理,但为什么心火不交,而相火也不下降呢?"

岐伯说:"只有君臣同德,天下才会得治。如果君火相交而相火下降,那么膀胱得到了火就能化水;如果君火分离而相火下降,那么膀胱

Qibo answered, "[Only when] the monarch and the ministers [share the same solidarity and] morality [can] the whole world [be well] governed. [When] monarch-fire communicates [with others], ministerial fire will descend and the bladder will get fire and transform water. [If] monarch-fire estranges [from others and] ministerial fire descends, the bladder gets fire but water [in it] is dry. Monarch-fire orders ministerial fire to manage [what is necessary], and ministerial fire depends on monarch-fire to govern [what is important]. [When] kidney [fire] has [the opportunity] to communicate with heart-fire and meet bladder-fire that descends, Yin and Yang will be of the same in nature. [In this case,] it is unnecessary to simply divide the kidney-Yin and the heart-Yang."

Shaoshi asked, "Are the achievement and loss in the bladder the same as that of the separation and combination of the heart and kidney?"

Qibo answered, "The bladder can be cold but cannot be too cold, can be hot but cannot be too hot. [If the bladder is] too cold, [it will cause] seminal emission; [if the bladder is] too hot, [it will cause] blockage. [This is] all caused by failure of the heart and kidney to interact with each other. That is why the most important [thing for] water and fire [to do is] to support [each other]."

Shaoshi said, "Excellent [explanation]!"

Chen Shiduo's comment, "The bladder is originally a water Fu-organ. But water stores fire. [If] there is no water, [the heart and the kidney] cannot communicate [with each other]; [if] there is no fire, [the heart and the kidney] also cannot communicate [with

得到了火,水反而会干燥。虽然君火依靠相火而行政,相火也必须借助君火而施治。只有当肾与心火相交,而包络之火又能下降,阴阳才会合而为一,这当然不能简单地将肾分为阴而将心分为阳了。"

少师问:"心肾的离合如此,膀胱的得失也是这样的吗?"

岐伯说:"膀胱可以寒冷,但是又不能太过寒冷;膀胱可以温热,但也不能太过温热。如果过于寒冷,就会导致遗精;如果过于温热,就会导致癃闭。这都是因为心肾不交所造成的后果。这就是水火重于既济的缘故。"

少师说:"好!"

陈士铎评论说:"膀胱本来是水腑。然而由于水中藏有火,所以如果没有水,心肾就不能相交,如果没有火,心肾也不能相交。所以心与肾这两个脏器都与膀胱之腑相通。如果膀胱不通,心肾又怎么能与之相交呢?心肾之所以能相交,正是因为其中藏有水火的缘故。"

each other]. *So the heart and the kidney are two Zang-organs* [*that*] *can communicate with the bladder* [*which is a*] *Fu-organ.* [*If*] *the bladder is obstructed, how* [*can it*] *communicate* [*with the heart and kidney*]? [*The reason why the bladder can*] *communicate with the heart and kidney* [*is that there are*] *water and fire stored* [*in it*]."

大肠金篇第三十四

【原文】

少师曰："金能生水，大肠属金，亦能生水乎？"

岐伯曰："大肠之金，阳金也。不能生水，且藉水以相生。"

少师曰："水何能生金哉？"

岐伯曰："水不生金而能养金，养即生也。"

少师曰："人身火多于水，安得水以养大肠乎？"

岐伯曰："大肠离水实无以养，而水苦无多，所异者，脾土生金，转输精液庶无干燥之虞。而后以肾水润之，便庆濡泽耳。是水土俱为大肠之父母也。"

少师曰："土生金，而大肠益燥何也？"

岐伯曰："土柔而大肠润，土刚而大肠燥矣。"

少师曰："土刚何以燥也？"

岐伯曰："土刚者，因火旺而刚也。土刚而生金更甚，然未免同火俱生，金喜土而畏火，虽生而实克矣。安得不燥哉。"

少师曰："水润金也，又善荡金者，何故欤？"

岐伯曰："大肠得真水而养，得邪水而荡也。邪正不两立，势必相遇而相争。邪旺而正不能敌，则冲激澎湃倾肠而泻矣。故大肠尤宜防水。防水者，防外来之水非防内存之水也。"

【英译】

Chapter 34
Large Intestine Metal

Shaoshi asked, "Metal can produce water and the large intestine belongs to metal. Is it able to produce water?"

Qibo answered, "Metal in the large intestine is Yang metal [that] cannot produce water and just depends on water to produce [metal]."

Shaoshi asked, "Why can water produce metal?"

Qibo answered, "Water cannot produce metal but can nourish metal. Nourishment is production."

Shaoshi asked, "[In] the human body, fire is more than water. How can water nourish the large intestine?"

Qibo answered, "[When] separating from water, the large intestine cannot be nourished. [In fact,] water is never excessive [and it is] hoped [that] spleen-metal produces metal and transfers essential fluid to avoid damage caused by dryness. [When this hope is realized,] kidney-water can moisten it and accomplish [the task of] moisture. That is why water and earth are the parents of the large intestine."

Shaoshi asked, "Earth produces metal. [But] why does the large intestine increasingly become dry?"

Qibo answered, "Earth is soft and the large intestine is moist. Earth is hard and the large intestine is [certainly] dry."

少师曰："人非水火不生，人日饮水，何以防之？"

岐伯曰："防水何若培土乎？土旺足以制水，土旺自能生金。制水不害邪水之侵，生金无愁真水之涸，自必火静而金安，可传导而变化也。"

少师曰："大肠无火，往往有传导变化而不能者，又何故欤？"

岐伯曰："大肠恶火又最喜火也。恶火者，恶阳火也。喜火者，喜阴火也。阴火不同，而肾中之阴火尤其所喜。喜火者，喜其火中之有水也。"

少师曰："肾火虽水中之火，然而克金，何以喜之？"

岐伯曰："肺肾子母也，气无时不通。肺与大肠为表里，肾气生肺，即生大肠也。大肠得肾中水火之气，始得司其开阖也。倘水火不入于大肠，开阖无权，何以传导变化乎！"

少师曰："善。"

陈士铎曰："大肠无水火，何以开阖？开阖既难，何以传导变化乎？可悟大肠必须于水火也。大肠无水火之真，即邪来犯之，故防邪仍宜润正耳。"

【今译】

少师问："金能生水，大肠属于金，也能生水吗？"

岐伯说："大肠在金是阳金，所以不能生水，只能暂时借助水来生金。"

Volume 4

Shaoshi asked, "Why [is the large intestine] dry [when] earth is hard?"

Qibo answered, "[The reason why] earth is hard [is that] fire is effulgent. [If] earth is hard, [it will] produce more metal. But [fire is] not necessarily to be produced together with fire [because] metal likes earth but fears fire. Although [it is] produced, in fact [it is] restricted. That is why it is dry."

Shaoshi asked, "Water moistens metal [but] also washes metal. Why?"

Qibo answered, "The large intestine [can be] nourished [when] getting genuine water and irritated [when] meeting evil water. Evil [Qi] and healthy [Qi] cannot coordinate with each other, but fight against each other [when] meeting. [If] evil [Qi] is exuberant and cannot be defeated by healthy [Qi], [it will] swash and surge, resulting in purgation of the [large] intestine. That is why the large intestine should prevent water. Preventing water [means] to prevent external water, not internal water."

Shaoshi asked, "Man cannot exist without water and fire and drinks water every day. How to prevent water?"

Qibo answered, "How can preventing water be the same as cultivating earth? [When] earth is prosperous, [it] can control water; [when] earth is prosperous, [it] can spontaneously produce metal. [The way that earth] controls water cannot be affected by invasion of evil water [and the way that earth] produces metal cannot be inhibited by exhaustion of genuine water. Naturally quietness of fire [ensures] peace of metal, promoting transportation [of waste] and transformation [of water and food]."

少师问："水怎么能生金呢?"

岐伯说："水不能生金,但能养金,养就是生的意思。"

少师问："人身中火多于水,怎么能获得水以养大肠呢?"

岐伯说："大肠如果离开了水,实际上就无法得到滋养了。而水是很难更多的,所不同的是脾土能生金,转而传输津液,所以就不会造成干燥的危害了,然后再用肾水予以滋润,这样就可以获得濡哺泽养了,所以水土均为大肠之父母。"

少师问："土能生金,但大肠为何又日益干燥呢?"

岐伯说："土柔软则大肠湿润,土坚硬则大肠干燥。"

少师问："土坚硬,为什么会造成大肠干燥呢?"

岐伯说："土之所以坚硬,是因为火旺盛而刚强。如果土坚硬,就更能生金,但却未免不与火一起生发,金喜欢土而畏惧火,虽然能生发,但实际上却是克制,怎么会不造成干燥呢?"

少师问："水滋润金,但又善于动荡金,为什么是这样的呢?"

岐伯说："大肠得到了真水才能得养,得到了邪水就会动荡,邪正两不立,相遇时势必又相争。如果邪气旺盛,正气就不能与之抗争,就会导致不断的冲激和激烈的动荡,整个大肠都会因之而泻。所以大肠尤其应当防水。所谓防水,就是预防外来之水,并不是预防内在之水。"

少师问："人没有了水火就不能生存,人每天都要饮水,又该如何预防呢?"

岐伯说："防水怎么能像培土呢? 如果土旺盛了,就足以制伏水;如果土旺盛了,就自然能生金。制水时就不用担心邪水的侵害,生金时

Shaoshi asked, "There is no fire in the large intestine. Usually [the large intestine is] unable to transport [waste] and transform [water and food]. What is the reason?"

Qibo answered, "The large intestine dislikes fire but also likes fire. The fire [that it] dislikes is Yang fire [and the fire that it] likes is Yin fire. [Different kinds of] Yin fire [are] different [in various ways]. Yin fire in the kidney [is the one that the large intestine] likes best. To like fire means to like water in fire."

Shaoshi asked, "Although in kidney-fire there is fire in water, [it] still restricts metal. Why [does it really] like?"

Qibo answered, "[The relationship between] the lung and the kidney [is just like that between] son and mother, [and therefore] Qi [in them] is never inhibited. The lung and the large intestine are externally and internally [related to each other]. Kidney-Qi promotes the lung, indicating [that it] promotes the large intestine. [Only when] the large intestine has obtained Qi from water and fire in the kidney [can it] begin [to accomplish the function of] opening and closing. If water and fire fail to enter the large intestine, [the large intestine is] not qualified [to perform its function of] opening and closing. [In this case,] how can [it] transport [waste] and transform [water and food]?"

Shaoshi said, "Excellent [explanation]!"

Chen Shiduo's comment, "[If] there is no water and fire in the large intestine, how [can it perform its function of] opening and closing? [If] opening and closing [are] difficult, how [can it] transport [waste] and transform [water and food]? [Such a fact]

也不用担忧真水的涸竭。火静则金自然就会安宁,传导和变化就自然能得以保证。"

少师问:"大肠没有火,往往不能传导和变化,这又是什么原因呢?"

岐伯说:"大肠厌恶火,但又最喜爱火。所厌恶的火,实际上是阳火;所喜爱的火,实际上是阴火。阴火各有不同,而肾中的阴火尤其是其所喜爱的。之所以喜爱火,就是因为火中有水。"

少师问:"肾火虽然是水中之火,但还是克金的,为什么还会喜爱它呢?"

岐伯说:"肺与肾实际上是子母关系,所以气无时不通。肺与大肠相为表里,所谓肾气生肺,实际上也是生大肠。大肠得到肾中的水火之气,才能实施其开合的功能。如果水火不入于大肠,大肠就无力开合了,又怎么能传导和变化呢?"

少师说:"好!"

陈士铎评论说:"如果大肠没有水火,又怎么能开合呢?既然难以开合,又怎么能继续传导和变化呢?由此可知,大肠必须有了水火才能开阖,才能传到和变化。如果大肠没有了水火的真气,邪气就会趁机侵犯,所以要防止邪气的入侵,依然需要滋润正气。"

inspires [*us that*] *there must be water and fire in the large intestine.* [*If*] *there is no genuine* [*Qi from*] *water and fire* [*in*] *the large intestine, evil will invade it. Thus the appropriate* [*way*] *to prevent* [*invasion of*] *evil* [*is*] *to moisten* [*and enrich*] *healthy* [*Qi*]."

小肠火篇第三十五

【原文】

少师曰："小肠属火乎？属水乎？"

岐伯曰："小肠与心为表里，与心同气，属火无疑。其体则为水之路，故小肠又属水也。"

少师曰："然则小肠居水火之间，乃不阴不阳之腑乎？"

岐伯曰："小肠属阳，不属阴也。兼属之水者，以其能导水也。水无火不化，小肠有火，故能化水。水不化火，而火且化水，是小肠属火明矣。惟小肠之火代心君以变化，心即分其火气以与小肠，始得导水以渗入于膀胱。然有心之火气、无肾之水气，则心肾不交，水火不合，水不能遽渗于膀胱矣。"

少师曰："斯又何故乎？"

岐伯曰："膀胱，水腑也，得火而化，亦必得水而亲。小肠之火欲通膀胱，必得肾中真水之气以相引，而后心肾会而水火济，可渗入亦可传出也。"

少师曰："肠为受盛之官，既容水谷，安在肠内无水，必藉肾水之通膀胱乎？"

岐伯曰："真水则存而不泄，邪水则走而不守也。小肠得肾之真水，故能化水谷而分清浊，不随水谷俱出也。此小肠所以必资于肾

Volume 4

【英译】

Chapter 35
Small Intestine Fire

Shaoshi asked, "Does the small intestine belongs to fire or water?"

Qibo answered, "The small intestine and the heart are externally and internally [related to each other]. Qi [in the small intestine is] the same [as that in] the heart, certainly belonging to fire. [However] the form [of the small intestine is] the path [in which] water flows. That is why the small intestine also belongs to water."

Shaoshi asked, "But the small intestine is located in between water and fire. Is it a Fu-organ of neither Yin nor Yang?"

Qibo answered, "The small intestine belongs to Yang, not belongs to Yin. [It] also belongs to water because it can transfer water. Without fire, water cannot be transformed. There is fire in the small intestine, that is why [it] can transform water. Water is unable to transform fire, but fire is able to transform water, proving [that] the small intestine belongs to fire. Only [when] fire in the small intestine transforms [water and food] on behalf of heart monarch [can] the heart share its fire-Qi to the small intestine and transfer water into the bladder. However [if] there is only fire-Qi in the heart but no water-Qi in the kidney, the heart and the

气耳。"

少师曰："善。"

陈士铎曰："小肠之火，有水以济之，故火不上焚，而水始下降也。火不上焚者，有水以引之也；水不下降者，有火以升也。有升有引，皆既济之道也。"

【今译】

少师问："小肠属于火还是属于水呢？"

岐伯说："小肠与心互为表里，也与心同气，无疑是属于火的。小肠的形体是水流行的通道，所以小肠也属于水。"

少师问："但是小肠位于水火之间，是不阴不阳之腑吗？"

岐伯说："小肠属于阳，不属于阴，同时也属于水，因为小肠能导水。水没有火就不能化生，小肠中有火，所以就能化水。水能不化火，而火则能化水，这就是小肠属火的明证。唯独小肠之火，可以代替心君行施变化，心即分其火气予小肠，这样才能引导水渗透到膀胱中。但是如果只有心之火气而没有肾之水气，心肾就不能相交，水火就不能相合，水就无法很快渗入膀胱中。"

少师问："这又是什么原因呢？"

岐伯说："因为膀胱是水腑，只有得到火才能得以气化，只有得到水才能得以亲近。小肠之火想通达膀胱，就必须得到肾中真水之气的引导。只有这样心肾才能相会，水火才能既济，才能发挥既能渗入又能

kidney cannot communicate [with each other] and water and fire cannot coordinate [with each other], [making it] impossible for water to infiltrate into the bladder."

Shaoshi asked, "What is the reason?"

Qibo answered, "The bladder, a water Fu-organ, transforms [Qi when] getting fire and is close [to the concerned organ when] getting water. [If] fire in the small intestine wants to penetrate through the bladder, [it] must get Qi from genuine water in the kidney to guide [it]. Only in this way [can] the heart and kidney communicate [with each other] and water and fire support [each other], either penetrating into [the heart and kidney] or draining out [of the heart and kidney]."

Shaoshi asked, "The [small] intestine is an organ of reception and contains water and food. Why is there no water in the [small] intestine? Does [it] have to depend on kidney-water to penetrate into the bladder?"

Qibo answered, "Genuine water only exists and never drains [while] evil water only runs wantonly and never keeps quiet. The small intestine obtains genuine water from the kidney. That is why [it] can transform water and food and separate the lucid and turbid, never excreting together with water and food. Thus the small intestine must be supported by kidney-Qi."

Shaoshi said, "Excellent [explanation]!"

Chen Shiduo's comment, "Fire in the small intestine is supported by water, that is why fire will not flame up and water

传出的功能。"

少师问："作为受盛之官,小肠既然能受纳水谷,为什么肠内反而没有水呢?难道还必须要借助肾水才能通达膀胱吗?"

岐伯说："真水只能贮存而不能排泄,邪水则只能恒流而不能保存。小肠只有得到了肾的真水,才能化水谷,才能分清浊,但却不会随着水谷而泄出,这就是为什么小肠必须要得到肾气的资助。"

少师说："好!"

陈士铎评论说："小肠之火,有水相济,所以火就不会沸腾上炎,这样水才能开始下降。火之所以不沸腾上炎,是因为有水的引导;水之所以不下降,是因为有火助其上升。有所上升,有所引导,这都是既济之道。"

begins to descend. Fire does not flame up [*because*] *there is water to guide it. Water does not descend* [*because*] *there is fire* [*to promote it*] *to rise up.* [*Promotion of*] *rising up and guidance* [*of flaming up*] *are the way of mutual support."*

命门真火篇第三十六

【原文】

少师曰："命门居水火中,属水乎? 属火乎?"

岐伯曰："命门,火也。无形有气,居两肾之间,能生水而亦藏于水也。"

少师曰："藏于水以生水,何也?"

岐伯曰："火非水不藏,无水则火沸矣。水非火不生,无火则水绝矣。水与火盖两相生而两相藏也。"

少师曰："命门之火,既与两肾相亲,宜与各脏腑疏矣?"

岐伯曰："命门为十二经之主。不止肾恃之为根,各脏腑无不相合也。"

少师曰："十二经皆有火也,何藉命门之生乎?"

岐伯曰："十二经之火皆后天之火也。后天之火非先天之火不化。十二经之火得命门先天之火则生生不息,而后可转输运动变化于无穷,此十二经所以皆仰望于命门,各倚之为根也。"

少师曰："命门之火气甚微,十二经皆来取资,尽为分给,不虞匮乏乎?"

岐伯曰："命门居水火中,水火相济,取之正无穷也。"

少师曰："水火非出于肾乎?"

岐伯曰："命门水火虽不全属于肾,亦不全离乎肾也。盖各经之水火均属后天,独肾中水火则属先天也。后天火易旺,先天火易衰。故命门火微,必须补火,而补火必须补肾,又必兼水火补之。正以命门之火

Volume 4

【英译】

Chapter 36
Genuine Fire in the Life Gate

Shaoshi asked, "The life gate is located in water and fire. Does [it] belong to water or fire?"

Qibo answered, "The life gate [belongs to] fire, invisible but with Qi, located between two kidneys, able to produce water and stay in water."

Shaoshi asked, "Why [does it] stay in water to produce water?"

Qibo answered, "Without water, fire cannot stay; without water, fire must blaze. Without fire, water cannot be produced; without fire, water must be exhausted. Water and fire depend on each other to produce and to exist."

Shaoshi asked, "Is it appropriate for fire in the life gate to be close to the two kidneys and estrange other Zang-organs and Fu-organs?"

Qibo answered, "The life gate is the governor of the twelve meridians. [It is] not only the root of the kidney[1], other Zang-organs and Fu-organs all coordinate [with it]."

Shaoshi asked, "There is fire in all the twelve meridians. Why do [they] all depend on the life gate to exist?"

Qibo answered, "Fire in all the twelve meridians is postnatal fire. Without innate fire, postnatal fire cannot be transformed. [Only when] fire from the twelve meridians has got innate fire from

可旺,而不可过旺也。火之过旺,水之过衰也。水衰不能济火,则火无所制,必焚沸于十二经,不受益而受损矣。故补火必须于水中补之。水中补火则命门与两肾有既济之欢,分布于十二经亦无未济之害也。"

少师曰:"命门之系人生死甚重,《内经》何以遗之?"

岐伯曰:"未尝遗也。主不明则十二官危。所谓主者,正指命门也。七节之旁有小心。小心者,亦指命门也。人特未悟耳。"

少师曰:"命门为主,前人未言何也?"

岐伯曰:"广成子云:窈窈冥冥,其中有神。恍恍惚惚,其中有气。亦指命门也。谁谓前人勿道哉。且命门居于肾,通于任督,更与丹田神室相接。存神于丹田,所以温命门也。守气于神室,所以养命门也。修仙之道无非温养命门耳。命门旺而十二经皆旺,命门衰而十二经皆衰也。命门生而气生,命门绝而气绝矣。"

少师曰:"善。"

陈士铎曰:"命门为十二经之主。《素问》不明言者,以主之难识耳。然不明言者,未尝不显言之也。无如世人不悟耳。经天师指示,而命门绝而不绝矣。秦火未焚之前,何故修命门者少,总由于不善读《内经》也。"

【今译】

少师问:"命门位于水火之中,到底是属于水呢还是属于火呢?"

岐伯说:"命门属于火,无形但有气,位于两肾之间,能生水,但也能藏于水中。"

the life gate [can it] exist forever, consequently transferring, transporting, moving and transforming all the time. That is why all the twelve meridians worship[2] the life gate and depend on [it as their] root."

Shaoshi asked, "Fire-Qi in the life gate is quite faint. [But] all the twelve meridians [try] to get [necessary] resource from [it and it also] tries the best to share [resource for them]. Could [it become] more faint?"

Qibo answered, "The life gate is located in water and fire, and water and fire support each other. [That is why its resource] can never be exhaustible."

Shaoshi asked, "Do water and fire not originate from the kidney?"

Qibo answered, "Not all water and fire in the life gate belong to the kidney, [but] not all [water and fire in the life gate] can separate from the kidney. [Because] water and fire from each meridian are postnatal, only water and fire in the kidney are innate. Postnatal fire is easy to blaze and innate fire is easy to debilitate. That is why fire in the life gate is faint and must be supplemented. In order to supplement fire, the kidney must be nourished [first] with the application of water and fire. [After supplementation,] fire in the life gate can be effulgent, but cannot be too effulgent. If fire is too effulgent, water will be debilitated. [If] water is debilitated, [it] cannot support fire. [If] fire is not controlled [by water], [it will] certainly burn the twelve meridians [which will] not benefit [from it] but be damaged [by it]. Thus supplementation of fire must be done in water. To supplement fire

少师问："火藏在水中但也能生水,这是什么道理呢?"

岐伯说："没有了水,火就不能藏在其中;没有了水,火就会沸腾起来。没有了火,水就不能生发;没有了火,水就会断绝。因为水与火是相生而又相藏的。"

少师问："命门之火既然与两肾亲近,那就应当与其他各脏腑疏远了?"

岐伯说："命门是十二经之主,不仅仅只是肾所依靠的根基,各脏腑也没有不与之相合的。"

少师问："十二经都有火,为什么唯独凭借命门而生呢?"

岐伯说："十二经之火都是后天之火,如果没有了先天之火,后天之火就不能变化。十二经之火只有得到了命门的先天之火,才能生生不息,然后才能转化、输送、运行和起动,这样就能变化于无穷了。所以十二经皆仰望于命门,皆以命门为其根基。"

少师问："起始命门之火气甚微,但十二经皆从中获取资助,如果全分给它们,难道命门不会有匮乏的问题吗?"

岐伯说："命门位于水火之中,而水火的相济则使其取资之无穷。"

少师问："水火不是从肾中生出的吗?"

岐伯说："虽然命门中的水火不全属于肾,但也不能全离开肾。因为各经的水火都属于后天之水火,惟独肾脏中的水火才属于先天之水火。后天之火易旺,而先天之火则易衰。所以命门之火衰微了,就必须补火,而要补火,就必须补肾,但同时又必须以水火相补。正因为命门之火可以旺盛,所以就不可使其过于旺盛。如果火过于旺盛,水就会过于衰微。水衰微了就不能济火,这样火就无法克制,其火势在十二经中必然会凶猛,这样十二经脉不仅不会受益,而且还会遭受损害。因此要

in water will support the life gate and the two kidneys. [As a result, water and fire will] spread to the twelve meridians for support, not for damage."

Shaoshi asked, "The life gate is so important to life and death of human beings. Why [is it] not recorded in [*Yellow Emperor's*] *Internal Canon* [*of Medicine*]?"

Qibo answered, "[It] is recorded [in the *Yellow Emperor's Internal Canon of Medicine*]. [In the *Internal Canon*, it says,] 'If the governor is not clear, all the twelve organs will be dangerous.' The so-called 'governor' just refers to the life gate. Beside the seven sections, there is a small heart. This small heart also refers to the life gate. People now still have not understood it yet."

Shaoshi asked, "Why people did not mention [it] before [that] the life gate is the governor?"

Qibo answered, "Guang Chengzi said, '[This place is] beautiful and quiet, there is spirit in it; [this place is] dark and vague, there is Qi in it.' 'This place' also refers to the life gate. Who says that people did not mention [it] before? Now that the life gate is located in the kidney and communicates with the conception vessel and governor vessel, also connected with Dantian (elixir field)[3] and spirit cabinet[4]. [When] spirit is stored in Dantian (elixir field), the life gate will be warmed; [when] Qi is kept in spirit cabinet, the life gate will be nourished. [Thus] the way for cultivating god is no more than warming and nourishing the life gate. [When] the life gate is prosperous, all the twelve meridians will be prosperous; [when] the life gate is debilitated, all the twelve meridians will be debilitated. [When] the life gate is promoted, Qi

补火，就必须在水中补。在水中补了火，命门与两肾就会获得既济之益，同时水火就会分布到十二经脉，就不会造成没有既济的危害。"

少师问："命门关系到人的生死，非常重要，这一点《内经》怎么就遗忘了呢？"

岐伯说："没有遗忘。《内经》所说的'主不明则十二官危'中的'主'，就是指的命门。'七节之旁有小心'中的'小心'，也是指的命门，人们现在还没有领悟到这一点啊！"

少师问："命门为主，但前人还未谈到，为什么呢？"

岐伯说："广成子说'窈窈冥冥，其中有神，恍恍惚惚，其中有气'，也是指的命门，谁说前人没有谈到命门呢？而且命门位于肾中，与任督二脉相贯通，更与丹田的神室相连接。因为神存于丹田，所以就温暖了命门。因为气固守于神室，所以就养育了命门。因此所谓的修仙之道，无非就是温暖和养育命门而已。如果命门旺盛了，十二经脉也会旺盛；如果命门衰弱了，十二经脉也会衰弱。如果命门生发了，气也就生发了；如果命门断绝了，气也就断绝了。"

少师说："好！"

陈士铎评论说："命门为十二经脉之主，《素问》没有明确地论述，因为命门对十二经脉的主管难以辨识。虽然没有明确地论述，但并不是没有明显地谈到，只是世人还无法领悟而已。经过天师的指导和说明，命门的问题似乎断绝了，但其实却没有断绝。秦始皇焚书坑儒之前，为什么研修命门的人就少呢？总的来说，主要是因为人们不善于读懂《内经》的基本精神而已。"

will be promoted; [when] the life gate is exhausted, Qi will be exhausted. "

Shaoshi said, "Excellent [explanation]!"

Chen Shiduo's comment, "The life gate is the governor of the twelve meridians. [In] Su Wen (Plain Conversation), [the life gate is] not thoroughly analyzed because it is difficult to understand. However, no thorough analysis [does not mean that it is] not clearly mentioned. [The only problem is that] people nowadays are unable to understand [it]. With the guidance of the Celestial Master, the life gate seems to have lost but actually not lost. Before [the incident of] burning [classical documents and books in] the Qin [dynasty], why few people well understood the life gate? Because [they] did not know how to read [Yellow Emperor's] Internal Canon [of Medicine]."

Notes

[1] Root of the kidney means that the kidney depends on the life gate.

[2] The word "worship" here means to depend on the life gate for existence and development.

[3] Please see notes in Chapter 22.

[4] Spirit cabinet also refers to Dantian (elixir field).

卷五

命门经主篇第三十七

【原文】

雷公问于岐伯曰:"十二经各有一主,主在何经?"

岐伯曰:"肾中之命门为十二经之主也。"

雷公曰:"十二经最神者,心也。宜心为主,不宜以肾中之命门为主也?"

岐伯曰:"以心为主,此主之所以不明也。主在肾之中,不在心之内。然而离心非主,离肾亦非主也。命门殆通心肾以为主乎。岂惟通心肾哉?五脏七腑无不共相贯通也。"

雷公曰:"其共相贯通者,何也?"

岐伯曰:"人非火不生,命门属火,先天之火也。十二经得命门之火始能生化,虽十二经未通于命门,亦命门之火原能通之也。"

雷公曰:"命门属火,宜与火相亲,何偏居于肾以亲水气耶?"

岐伯曰:"肾火,无形之火也;肾水,无形之水也。有形之火,水能克之,无形之火,水能生之。火克于水者,有形之水也。火生于水者,无形之水也。然而无形之火偏能生无形之水,故火不藏于火,转藏于水。所谓一阳陷于二阴之间也。

人身先生命门而后生心。心生肺,肺生脾,脾生肝,肝生肾,相合而

Volume 5
【英译】

Chapter 37
The Life Gate [Is] the Governor of Meridians

Leigong asked Qibo, "[Among] the twelve meridians, each has a governor. Which meridian is the governor in?"

Qibo answered, "The life gate in the kidney is the governor of the twelve meridians."

Leigong asked, "The most important [among] the twelve meridians is the heart. The heart should be the governor. Is it inappropriate for the life gate in the kidney to be the governor?"

Qibo answered, "[If] taking the heart as the governor, such a governor is unclear. [In fact,] the governor is in the kidney, not in the heart. However, [if it] departs from the heart, [it is] not the governor; [if it] departs from the kidney, [it is] also not the governor. [Only when] the life gate is connected with both the heart and the kidney, can it be the governor. [In fact, the life gate is] not only connected with the heart and the kidney, but also with the five Zang-organs and seven Fu-organs."

Leigong asked, "Why [is the life gate also] connected with all [the other organs]?"

Qibo answered, "Without fire human beings cannot exist. The life gate belongs to fire and is innate fire. [Only when] getting fire from the life gate, can the twelve meridians exist and transform.

相生,亦相克而相生也。十二经非命门不生,正不可以生克而拘视之也。故心得命门,而神明应物也;肝得命门,而谋虑也;胆得命门,而决断也;胃得命门,而受纳也;脾得命门,而转输也;肺得命门,而治节也;大肠得命门,而传导也;小肠得命门,而布化也;肾得命门,而作强也;三焦得命门,而决渎也;膀胱得命门,而畜泄也。是十二经为主之官,而命门为十二官之主。有此主则十二官治,无此主则十二官亡矣。

命门为主,供十二官之取资。其火易衰,其火亦易旺,然衰乃真衰,旺乃假旺。先天之火非先天之水不生,水中补火,则真衰者不衰矣。火中补水,则假旺者不旺矣。见其衰,补火而不济之以水,则火益微;见其旺,泻火而不济之以水,则火益炽。"

雷公曰:"何道之渺乎,非天师又孰能知之。"

陈士铎曰:"命门在心肾之中,又何说之有,无如世人未知也。此篇讲得畅快,非无主之文。"

【今译】

雷公请问岐伯说:"十二经脉各有其主,其主在哪一经呢?"

岐伯说:"肾中的命门就是十二经脉之主。"

雷公说:"十二经中最为神圣的就是心经,所以心应当是十二经脉之主,不应当以肾中的命门作为十二经脉之主吧。"

岐伯说:"如果以心为主,那么十二经脉之主就不清晰了。事实上,十二经脉之主在肾之中,并不在心内。当然,离开了心就不能成为

Volume 5

Although the twelve meridians are not necessarily connected with the life gate, fire in the life gate is originally connected [with all the twelve meridians]."

Leigong asked,"The life gate belongs to fire and is appropriate to be close to fire. [But] why [is it] located in the kidney and close to water-Qi?"

Qibo answered, "Kidney-fire is invisible fire and kidney-water is invisible water. Visible fire can be restricted by water [while] invisible fire can be produced by water. Water [that can] restrict fire is visible water [while] water [that can be] produced by fire is invisible water. However, invisible fire also can produce invisible water. That is why fire cannot store in fire [itself], but transferring it to store in water. That is what one Yang stays in between two Yin[1].

[In] the human body, the life gate is produced earlier than the heart. The heart produces the lung, the lung produces the spleen, the spleen produces the liver and the liver produces the kidney, [all of which] combine with each other and produce each other as well as restrict each other and produce each other[2]. Without the life gate, the twelve meridians cannot exist. Thus [the activities of] production and restriction [among the five elements] cannot be only used to analyze [the life gate]. That is why [only when] the heart is connected with the life gate can spirit and brightness[3] correspond to all things; [only when] the liver is connected with the life gate can there be strategy and consideration[4]; [only when] the gallbladder is connected with the life gate can decision be made; [only when] the stomach is connected with the life gate can there be

其主了，离开了肾也不能成为其主了。难道只有贯通了心肾命门才能成为其主吗？需要贯通又岂止于心肾呢？其实五脏七腑，没有不需要贯通的。"

雷公说："为什么要与五脏七腑贯通呢？"

岐伯说："人离开了火就不能生存。命门属于火，而且是先天之火。十二经脉只有得到了命门之火，才能够生发和传化。虽然十二经脉不一定都要与命门相通，但命门之火本来就与之相通的。"

雷公说："命门属火，应当与火亲近，但为什么命门却偏居于肾而亲近于水呢？"

岐伯说："肾火是无形之火，肾水是无形之水。有形之火，水可以克制；无形之火，水能够生发。克制火的水，是有形之水；从水中生的火，是无形之水。然而，无形之火恰好能够生发无形之水，所以火不藏在火中，转而藏在水中，这就是所说的一阳沉陷在二个阴之间的意思。在人体中，首先生成的是命门，然后心才生成。心生肺，肺生脾，脾生肝，肝生肾，彼此之间既相合又相生，但也是既相克又相生。没有命门，十二经脉就不能生成，所以不能仅仅以生克来对其加以观察和分析。所以心得到了命门的资助，神明才能应物；肝得到了命门的资助，才能谋划和思虑；胆得到了命门的资助，才能判断和决定；胃得到了命门的资助，才能受纳水谷；脾得到了命门的资助，才能转化和输布水谷精微；肺得到了命门的资助，才能治理和调节水道；大肠得到了命门的资助，才能传输和导入糟粕；小肠得到了命门的资助，才能输布和传化水谷精华；肾得到了命门的资助，才能成为有技能又强壮的器官；三焦得到了

Volume 5

reception; [only when] the spleen is connected with the life gate can transference [be accomplished]; [only when] the lung is connected with the life gate can regulation [be fulfilled]; [only when] the large intestine is connected with the life gate can transportation and guidance [be realized]; [only when] the small intestine is connected with the life gate can dissemination and transformation [be made]; [only when] the kidney is connected with the life gate can [it become] strong; [only when] the triple energizer is connected with the life gate can [the way in which water flows be] adjusted; [only when] the bladder is connected with the life gate can [water be] amassed and excreted. [Such a connection] makes the twelve meridians [as] the officials [under the leadership of the monarch] and the life gate [as] the governor of these twelve officials. With such a governor[5], these twelve officials[6] are able to manage [what they should do]. Without such a governor, these twelve officials will lose [their ability to manage what they should do].

As the governor, the life gate provides the twelve officials necessary resources. [In the life gate] fire is easy to debilitate and also easy to blaze. However, to debilitate is true but to blaze is false. Without innate water, innate fire cannot be produced. To supplement fire in water will enable truely debilitated [fire] not to debilitate; to supplement water in fire will enable falsely blazing [fire] not to blaze. Debilitation [of fire indicates that] fire is not supplemented with water, and therefore making fire more faint; blazing [of fire indicates that] fire is purged with water, and therefore making fire more blazing."

命门的资助，才能开启和贯通水道；膀胱得到了命门的资助，才能储蓄和排泄水液。这样十二经脉就成为主子的下属官员了，而命门就成为十二位官员的主子了。有了命门这个主子，十二经脉这些官员才能履行其治理的职责。如果没有命门这个主子，十二经脉这些官员就会亡失了。命门作为主子，就能为十二经脉这些官员提供资助，其火既易于衰微，也易于旺盛。衰微才是真正的衰微，旺盛则是虚假的旺盛。如果没有先天之水，先天之火就不能生发。如果在水中补了火，真正衰微的就不会衰微了；如果在火中补了水，虚假旺盛的也就不会旺盛了。看到火衰微了，只是单纯地补火而不是用水予以相济，那么火就会更加衰微；见到火旺盛了，只是单纯地泻火而不是用水予以相济，那么火就会更加旺盛了。"

雷公说："这个道理可真妙啊！除了天师，谁还能懂得这个道理呢？"

陈士铎评论说："命门在心肾之中，怎么才能说清楚呢？可惜的是世人对此并不了解。这一篇文章讲得简明扼要，并非没有主题。"

Volume 5

Leigong said,"How miraculous it is! Nobody can understand it except the Celestial Master!"

Chen Shiduo's comment, " The life gate [is located] in the heart and kidney. How to explain its existence? [Unfortunately] almost nobody knows [it] in this world. The discussion in this chapter is excellent. [It is] not an article without any theme."

Notes

[1] This is a description about the structure of Kan Gua (坎卦, Kan Diagram). Please see [2] in Chapter 7.

[2] The word "produce" in this passage means "promote" or "support".

[3] The so-called "spirit and brightness" actually refer to mind and intelligence.

[4] The so-called "strategy and consideration" actually refer to thought and analysis.

[5] Governor here refers to the life gate.

[6] Twelve officials here refer to the twelve meridians.

五行生克篇第三十八

【原文】

雷公问于岐伯曰："余读《内经》载五行甚详，其旨尽之乎?"

岐伯曰："五行之理，又何易穷哉。"

雷公曰："盍不尽言之?"

岐伯曰："谈天乎? 谈地乎? 谈人乎?"

雷公曰："请言人之五行。"

岐伯曰："心、肝、脾、肺、肾配火、木、土、金、水，非人身之五行乎?"

雷公曰："请言其变。"

岐伯曰："变则又何能尽哉。试言其生克。生克之变者，生中克也，克中生也。生不全生也，克不全克也，生畏克而不敢生也，克畏生而不敢克也。"

雷公曰："何以见生中之克乎?"

岐伯曰："肾生肝，肾中无水，水涸而火腾矣，肝木受焚，肾何生乎? 肝生心，肝中无水，水燥而木焦矣，心火无烟，肝何生乎? 心君火也，包络相火也，二火无水将自炎也，土不得火之生，反得火之害矣。脾生肺金也，土中无水，于土何以生物，烁石流金，不生金反克金矣。肺生肾水也，金中无水，死金何以出泉? 崩炉飞汞，不生水反克水矣。盖五行多水则不生，五行无水亦不生也。"

【英译】

Chapter 38
Production and Restriction in the Five Elements

Leigong asked Qibo, "I have read [*Yellow Emperor's*] *Internal Canon* [*of Medicine*]. The discussion about the five elements is quite thorough. Are the main ideas all mentioned [in it]?"

Qibo asked, "The theory about the five elements is not so easy to be mentioned completely."

Leigong asked, "Why can [it] not be discussed completely?"

Qibo said, "To discuss about the sky, or about the earth, or about man?"

Leigong said, "Please talk about [the relationship between] man and the five elements."

Qibo answered, "The heart, the liver, the spleen, the lung and the kidney match with fire, wood, earth, metal and water. Are they not the five elements in the human body?"

Leigong said: "Please explain their changes."

Qibo said: "How can the changes be completely mentioned? [Please let me] try to talk about production and restriction. The changes in production and restriction [indicate that] there is restriction in production and there is production in restriction. Production is not just production and restriction is not just restriction. [When] production fears restriction, [it] dares not to produce; [when] restriction fears production, [it] dares not to

雷公曰:"何以见克中之生乎?"

岐伯曰:"肝克土,土得木以疏通则土有生气矣。脾克水,水得土而畜积则土有生基矣。肾克火,火得水以相济,则火有神光矣。心克金,然肺金必得心火以煅炼也。肺克木,然肝木必得肺金以斫削也。非皆克以生之乎?"

雷公曰:"请言生不全生。"

岐伯曰:"生不全生者,专言肾水也.各脏腑无不取资于肾。心得肾水而神明焕发也;脾得肾水而精微化导也;肺得肾水而清肃下行也;肝得肾水而谋虑决断也。七腑亦无不得肾水而布化也。然而取资多者分给必少矣。亲于此者疏于彼,厚于上者薄于下,此生之所以难全也。"

雷公曰:"请言克不全克。"

岐伯曰:"克不全克者,专言肾火也。肾火易动难静,易逆难顺,易上难下,故一动则无不动矣,一逆则无不逆矣,一上则无不上矣。腾于心,躁烦矣;入于脾,干涸矣;升于肺,喘嗽矣;流于肝,焚烧矣;冲击于七腑,燥渴矣。虽然肾火乃雷火也,亦龙火也。龙雷之火其性虽猛,然聚则力专,分则势散,无乎不克,反无乎全克矣。"

雷公曰:"生畏克而不敢生者若何?"

岐伯曰:"肝木生心火也,而肺金太旺,肝畏肺克不敢生心,则心气转弱,金克肝木矣。心火生胃土也,而肾水太旺不敢生胃,则胃气更虚,水侵胃土矣。心包之火生脾土也,而肾水过泛不敢生脾,则脾气加困,水欺脾土矣。脾胃之土生肺金也,而肝木过刚,脾胃畏肝不敢生肺,则肺气愈损,木侮脾胃矣。肺金生肾水也,而心火过炎,肺畏心克,不敢生

restrict."

Leigong asked,"How to find restriction in production?"

Qibo answered, "The kidney produces[1] the liver. [If] there is no water in the kidney, water will dry up, fire will blaze and liver-wood will be burnt. [If this happens,] how can the kidney produce [the liver]? The liver produces the heart. [If] there is no water in the liver, water will be dry, wood will be scorched and heart-fire will have no smoke. [If this happens,] how can the liver produce [the heart]? The heart [belongs to] monarch-fire and the pericardium [belongs to] ministerial fire. [If] there is no water, these two [kinds of] fire will blaze spontaneously. [As a result,] earth fails to be produced by fire, but is damaged by fire. The spleen produces lung-metal. [If] there is no water in earth, how can earth produce all things? [On the contrary, it will] melt stone and metal, and, instead of producing metal, [it will] restrict metal. The lung produces kidney-water. [If] there is no water in metal, how can dead metal come out of the spring[2]? [When] the stove is broken and sand is flying, water cannot be produced, instead, water will be restricted. Because [if] there is too much water, the five elements cannot exist; [if] there is no water, the five elements cannot also exist."

Leigong asked,"How to understand production in restriction?"

Qibo answered, "The liver restricts earth. [When] earth has acquired wood, [it can] unobstruct [itself] and there will be vital Qi in earth. The spleen restricts water. [When] water has acquired earth, [it will] amass [itself] and there will be opportunity for earth to exist. The kidney restricts fire. [When] fire has acquired

肾,则肾气益枯,火刑肺金矣。肾水生肝木也,而脾胃过燥,肾畏脾胃之土,不敢生肝,则肝气更凋,土制肾水矣。"

雷公曰:"何法以制之乎?"

岐伯曰:"制克以遂其生,则生不畏克。助生而忘其克,则克即为生。"

雷公曰:"善。克畏生而不敢克者,又若何?"

岐伯曰:"肝木之盛由于肾水之旺也,木旺而肺气自衰,柔金安能克刚木乎?脾胃土盛由于心火之旺也,土旺而肝气自弱,僵木能克焦土乎?肾水之盛由肺金之旺也,水旺而脾土自微,浅土能克湍水乎?心火之盛,由于肝木乏旺也,火旺而肾气必虚,弱水能克烈火乎?肺金之盛由于脾土之旺也,金盛而心气自怯,寒火能克顽金乎?"

雷公曰:"何法以制之?"

岐伯曰:"救其生不必制其克,则弱多为强。因其克反更培其生则衰转为盛。"

雷公曰:"善。"

陈士铎曰:"五行生克,本不可颠倒。不可颠倒而颠倒者,言生克之变也。篇中专言其变,而变不可穷矣。当细细观之。"

【今译】

雷公请问岐伯:"我读《内经》时,发现对五行的记载颇为详尽。其主旨是否也细致地讲述了呢?"

water, [it will be] supplemented and there will be great effulgence in fire. The heart restricts metal. However, [only when] lung-metal has acquired heart-fire can it train itself. The lung restricts wood. [Only when] liver-wood has acquired lung-metal can it reduce itself. So not all restriction ensures production."

Leigong asked, "Please explain [that] production is not all production."

Qibo answered, "[The idea that] production is not all production just talks about kidney-water, [from which] all the Zang-organs and Fu-organs get necessary resource. [Only when] the heart has got water from the kidney can Shen Ming[3] be cultivated; [only when] the spleen has got water from the kidney can essential nutrients[4] be transformed and transferred; [only when] the lung has got water from the kidney can it become lucid and descend; [only when] the liver has got water from the kidney can strategy and decision be made. [Among] the seven Fu-organs, every one must get water from the kidney to disseminate and transform [it]. However, [if one has] obtained more resource, [it will] certainly share less [with others]. [If one is] close to this side, [it] must estrange the next side; [if one] emphasizes the upper, [it will] certainly neglect the lower. That is why production is difficult to be perfect."

Leigong asked, "Please explain [that] restriction is not complete restriction."

Qibo answered, "[The idea that] restriction is not absolute restriction actually talks about kidney-fire. Kidney-fire is easy to be active but difficult to be quiet, easy to move reversely but difficult

岐伯说：“对五行之理的论述，怎么可能很容易地道尽呢？”

雷公说：“为何不能道尽呢？”

岐伯说：“是想从天说起呢？还是从地说起呢？还是从人说起呢？”

雷公说：“请从人身的五行说起吧。”

岐伯说：“人体的心、肝、脾、肺、肾配以五行的火、木、土、金、水，这不就是人身的五行吗？”

雷公说：“请说明其中的变化。”

岐伯说：“其中的变化又怎么能够说尽呢？那就先试着说说五行的生克变化吧。五行的生克变化，就是生中有克，克中有生，生并不全生，克也并不全克。如果生畏惧克，就不敢生了；如果克畏惧生，就不敢克了。”

雷公说：“怎么理解生中之克呢？”

岐伯说：“肾能生肝，如果肾中没有了水，水就会干涸，火就会沸腾，肝木就会遭受焚烧，肾又怎么能生肝呢？肝能生心，如果肝中没有了水，水就会枯燥，木就会枯焦，心火中没有烟，肝又怎么能生出来呢？心是君火，包络是相火，如果这两种火没有了水，就将自行上炎。如果土得不到火的资生，就会遭受火的伤害。脾能生肺金，如果土中没有了水，干燥的土又怎么能生发万物呢？如果石被烧得烁化了，如果金被烧的液化了，不但不能生金，反而会克金。肺能生肾水，如果金中没有水，僵死之金又怎么能生出泉水呢？如果炉崩塌、汞飞散，就会导致不生水反克水的后果。所以五行多水则不能生，五行无水也不能生。”

to move normally, easy to ascend but difficult to descend. That is why once [it begins] to move, [it is] difficult to stop; once [it begins to move] reversely, [it will] never [move] normally; once [it begins] to ascend, [it will] never descend. [When fire] flames up to the heart, [there will be] vexation and restlessness; [when fire] enters the spleen, [there will be] dryness and witheredness; [when fire] rises up to the lung, [there will be] panting and cough; [when fire] runs into the liver, [there will be] combusting and burning; [when fire] rushes into the seven Fu-organs, [there will be] dryness and thirst. Although kidney-fire is thundery fire, [it is] also Loong[5] fire. [Although] thundery and Loong fire is quite fierce, [its] power is concentrated [when it] accumulates and slack [when it] disperses. [In fact there is] nothing [that] cannot be restriced [by fire] and [there is] also nothing [that] can be completely restricted [by fire]."

Leigong asked, "Why [is there] production [that] fears restriction and dares not to produce?"

Qibo answered, "Liver-fire produces heart-fire. [If] lung-metal is too effulgent, the liver fears [to be] restricted [by] the lung and dares not to produce heart [-fire]. [As a result,] heart-Qi [will be] weakened and metal [will] restrict liver-wood. Heart-fire produces stomach-earth. [If] kidney-water is too flooding, [heart-fire] fears to produce stomach [-earth]. [As a result,] stomach-Qi [will be] more weakened and [kidney-] water [will] invade stomach-earth. Pericardium-fire produces spleen-earth. If kidney-water is overflowing, [pericardium-fire] dares not to produce spleen [-earth]. [As a result,] spleen-Qi [will be] encumbered and

雷公说："怎么理解克中之生呢？"

岐伯说："肝能克土,土只有得到木才能疏通,这样土才能有生气。脾能克水,水只有得到土才会积蓄,这样土才能有生发的根基。肾能克火,火只有得到水才能相济,这样火才会有神光。心能克金,但肺金只有得到了心火才能得以煅炼。肺能克木,但肝木只有得到了肺金才能砍伐成材,才能削切成器。这不就是克而为生的体现吗?"

雷公说："请说明何谓生不全生。"

岐伯说："所谓生不全生,是专门讲肾水的。各个脏腑没有不从肾中获取资助的。当心得到肾水时,神明才会焕发;当脾得到肾水时,精微才能得以传化和传导;当肺得到肾水时,才能开始清肃和下行;当肝得到肾水时,才会进行谋虑和决断。七腑之中,也没有任何一个不是因为得到了肾水才能进行输布和传化。然而获取得多了,分给的机会就必然会少了。所以亲近于此的,就必然会疏远于彼。对上面优厚的,对下面就必然会轻薄。这就是为什么生发难以完全实现。"

雷公说："请说明何谓克不全克。"

岐伯说："所谓克不全克,只要讲的是肾中之火。肾火易搏动而难宁静,易逆行而难顺行,易上行难下行,所以只要搏动就没有能宁静的,只要一逆行就没有不逆行的,只要一上行就没有不上行的。如果肾火升腾到了心,就会导致烦躁;如果进入到脾,就会造成干涸;如果升入到肺,就会引起咳喘;如果流入肝中,就会引发焚烧;如果冲击了七腑,就会引起干燥和烦渴。虽然肾火是雷火,但也是龙火。龙雷之火,其性虽然猛烈,但是聚集时其力还是专一的,分开时其势就会涣散,虽然没有

[kidney-] water [will] bully spleen-earth. Spleen [-earth] and stomach-earth produce lung-metal. If liver-wood is too hard, spleen [-earth] and stomach [-earth] dare not produce lung [-metal]. [As a result,] lung-Qi [will be] damaged more seriously and [liver-] wood [will] insult spleen [-earth] and stomach [-earth]. Lung-metal produces kidney-water. If heart-fire is too blazing, lung [-metal] fears [to be] restricted [by] heart [-fire] and dares not to produce kidney [-water]. [As a result,] kidney-Qi [will be] withered increasingly and [heart-] fire [will] punish lung-metal. Kidney-water produces liver-wood. If spleen [-earth] and stomach [-earth] are too dry, kidney [-water] fears earth in the spleen and stomach and dares not to produce liver [-wood]. [As a result,] liver-Qi [will be] more withered and earth [in the spleen and stomach will] control kidney-water."

Leigong asked,"How to subdue it?"

Qibo answered, "[Only when] restriction [is] subdued [can] production [be] ensured. [When] production [is ensured, it will] not fear restriction. [Measures should be taken] to assist production [and enable it] to forget restriction. [In such a way] restriction [will] change into production."

Leigong asked, "Good! [If] restriction fears production and dares not to restrict, what will happen?"

Qibo answered, "Exuberance of liver-wood is caused by kidney-water [that is] surging. [When liver-] wood is exuberant, lung-Qi [will be] debilitated. How can soft metal restrict hard wood? Exuberance of earth [in] the spleen and stomach is due to blazing of heart-fire. [When] earth [in the spleen and stomach is] exuberant,

不能克制的,但却没有能够被完全克制的。"

雷公说:"生惧怕克制而不敢生的,又会是怎样的呢?"

岐伯说:"肝木生心火,如果肺金太旺,肝木就会畏惧肺金的克制,就不敢再生心了,心气就会因此而转弱,肺金就开始克制肝木了。心火生胃土,如果肾水太旺,就不敢生胃了,胃气就会因此而变得更虚,肾水就会借机而侵犯胃土。心包之火生脾土,如果肾水太过泛滥,就不敢生脾了,脾气就会因此而遭受困扰,肾水就会借机而欺侮脾土。脾胃之土生肺金,如果肝木太过刚硬,脾胃就会畏惧肝的克制,也就不敢生肺了,肺气就会因此而遭受更大的损害,肝木也会借机而欺辱脾胃。肺金生肾水,如果心火太过沸腾,肺就会畏惧心的克制,也就不敢生肾了,肾气就会因此而日益枯竭,心火就会借机而刑伐肺金。肾水生肝木,如果脾胃太过干燥,肾就会畏惧脾胃之土,就不敢生肝了,肝气就会因此而更加凋零,土就会借机而克制肾水。"

雷公说:"可用什么方法予以控制呢?"

岐伯说:"只有通过控制和克制,才能使其生发,这样的生发就会畏惧克制了。只有通过资助生发,才能使之淡忘其克制,这样克制就能转而为生发了。"

雷公说:"好! 由于克制畏惧生发,因而就不敢克制了。如此又会怎样呢?"

岐伯说:"肝木之所以旺盛,就是因为肾水旺盛。一旦木旺了,肺气就会自行衰弱,柔软的金又怎么能克制木呢? 脾胃之所以土旺盛,就是因为心火旺盛。一旦土气旺盛,肝气就会自行衰弱,在这种情况下僵

liver-Qi [is] spontaneously weakened. How can hard wood restrict scorched earth? Exuberance of kidney-water is due to effulgence of lung-metal. [When kidney-] water is flooding, spleen-earth [will be] naturally depleted. How can poor earth restrict turbulent water? Exuberance of heart-fire is due to prosperity of liver-wood. [When heart-] fire is exuberant, kidney-Qi must [be] weakened. How can weakened water restrict blazing fire? Exuberance of lung-metal is due to fertility of spleen-earth. [When lung-] metal is exuberant, heart-Qi [will be] spontaneously weakened. How can cold fire restrict hard [and strong] metal?"

Leigong asked, "How to control it?"

Qibo answered, "To assist production is unnecessary to control restriction. In this way, weakness [will] eventually become strong because [the power of] restriction can strengthen [the power of] production. [That is why] weakness can develop into exuberance."

Leigong said, "Excellent [explanation]!"

Chen Shiduo's comment, "Production and restriction in the five elements originally cannot be reversed. [The reason why the activities that] cannot be reversed are now reversed [is] to talk about the changes of production and restriction. This chapter mainly talks about changes, but changes are infinite. [So we] should carefully read it."

Notes

[1] In this chapter, the word "produce" mainly means promotion or support.

木能克制焦土吗？肾水之所以旺盛，就是因为肺金旺盛。一旦水气旺盛，脾土就会自行衰薄，在这种情况下衰薄的土能克制湍急的水吗？心火之所以旺盛，就是因为肝木旺盛。一旦火气旺盛，肾气就必然虚弱，在这种情况下虚弱的水能克制烈火吗？肺金之所以旺盛，就是因为脾土旺盛，金气旺则心气自然就会变得懦弱，在这种情况下寒火能克制顽金吗？"

雷公说："用什么方法才能控制呢？"

岐伯说："要救其生发，就不必对其进行控制和克制了，这样弱就会变强。同时，由于克制之力，就更有利于增强其培育和滋生了。这样衰就可以转变为盛了。"

雷公说："好！"

陈士铎评论说："五行的生克，本来是不可颠倒的。不能颠倒而又颠倒了，实际上说的就是生克的变化。本篇专门谈论生克的变化，而变化也是不可穷尽的。应当仔细观察。"

Volume 5

〔2〕 In this sentence，"dead" refers to water that cannot flow；"metal" refers to the lung which is the upper source of water；"spring" refers to the kidney which is the lower source of water.

〔3〕 Shen Ming（神明）literally means spiritual brightness and actually means spirit，intelligence and right way of thinking.

〔4〕 Essential nutrients refer to the best part of water and food that are transformed by the spleen and absorbed mainly by the small intestine.

〔5〕 Please see 〔3〕 in Chapter 26.

小心真主篇第三十九

【原文】

为当问于岐伯曰："物之生也,生于阳。物之成也,成于阴。阳,火也;阴,水也。二者在身藏于何物乎?"

岐伯曰："大哉问也。阴阳有先后天之殊也,后天之阴阳藏于各脏腑,先天之阴阳藏于命门。"

为当曰："命门何物也?"

岐伯曰："命门者,水火之源。水者,阴中之水也;火者,阴中之火也。"

为当曰："水火均属阴,是命门藏阴不藏阳也。其藏阳又何所乎?"

岐伯曰："命门,藏阴即藏阳也。"

为当曰："其藏阴即藏阳之义何居?"

岐伯曰："阴中之水者,真水也;阴中之火者,真火也。真火者,真水之所生;真水者,真火之所生也。水生于火者,火中有阳也。火生于水者,水中有阳也。故命门之火,谓之原气。命门之水,谓之原精。精旺则体强,气旺则形壮。命门水火实藏阴阳,所以为十二经之主也。主者,即十二官之化源也。命门之精气尽,则水火两亡,阴阳间隔,真息不调,人病辄死矣。"

为当曰："阴阳有偏胜,何也?"

Volume 5

【英译】

Chapter 39
The Small Heart [Is] the Genuine Governor

Wei Dang[1] asked Qibo, "The production of [all] things depends on Yang. The development of [all] things depends on Yin. Yang is fire and Yin is water. Where are they located in the human body?"

Qibo answered, "A great question! Yin and Yang are either innate or postnatal. The postnatal Yin and Yang are located in the Zang-organs and Fu-organs [while] the innate Yin and Yang are located in the life gate."

Wei Dang asked, "What is the life gate?"

Qibo answered, "The life gate is the source of water and fire. [The so-called] water refers to water in Yin and [the so-called] fire refers to fire in Yin."

Wei Dang asked, "Both water and fire belong to Yin because the life gate stores Yin but not stores Yang. Where is Yang stored then?"

Qibo answered, "The life gate stores Yin and also Yang."

Wei Dang asked, "What [does it] mean [that the life gate] stores Yin and also Yang?"

岐伯曰:"阴胜者,非阴盛也,命门火微也。阳胜者,非阳盛也,命门水竭也。"

为当曰:"阴胜在下阳胜在上者,何也?"

岐伯曰:"阴胜于下者,水竭其源则阴不归阳矣。阳胜于上者,火衰其本则阳不归阴矣。阳不归阴,则火炎于上而不降。阴不归阳,则水沉于下而不升。可见命门为水火之府也,阴阳之宅也,精气之根也,死生之窦也。"

为当曰:"命门为十二官之主寄于何脏?"

岐伯曰:"七节之旁中有小心,小心即命门也。"

为当曰:"鬲肓之上,中有父母,非小心之谓软?"

岐伯曰:"鬲肓之上,中有父母者,言三焦包络也,非言小心也。小心在心之下,肾之中。"

陈士铎曰:"小心在心肾之中,乃阴阳之中也。阴无阳气则火不生,阳无阴气则水不长。世人错认小心在膈肓之上,此命门真主不明也。谁知小心即命门哉?"

【今译】

为当请问岐伯:"万物的发生,生发于阳;万物的形成,形成于阴。阳是火,阴是水。在人体中,阴和阳这两个元素藏在何处?"

岐伯说:"你提的真是个大问题!阴阳有先天和后天的区别。后天阴阳藏在各个脏腑之中,先天阴阳藏在命门之中。"

Volume 5

Qibo answered, "Water in Yin is the genuine water and fire in Yin is the genuine fire. The genuine fire is produced by genuine water and the genuine water is produced by the genuine fire. [The fact that] water is produced by fire [indicates that] there is Yang in fire [and that] fire is produced by water [indicates that] there is Yang in water. Thus fire in the life gate is called original Qi and water in the life gate is called original essence. [When] essence is exuberant, the body is strong; [when] Qi is exuberant, the body is sturdy. In fact water and fire in the life gate store Yin and Yang, and therefore are the governors of the twelve meridians. [The so-called] governor refers to the transformation source of the twelve organs. [When] essential Qi in the life gate is exhausted, water and fire [will] perish. [If] Yin and Yang are separated from each other, the genuine Qi [will be] imbalanced and man [will contract] disease and die."

Wei Dang asked, "Why are Yin and Yang inclined to exuberance?"

Qibo answered, "[If] Yin [is] inclined to exuberance, [it is actually] not exuberance of Yin, but faintness of fire in the life gate. [If] Yang [is] inclined to exuberance, [it is actually] not exuberance of Yang, but exhaustion of water in the life gate."

Wei Dang asked, "Why is exuberant Yin in the lower while exuberant Yang is in the upper?"

Qibo answered, "[When] Yin is exuberant in the lower, the

为当问："什么是命门呢?"

岐伯说："命门是水火之源。水是阴中之水,火是阴中之火。"

为当问："水火均属阴,那么命门就藏阴而不藏阳了。阳该藏在何处呢?"

岐伯说："命门藏阴,但也藏阳。"

为当问："命门藏阴也藏阳的意义在哪里呢?"

岐伯说："阴中之水是真水,阴中之火是真火。真火是由真水所生的,真水是由真火所主的。水生于火,所以火中是有阳的;火生于水,所以水中也是有阳的。所以命门之火称为原气,命门之水称为原精。当精气旺盛的时候,身体就会变得强健;当原气旺盛的时候,身形就会变得强壮。命门中的水火,其实就藏有阴阳,所以就成为十二经脉之主了。所谓主,指的是十二经脉化生的源泉。如果命门的精气耗尽了,水火就会同时消亡。当阴阳相互发生间隔,真气衰微,气息不调,人就会突发死亡。"

为当问："阴阳有偏胜之势,这是什么原因呢?"

岐伯说："阴胜,并不只是阴的旺盛,而是命门之火的衰微所致;阳胜并不只是阳的旺盛,而是命门之水枯竭所致。"

为当问："阴胜在下而阳胜在上,这又是什么原因呢?"

岐伯说："阴胜之所以在下,是因为水源的枯竭而导致阴不能归于阳;阳胜之所以在上,是因为火之本源的衰竭而导致阳不能归于阴。阳不能归于阴,火就会上炎而不能下降;阴不能归于阳,水就会沉于下而不能上升。可见,命门就是水火之府,就是阴阳之宅,就是精气之根,就

Volume 5

source of water [will be] exhausted and Yang cannot be attached to Yin. [If] Yang cannot be attached to Yin, fire [will] flame up and cannot descend; [if] Yin cannot be attached to Yang, water [will] descend and cannot rise up. [It is] proved [that] the life gate is the palace of water and fire, the cabinet of Yin and Yang, the root of essential Qi and the gate of life and death."

Wei Dang asked, "The life gate is the governor of the twelve organs. In which organ does it stay?"

Qibo answered, "There is a small heart beside the seven sections[2]. The [so-called] small heart refers to the life gate."

Wei Dang asked, "Above the diaphragm are parents[3]. Is it not the small heart?"

Qibo said, "[The saying that] above the diaphragm are parents refers to the triple energizer and pericardium, not the small heart. The small heart [is located] below the heart and in the kidney."

Chen Shiduo's comment, "The small heart [is located] in between the heart and kidney, [that is to say it is located] in between Yin and Yang. [If] there is no Yang Qi in Yin, fire cannot be produced; [if] there is no Yin Qi in Yang, water cannot be produced. People in this world misdeems [that] the small heart [is located] above the diaphragm because [they are] unclear [that] the life gate is the genuine governor. Who knows [that] the small heart is [actually] the life gate?"

是死生之门户。"

为当问："命门是十二经脉之主，位居于哪一脏呢？"

岐伯说："命门位居于七节的旁边，其中有一小心，这个小心就是命门。"

为当问："隔膜和膏肓之上，有父有母，这难道不是小心吗？"

岐伯说："隔膜和膏肓之上，其中是有父有母，指的是三焦和包络，不是指的小心。小心位于心之下而肾之中。"

陈士铎评论说："小心位于心肾之中，也就是在阴阳之中。阴中如果没有阳气，火就不能生；阳中如果没有阴气，水就不能长。世人误以为小心就在隔膜和膏肓之上，这是因为不明白命门这一真主的道理。如果不明白这一道理，又怎么能知道小心就是命门呢？"

Volume 5

Notes

[1] Wei Dang (为当) was the minister of Yellow Emperor.

[2] The seven sections refer to the seven vertebrae above the coccygeal vertebra.

[3] Parents here refer to the triple energizer and pericardium.

水不克火篇第四十

【原文】

大封司马问于岐伯曰："水克火者也，人有饮水而火不解者，岂火不能制水乎？"

岐伯曰："人生于火，养于水。水养火者，先天之真水也。水克火者，后天之邪水也。饮水而火热不解者，外水不能救内火也。"

大封司马曰："余终不解其义，幸明示之。"

岐伯曰："天开于子，地辟于丑，人生于寅，寅实有火也。天地以阳气为生，以阴气为杀。阳即火，阴即水也。然而火不同，有形之火，离火也。无形之火，乾火也。有形之火，水之所克。无形之火，水之所生。饮水而火不解者，无形之火得有形之水而不相入也。岂惟不能解，且有激之而火炽者。"

大封司马曰："然则水不可饮乎？"

岐伯曰："水可少饮以解燥，不可畅饮以解氛。"

大封司马曰："此何故乎？"

岐伯曰："无形之火旺，则有形之火微。无形之火衰则有形之火盛。火得水反炽，必多饮水也，水多则无形之火因之益微矣。无形之火微，而有形之火愈增酷烈之势，此外水之所以不能救内火，非水之不克火也。"

Volume 5

【英译】

Chapter 40
Inability of Water to Restrict Fire

Dafeng Sima[1] asked Qibo, "[When] water restricts fire, fire cannot be resolved [after] drinking water. Does [it indicate that] fire cannot control water?"

Qibo answered, "Man depend on fire to live and water to nourish. The water [that] nourishes fire is the innate water. The water [that] restricts fire is the postnatal water [which is] evil water. [If] fire and heat cannot be resolved [after] drinking water, [it indicates that] external water cannot save internal fire."

Dafeng Sima said, "I still could not understand it. Please explain it [for me]."

Qibo answered, "The sky was separated at [the time of] Zi (23:00 – 1:00), the earth was separated at [the time of] Chou (1:00 – 3:00) and a man was born at [the time of] Yin (3:00 – 5:00). [In the time of] Yin (3:00 – 5:00), there is fire [in it]. [In] the sky and earth, Yang Qi [is responsible for] production and Yin Qi [is responsible for] killing. Yang is fire and Yin is water. However fire is different. Visible fire is Li[2] fire [and] invisible fire is Qian[3] fire. Visible fire can be restricted by water [while] invisible fire is produced by water. [If] fire is not resolved [after] drinking water, [it is due to] inability of invisible fire and visible water to coordinate [with each other]. [It is] not only unable to resolve

大封司马曰："何以治之？"

岐伯曰："补先天无形之水，则无形之火自息矣，不可见其火热，饮水不解，劝多饮以速亡也。"

陈士铎曰："水分有形无形，何疑于水哉？水克有形之火，难克无形之火，故水不可饮也。说得端然实理，非泛然而论也。"

【今译】

大封司马请问岐伯："水能克火，有人饮了水但火却不能解除的，这岂不是水不能克火吗？"

岐伯说："人虽然生于火，但却要依靠水来滋养。水能滋养火的，是先天之真水；水能克制火的，是后天的邪气之水。饮水之后但火却不能解除的，这是因为外水不能救内火的缘故。"

大封司马说："我还是不理解这个意思，请再予以详细说明。"

岐伯说："天开于子时，地辟于丑时，人生于寅时，而寅时其实是有火的。天地以阳气为生发之机，以阴气为消杀之际。阳是火，阴是水。但火则各有不同。有形之火，是离火；无形之火，是乾火。有形之火是可以由水来克制的。无形之火是可以由水来生发的。饮水后火却不能解除的，这是无形之火得到了有形之水，却不相融入的缘故。在这种情况下，饮水不仅不能解除火，而且还会激发火，从而使火更加炽热。"

大封司马问："这是不是意味着不能饮水呢？"

岐伯说："可以少量饮水以消解燥热，但却不能通过畅饮来解除

[thirst], but also stimulate [fire] to blaze."

Dafeng Sima asked, "[Does it mean that] water cannot be drunken?"

Qibo answered, "Water can be drunken less to resolve thirst but cannot drunken more to resolve heat."

Dafeng Sima asked, "What is the reason?"

Qibo answered, "[When] invisible fire is effulgent, visible fire is faint; [when] invisible fire is debilitated, visible fire is exuberant. [When] fire has got water, [it will be] blazing and more water should be drunken. [When] more water [is drunken], invisible fire [will become] more faint. [When] invisible fire is faint, visible fire [will] increasingly flame and blaze. That is why external water cannot save internal fire. [It does not mean that] water cannot restrict fire."

Dafeng Sima asked, "How to treat it?"

Qibo answered, "[When] the innate invisible water is supplemented, invisible fire [will] distinguish spontaneously. [If] heat cannot be resolved by drinking water, [you] cannot persuade [the patient] to drink more water [because it may] hasten demise."

Chen Shiduo's comment, "Water can be divided into visible water and invisible water. Why [is there] doubt about water? Water can restrict visible fire and cannot restrict invisible fire. That is why [it is forbidden] to drink [more] water. This analysis is clear and reasonable, not just a general discussion."

火热。"

大封司马问："这是什么原因呢？"

岐伯说："如果无形之火旺盛了，有形之火就会衰微；如果无形之火衰微了，有形之火就会旺盛。火得到了水，反而炽热，这必然是饮水过多的缘故。如果饮水过多，无形之火就会日益衰微。如果无形之火衰微了，有形之火的酷烈之势就会日益增强，这就是为什么外水不能救内火，并不是水不能克火的缘故。"

大封司马问："用什么方法可以治疗呢？"

岐伯说："只要补益了先天的无形之水，无形之火就会自行解除。火热是不可以出现的，通过饮水是不能解除的。如果劝病人多饮水，就会导致其快速的死亡。"

陈士铎评论说："水可分为有形之水与无形之水，怎么能怀疑水呢？水可以克制有形之火，但却难以克制无形之火，所以是不能过多饮水的。本文谈的颇为实实在在，并非泛泛而论。"

Notes

[1] Dafeng Sima（大封司马）was the title of an official in ancient China.

[2] Li（离）refers to Li Gua（离卦，Li Diagram），the sixth diagram in the *Yi Jing*（《易经》），representing fire.

[3] Please see [2] in Chapter 14.

三关升降篇第四十一

【原文】

巫咸问曰："人身三关在何经乎？"

岐伯曰："三关者，河车之关也。上玉枕，中肾脊、下尾闾。"

巫咸曰："三关何故关人生死乎？"

岐伯曰："关人生死，故名曰关。"

巫咸曰："请问生死之义。"

岐伯曰："命门者，水中火也。水火之中实藏先天之气，脾胃之气后天之气也。先天之气不交于后天，则先天之气不长。后天之气不交于先天，则后天之气不化。二气必昼夜交，而后生生不息也。然而后天之气必得先天之气先交而后生。而先天之气必由下而上，升降诸脾胃，以分散于各脏腑。三关者，先天之气所行之径道也。气旺则升降无碍，气衰则阻，阻则人病矣。"

巫咸曰："气衰安旺乎？"

岐伯曰："助命门之火，益肾阴之水，则气自旺矣。"

巫咸曰："善。"

陈士铎曰："人有三关，故可生可死。然生死实在先天，不在后天也。篇中讲后天返死而生，非爱生而恶死。人能长守先天，何恶先天之

Volume 5

【英译】

Chapter 41
Ascendance and Descendence of the Three Passes

Wuxian[1] asked, "In which meridian are the three passes located?"

Qibo answered, "The three passes are the passes in Heche[2]. [The one in] the upper [is] Yuzhen[3], [the one in] the middle [is] Zhongji[4] [and the one in] the lower [is] Weilü[5]."

Wuxian asked, "Why are the three passes related to life and death of human beings?"

Qibo answered, "[Because it is] related to life and death of human beings, that is why it is called pass."

Wuxian asked, "What is the meaning of life and death?"

Qibo answered, "The life gate is fire in water. In fact there is innate Qi in water and fire. Qi in the spleen and stomach is postnatal Qi. [If] innate Qi does not coordinate with postnatal Qi, it cannot grow; [if] postnatal Qi does not coordinate with innate Qi, it cannot transform. [Only when these] two [kinds of] Qi coordinate with each other day and night can [they] exist eternally. Besides, [only when] postnatal Qi coordinates with innate Qi [can it] grow. Furthermore, [only when] innate Qi rises from the lower to the upper and then descends to the spleen and stomach [can it] spread to each Zang-organ and Fu-organ. The three passes are the roads for innate Qi to flow. [When] Qi is strong, there is no block

能死乎?"

【今译】

巫咸问道:"人身的三关位于哪条经脉?"

岐伯说:"所谓三关,指的是河车中的三关,包括上部的玉枕关,中部的肾脊关和下部的尾闾关。"

巫咸问:"三关为什么会关系到人的生死呢?"

岐伯说:"因为关系到人的生死,所以才称其为关。"

巫咸说:"请问生死的含义是什么呢?"

岐伯说:"命门是水中之火。水火之中实际上隐藏有先天之气。脾胃中的气是后天之气。如果先天之气不与后天之气相交,先天之气就不能得以长;如果后天之气不与先天之气相交,后天之气就不能得以化。所以先天之气与后天之气必须昼夜相交,只有如此才能生生不息。就后天之气而言,必须先与先天之气相交,才能得以生发。就先天之气而言,必然由下向上升发,然后再降到脾胃,才能因此而分散到各个脏腑。而三关,则是先天之气运行时所必须通过的路径。所以如果气旺,其上升和下降都不会有任何障碍。但如果气衰了,其上升和下降都会受阻,受阻后就会引发疾病。"

巫咸问:"如果气衰弱了,怎么才能使其旺盛呢?"

岐伯说:"只有通过资助命门之火和补益肾阴之水,气才会自行旺盛。"

巫咸说:"好!"

in ascending and descending. [When] Qi is debilitated, [there will be] block [in Qi movement] and block [in Qi movement will] cause disease."

Wuxian asked, "How to invigorate Qi [when it is] debilitated?"

Qibo answered, "[Only when] fire in the life gate is assisted and water in kidney Yin is replenished [can] Qi invigorate spontaneously."

Wuxian said, "Excellent [explanation]! "

Chen Shiduo's comment, "There are three passes in the human body and therefore there is life and death. However life and death actually depend on the innate, not the postnatal. This chapter talks about resuscitation from death, not just loving life and detesting death. [If] man can hold fast to the innate, how could there be worry about death of the postnatal?"

Notes

[1] Wuxian (巫咸) was a minister of Yellow Emperor.

[2] Heche (河车), literally river cart, is a concept in alchemy which refers to genuine Qi stored in the kidneys that are regarded as the palaces of water. In the human body, there are two kidneys located in the left and right sides of the waist, like the sun and the moon moving side by side in the sky, and also like two wheels in the cart. That is why this concept is so named.

[3] Yuzhen (玉枕), literally jade pillow, refers to the protruding tip of the occipital bone.

[4] Shenji (肾脊), literally kidney and spine, refers to the region

陈士铎评论说:"人有三关,所以才会有生有死。但生死实际上取决于先天,而不是后天。本文中谈到后天能去死而复生,这不是爱好生厌恶死的意思。如果人能一直固守先天,怎么会恐惧先天能导致死亡呢?"

between the scapulae.

    ［5］ Weilü （尾闾）, literally tail middle，refers to the lowest region of the backbone.

表微篇第四十二

【原文】

奚仲问于岐伯曰："天师《阴阳别论》中有阴结、阳结之言。结在脏乎？抑结在腑乎？"

岐伯曰："合脏腑言之也。"

奚仲曰："脏阴腑阳，阴结在脏，阳结在腑乎？"

岐伯曰："阴结阳结者，言阴阳之气结也。合脏腑言之，非阳结而阴不结，阴结而阳不结也。阴阳之道，彼此相根，独阳不结，独阴亦不结也。"

奚仲曰："《阴阳别论》中，又有刚与刚之言。言脏乎？言腑乎？"

岐伯曰："专言脏腑也，阴阳气不和，脏腑有过刚之失，两刚相遇，阳过旺阴不相接也。"

奚仲曰："脏之刚乎？抑腑之刚乎？"

岐伯曰："脏刚传腑，则刚在脏也。腑刚传脏，则刚在腑也。"

奚仲曰："《阴阳别论》中又有阴搏阳搏之言，亦言脏腑乎？"

岐伯曰："阴搏阳搏者言十二经之脉，非言脏腑也。虽然十二脏腑之阴阳不和，而后十二经脉始现阴阳之搏，否则搏之象不现于脉也。然则阴搏阳搏，言脉而即言脏腑也。"

奚仲曰："善。"

Volume 5

【英译】

Chapter 42
External Faintness

Xizhong[1] asked Qibo, "In Celestial Master's Special Discussion about Yin and Yang, there are [concepts about] Yin connection and Yang connection. Is such connection in the Zang-organs or the Fu-organs?"

Qibo answered, "[Such a] discussion is combined with the Zang-organs and Fu-organs."

Xizhong asked, "The Zang-organs [belong to] Yin and the Fu-organs [belong to] Yang. Is Yin connection in the Zang-organs and Yang connection in the Fu-organs?"

Qibo answered, "[The so-called] Yin connection and Yang connection refer to Qi connection in Yin and Yang. [In terms of] combination with the Zang-organs and Fu-organs, [it does] not mean [that there is] no Yin connection [when there is] Yang connection [and there is] no Yang connection [when there is] Yin connection. The law of Yin and Yang [indicates that they] depend on each other. [Thus] neither isolated Yang nor isolated Yin can connect [with each other].

Xizhong asked, "In *Special Discussion about Yin and Yang*, there is [discussion about] hardness and hardness. Does [it] refer to the Zang-organs or Fu-organs?"

Qibo answered, "[It] just refers to the Zang-organs or Fu-

陈士铎曰："阴结、阳结、阴搏、阳搏,俱讲得微妙。"

【今译】

　　奚仲请问岐伯:"在《阴阳别论》中,天师谈到了阴结和阳结的问题。到底是结在脏呢? 还是结在腑呢?"

　　岐伯说:"我是将脏腑融合在一起而谈的。"

　　奚仲说:"脏是阴,腑是阳,是不是阴结在脏而阳结在腑呢?"

　　岐伯说:"所谓阴结与阳结,说的是阴阳之气的交结。就脏腑融合在一起来说,并不是阳结而阴不结,也不是阴结而阳不结。所谓阴阳之道,说的就是彼此相互为根,所以独阳不能结,独阴也不能结。"

　　奚仲说:"在《阴阳别论》中,又有'刚与刚'之说,是说脏呢? 还是说腑呢?"

　　岐伯说:"是专门说脏腑的。如果阴阳之气不和,脏腑就会有太过刚硬的过失。脏的刚硬与腑的刚硬相遇,阳就会过旺,阴就不能与之相接。"

　　奚仲说:"到底是脏刚硬呢? 还是腑刚硬呢?"

　　岐伯说:"如果脏刚硬了,并且传给了腑,那么刚硬的发生就在于脏;如果腑刚硬了,并且传给了脏,那么刚硬的发生就在于腑。"

　　奚仲说:"《阴阳别论》中又有阴搏、阳搏之说,说的也是脏腑吗?"

　　岐伯说:"所谓阴搏和阳搏,说的是十二经脉,不是脏腑。如果十二脏腑中的阴阳不和,十二经脉就会出现阴搏和阳搏。否则搏结的现象就不会出现在经脉上。所以阴搏阳搏之说,既是说经脉,也是说

organs. [If] Qi in Yin and Yang is in disharmony, there is error of excessive hardness in the Zang-organs or Fu-organs. [When] double hardness meets with each other, Yin cannot connect [with others if] Yang is too exuberant. "

Xizhong asked, "Is [it] hardness of the Zang-organs or hardness of the Fu-organs?"

Qibo answered, "[If] hardness of the Zang-organs is transferred to the Fu-organs, the hardness is in the the Zang-organs; [if] hardness of the Fu-organs is transferred to the Zang-organs, the hardness is in the Fu-organs. "

Xizhong asked, "In *Special Discussion about Yin and Yang*, there is [discussion about] Yin contention and Yang contention. Does [it] refer to the Zang-organs or Fu-organs?"

Qibo answered, "[The so-called] Yin contention and Yang connection refer to the twelve meridians, not just the Zang-organs or Fu-organs. However, [only when] Yin and Yang in the twelve Zang-organs or Fu-organs are in disharmony can Yin and Yang in the twelve meridians begin to contend [with each other]. Otherwise the phenomenon of contention will not appear in the pulse. Thus Yin contention and Yang contention refer to the meridians and also the Zang-organs or Fu-organs. "

Xizhong said, "Excellent [explanation]!"

Chen Shiduo's comment, " The discussion about Yin connection, Yang connection, Yin contention and Yang contention is thorough and excellent."

脏腑。"

奚仲说："好！"

陈士铎评论说："阴结、阳结、阴搏、阳搏，都讲得很细微而精妙。"

Volume 5

Notes

［1］ Xizhong（奚仲）was a minister of Yellow Emperor who created cart.

呼吸篇第四十三

【原文】

雷公问于岐伯曰："人气之呼吸应天地之呼吸乎？"

岐伯曰："天地人同之。"

雷公曰："心肺主呼，肾肝主吸，是呼出乃心肺也，吸入乃肾肝也。何有时呼出不属心肺而属肾肝，吸入不属肾肝而属心肺乎？"

岐伯曰："一呼不再呼，一吸不再吸，故呼中有吸，吸中有呼也。"

雷公曰："请悉言之。"

岐伯曰："呼出者，阳气之出也。吸入者，阴气之入也。故呼应天，而吸应地。呼不再呼，呼中有吸也。吸不再吸，吸中有呼也。故呼应天而亦应地，吸应地而亦应天。所以呼出心也、肺也，从天言之也；吸入肾也、肝也，从地言之也。呼出肾也、肝也，从地言之也；吸入心也、肺也，从天言之也。盖独阳不生，呼中有吸者，阳中有阴也；独阴不长，吸中有呼者，阴中有阳也。天之气不降则地之气不升。地之气不升则天之气不降。天之气下降者，即天之气呼出也。地之气上升者，即地之气吸入也。故呼出心肺，阳气也，而肾肝阴气辄随阳而俱出矣。吸入肾肝，阴气也，而心肺阳气辄随阴而俱入矣。所以阴阳之气，虽有呼吸而阴阳之根无间隔也。呼吸之间虽有出入而阴阳之本无两歧也。"

雷公曰："善。"

Volume 5

【英译】

Chapter 43
Inhalation and Exhalation

Leigong asked Qibo, "Do exhalation and inhalation of human beings correspond to that of the sky and earth?"

Qibo answered, "The sky, earth and human beings are the same."

Leigong asked, "The heart and lung govern exhalation, the kidney and liver govern inhalation. Therefore exhalation is related to the heart and lung, inhalation is related to the kidney and liver. Why sometimes is exhalation not related to the heart and lung but related to the kidney and liver, and inhalation not related to the kidney and liver but related to the heart and lung?"

Qibo answered, "Once [there is] exhalation [there] cannot [be] exhalation again; once [there is] inhalation [there] cannot [be] inhalation again. Thus there is inhalation in exhalation and exhalation in inhalation."

Leigong asked, "Please explain in detail."

Qibo answered, "Exhalation is outflow of Yang Qi and inhalation is inflow of Yin Qi. Therefore exhalation corresponds to the sky and inhalation corresponds to the earth. Once [there is] exhalation [there] cannot [be] exhalation again, [indicating that] there is inhalation in exhalation; once [there is] inhalation [there]

陈士铎曰："呼中有吸，吸中有呼，是一是二，人可参天地也。"

【今译】

雷公请问岐伯："人的呼吸对应于天地的呼吸吗?"

岐伯说："天、地、人的呼吸是相同的。"

雷公说："心肺主呼气，肾肝主吸气，所以呼出气是由心肺主持的，吸入气是由肾肝主持的。为什么有时呼出之气不属于心肺，而属于肾肝呢? 为什么有时吸入之气不属于肾肝，而属于心肺呢?"

岐伯说："呼吸的时候，一旦呼出气就不能再继续呼出，一旦吸入气后也不能再继续吸入，所以呼出中有吸入，吸入中也有呼出。"

雷公说："请予以详细说明。"

岐伯说："呼出的气是阳气的排出，吸入的气是阴气纳入。所以呼出之气对应于天，而吸入之气则对应于地。因此，一旦呼出气之后就不能再呼出了，因为呼出中也有吸入;一旦吸入之后也不能再吸入，因为吸入中也有呼出。因此呼出之气既对应于天，也对应于地;而吸入之气既对应于地，也对应于天。所以，呼出气与心和肺有关，这是就天而言的;而吸入则与肾和肝有关，这是就地而言的。呼出与肾和肝有关，这是就地而言的;而吸入则与心和肺有关，这是就天而言的。因为孤阳不生，所以呼出之中有吸入，就是阳中有阴的体现;由于孤阴不长，所以吸入之中有呼出，就是阴中有阳的体现。如果苍天之气不降，大地之气就不能上升;如果大地之气不升，苍天之气也不能下降。如果苍天之气下降，实际上就是苍天之气的呼出;如果大地之气上升，实际上就是大地

cannot [be] inhalation again, [indicating that] there is exhalation in inhalation. That is why exhalation corresponds to the sky and also to the earth and inhalation corresponds to the earth and also to the sky. For this reason, exhalation originates from the heart and lung in terms of the sky; inhalation originates from the kidney and liver in terms of the earth. [That is to say that] exhalation starts from the kidney and liver in terms of the earth and inhalation starts from the heart and lung in terms of the sky. Because isolated Yang cannot exist and therefore there is inhalation in exhalation and there is Yin in Yang; [for] isolated Yin cannot grow and therefore there is exhalation in inhalation and there is Yang in Yin. [If] Qi in the sky does not descend, Qi in the earth is unable to rise; [if] Qi in the earth does not rise, Qi in the sky is unable to descend. [The fact that] Qi in the sky descends indicates [that] Qi in the sky exhales [and that] Qi in the earth rises indicates [that] Qi in the earth inhales. Thus [Qi] exhales from the heart and lung is Yang Qi, and Yin Qi from the kidney and liver flows out together with Yang [Qi]; [Qi that] inhales into the kidney and liver is Yin Qi, and Yang Qi from the heart and lung flows into [the body] together with Yin [Qi]. Although there is exhalation and inhalation [of Qi in Yin and Yang], there is no interval in the root of Yin and Yang; [although] there is outflow and inflow in exhalation and inhalation, there is no difference in the root of Yin and Yang. "

Leigong said, "Excellent [explanation]!"

Chen Shiduo's comment, "There is inhalation in exhalation and

之气的吸入。所以由心和肺而呼出的气,就是阳气,肝和肾中的阴气也会随着阳气而一同出来;由肝和肾而吸入的气,就是阴气,心和肺中的阳气也会随着阴气而一同进入。所以,虽然阴阳之气有呼出也有吸入,但是阴阳之根却没有任何的间隔;虽然呼吸之间既有出来也有进入,但是阴阳之本却不存在实质差异。"

雷公说:"好!"

陈士铎评论说:"呼出中有吸入,吸入中有呼出。这种情况既可以视为一,也可以看作二,因为人是可以与天地相应的。"

there is exhalation in inhalation. [It seems] to be one [but actually] are two, [indicating that] man can integrate with the sky and earth."

脉动篇第四十四

【原文】

雷公问于岐伯曰："手太阴肺、足阳明胃、足少阴肾，三经之脉常动不休者何也?"

岐伯曰："脉之常动不休者，不止肺、胃、肾也。"

雷公曰："何以见之?"

岐伯曰："四末阴阳之会者，气之大络也。四街者，气之曲径也。周流一身，昼夜环转，气无一息之止，脉无一晷之停也。肺、胃、肾脉独动者，胜于各脏腑耳。非三经之气独动不休也。夫气之在脉也，有清气中之，有浊气中之，邪气中之也。清气中在上，浊气中在下，此皆客气也。见于脉中，决于气口。气口虚，补而实之，气口盛，泻而泄之。"

雷公曰："十二经动脉之穴可悉举之乎?"

岐伯曰："手厥阴心包经，动脉在手之劳宫也。手太阴肺经，动脉在手之太渊也。手少阴心经，动脉在手之阴郄也。足太阴脾经，动脉在腹冲门也。足厥阴肝经，动脉在足之太冲也。足少阴肾经，动脉在足之太溪也。手少阳三焦经，动脉在面之和髎也。手太阳小肠经，动脉在项之天窗也。手阳明大肠经，动脉在手之阳溪也。足太阳膀胱经，动脉在足之委中也。足少阳胆经，动脉在足之悬钟也。足阳明胃经，动脉在足之冲阳也。各经时动时止，不若胃为六腑之原，肺为五脏之主，肾为十

Volume 5

【英译】

Chapter 44
Merdian Movement

Leigong asked Qibo, "Why do the three meridians, the lung meridian of hand-Taiyin, the stomach meridian of foot-Yangming and the kidney meridian of foot-Shaoyin, often move and never stop?"

Qibo answered, "The meridians [that] always move and never stop are not just [that of] the lung, the stomach and the kidney."

Leigong asked, "What is the reason?"

Qibo answered, "Communication of Yin [Qi] and Yang [Qi] at the distal regions of the four limbs [are] the large collaterals of Qi. The four streets[1] [are] the roads [along which] Qi moves. [Qi] flows in the whole body day and night. [In flowing,] Qi never stops and meridians never cease. [Among all the meridians, there are] only pulsations in the lung, stomach and kidney meridians, quite outripping the other meridians. [In fact there are] not only constant pulsations in these three meridians. Qi [is flowing] in the meridians, [during which] evil Qi invades, and so do lucid Qi and turbid Qi. [Usually] evil Qi invades the middle [parts of the meridians], lucid Qi invades the upper [parts of the meridians] and turbid Qi invades the lower [parts of the meridians], all [of which] are evil Qi. [Invasion is] seen in the meridians and made at Qikou[2]. [If the meridian at] Qikou is weak, [it should be]

二经之海,各常动不休也。"

陈士铎曰:"讲脉之动处,俱有条理,非无因之文也。"

【今译】

雷公请问岐伯:"手太阴肺经、足阳明胃经、足少阴肾经,这三条经脉经常搏动而不休,这是为什么呢?"

岐伯说:"经脉经常搏动而不休,这种情况并不仅限于肺经、胃经和肾经。"

雷公说:"为什么会这样呢?"

岐伯说:"阴阳在四肢的交会之处,是气的大络。人体的四大气街(即头部、胸部、腹部和胫部),是气蜿蜒运行的路径。气在人体循环往复地流行,昼夜环转不休,所以气的运行一分一秒都不会停止,经脉的循行也没有一时一刻的停止。但只有肺经、胃经和肾经的脉搏跳动不止,所以其运动胜于各个脏腑的脉象,并非只有这三条经脉之气才能独自运动不息。当气在脉中的时候,有时会遭受清气的侵袭,有时会遭受浊气的侵害,有时会遭受邪气的攻击。清邪侵袭人体之上,浊邪侵害人体之下,这都是外来之邪气。其对人体的侵害体现在脉中,开始于气口。如果气口虚弱,可以通过补法予以充实;如果气口旺盛,可以通过泻法予以减少。"

雷公说:"可以列举出十二经动脉的穴位吗?"

岐伯说:"手厥阴心包经,其动脉位于手心中的劳宫穴;手太阴肺

strengthened by tonification; [if the meridian at] Qikou is strong, [it should be] reduced through purgation."

Leigong asked, "Could the acupoints at the pulsations of the twelve meridians be listed?"

Qibo answered, "The pulsation of the pericardium meridian of hand-Jueyin [is located] in [the acupoint named] Laogong (PC 8) in the palm; the pulsation of the lung meridian of hand-Taiyin [is located] in [the acupoint named] Taiyuan (LU 9) at the wrist; the pulsation of the heart meridian of hand-Shaoyin [is located] in [the acupoint named] Yinxi (HT 6) at hand; the pulsation of the spleen meridian of foot-Taiyin [is located] in [the acupoint named] Chongmen (SP 12) at the abdomen; the pulsation of the liver meridian of hand-Jueyin [is located] in [the acupoint named] Taichong (LR 3) at the foot; the pulsation of the kidney meridian of foot-Shaoyin [is located] in [the acupoint named] Taixi (KI 3) at the foot; the pulsation of the triple energizer meridian of hand-Shaoyang [is located] in [the acupoint named] Heliao (TE 22) at the face; the pulsation of the small intestine meridian of hand-Taiyang [is located] in [the acupoint named] Tianchuang (SI 16) at the neck; the pulsation of the large intestine meridian of hand-Yangming [is located] in [the acupoint named] Yangxi (LI 5) at the hand; the pulsation of the bladder meridian of foot-Taiyang [is located] in [the acupoint named] Weizhong (BL 40) at the foot; the pulsation of the gallbladder meridian of foot-Shaoyang [is located] in [the acupoint named] Xuanzhong (GB 39) at the foot; and the pulsation of the stomach meridian of foot-Yangming [is located] in [the acupoint named] Chongyang (ST 42) at the foot.

经,其动脉位于手腕部的太渊穴;手少阴心经,其动脉位于手部的阴郄穴;足太阴脾经,其动脉位于腹部的冲门穴;足厥阴肝经,其动脉位于足部的太冲穴;足少阴肾经,其动脉位于足部的太溪穴;手少阳三焦经,其动脉位于面部的和髎穴;手太阳小肠经,其动脉位于项部的天窗穴;手阳明大肠经,其动脉位于手部的阳溪穴;足太阳膀胱经,其动脉位于足部的委中穴;足少阳胆经,其动脉位于足部的悬钟穴;足阳明胃经,其动脉位于足部的冲阳穴。各条经脉有时搏动有时停止,而不像作为六腑之原的胃经、作为五脏之主的太阴肺经和作为十二经之海的少阴肾经,经常搏动而不休。"

陈士铎评论说:"本文所谈到的有关经脉搏动之处,都很有条理,并不是没有因由的论述。"

Each ⌈of these⌉ meridians now move and then cease, not just like the stomach ⌈meridian which is⌉ the source of the six Fu-organs, the lung ⌈meridian which is⌉ the governor of the five Zang-organs and the kidney ⌈meridian which is⌉ the sea of the twelve meridians ⌈that⌉ constantly move and never stop. "

Chen Shiduo's comment, "Description about the places ⌈where⌉ the meridians pulsate is quite reasonable, absolutely no fabrication."

Notes

⌈1⌉ Street here refers to Qi Street, please see ⌈12⌉ in Chapter 17.

⌈2⌉ Qikou (气口), literally orifice of Qi, also known as Cunkou (寸口, literally inch orifice) and Maikou (脉口, literally vessel or meridian orifice), is located in the place at the wrist where the radial artery pulsates.

瞳子散大篇第四十五

【原文】

云师问于岐伯曰："目病，瞳子散大者何也？"

岐伯曰："必得之内热多饮也。"

云师曰："世人好饮亦常耳，未见瞳子皆散大也。"

岐伯白："内热者，气血之虚也。气血虚，则精耗矣。五脏六腑之精皆上注于目，瞳子尤精之所注也。精注瞳子，而目明，精不注瞳子，而目暗。今瞳子散大则视物必无准矣，"

云师曰："然往往视小为大也。"

岐伯曰："瞳子之系通于脑。脑热则瞳子亦热，热极而瞳子散大矣。夫瞳子之精，神水也。得脑气之热，则水中无非火气，火欲爆而光不收，安得不散大乎？"

云师曰："何火之虐乎？"

岐伯曰："必饮火酒兼食辛热之味也。火酒大热，得辛热之味以助之则益热矣。且辛之气散，而火酒者，气酒也，亦主散。况火酒至阳之味，阳之味必升于头面，火热之毒真归于脑中矣。脑中之精，最恶散而最易散也。得火酒辛热之气，有随入随散者，脑气既散于中，而瞳子散大应于外矣。彼气血未虚者，脑气尚不至尽散也，故瞳子亦无散大之象。然目则未有不昏者也。"

Volume 5

【英译】

Chapter 45
Dilation of Pupils

Yunshi asked Qibo, "Why are the pupils dilated [when] the eye is in disorder?"

Qibo answered, "[It] must be caused by internal heat and excessive drinking [of water]."

Yunshi said, "[It is] quite normal [that] people in this world like to drink water. [I have] never seen any dilation of pupils [due to drinking water]."

Qibo said, "Internal heat [indicates] deficiency of Qi and blood. Deficiency of Qi and blood will [cause] exhaustion of essence. Essence from the five Zang-organs and six Fu-organs all rises up to infuse into the eyes. The pupils are the major areas [into which] essence infuses. [When] essence has infused into the pupils, the eyes are bright; [if] essence does not infuse into the pupils, the eyes will be dull. Now the pupils are dilated, [the eyes] certainly cannot see things clearly."

Yunshi said, "However small [things are] often seen as large."

Qibo said, "The pupils are connected with the brains. [If there is] heat [in] the brains, [there is] also heat [in] the pupils. [If there is] extreme heat [in the pupils], the pupils [will be] dilated. Essence in the pupils is spiritual water. [If the pupils are] affected

云师曰："善。"

陈士铎曰："瞳子散大,不止于酒。大约肾水不足,亦能散大。然水之不足,乃火之有余也。益其阴而火降,火降而散大者不散大也。不可悟火之虐乎?必认作火酒之一者,尚非至理。"

【今译】

云师请问岐伯:"眼病一旦发生,瞳子就会散大,这是什么原因呢?"

岐伯说:"这当然是体内有热又饮水过多的原因。"

云师说:"世人喜欢饮水也是常事,但并没有见到瞳子都会因此而散大。"

岐伯说:"体内一旦发热,气血就会虚弱。气血一旦虚弱,精气就会耗散。五脏六腑的精气都会向上注入眼睛,瞳子尤其是精气的注入之处。精气注入瞳子后,眼睛就会明亮。如果精气不能注入瞳子,眼睛就会昏暗。一旦瞳子散大,眼睛自然就无法准确地观察事物了。"

云师说:"但眼睛则往往将小的东西看成大的东西。"

岐伯说:"瞳子的脉落与大脑相连通。如果大脑发热了,瞳子也会发热,一旦热到了极点,瞳子就会散大。瞳子之精,就是神水。如果脑中有热气,水中无非都是火气。如果脑中之火将要爆发,目光就难以收拢,怎么能不散大呢?"

云师说:"火为什么如此肆虐呢?"

by heat from the brains, there must be fire-Qi in [spiritual] water. [When] fire tends to blaze, the vision cannot be restrained. How can [the pupils] not [be] dilated [under such a condition]?"

Yunshi asked, "Why fire is so rampant?"

Qibo answered, "[It is] certainly [due to] drinking strong alcohol and pungent food. [There is] great heat in strong alcholol. [When] assisted by pungent food, heat [in it will] greatly increase. Besides, pungent [taste will] disperse Qi. Strong alcohol is Qi-alcohol and also disperses [Qi]. Furthermore, [there is] the taste of great Yang in strong alcohol and the taste of great Yang must rise up to the head and face. [In this case,] toxin of fire and heat will directly enter the brains. Essence in the brains detests dispersion but is very easy to be dispersed. [When] affected by Qi from strong alcohol and pungent heat, [essence in the brain will] now enter and then dissipate. [Since essential] Qi dissipates in the brains, the pupils in the external [will certainly] dilate in corresponding to it. [For] those [whose] Qi and blood are not deficient, [essential] Qi in the brains will not completely dissipate. That is why there are no signs of dilation concerning the pupils. However, the eyes are still inevitably dull."

Yunshi said, "Excellent [explanation]!"

Chen Shiduo's comment, "Dilation of the pupils is not only caused by alcohol. Generally speaking, insufficiency of kidney-water will also cause dilation [of the pupils]. However, insufficiency of water also indicates excessive fire. To replenish [kidney-] Yin will

岐伯说:"这当然与饮用了火性酒又吃了辛热性的食物有关。火性酒太热,又受到辛热性食物的影响,热度就会更高了。况且辛味食物会使气散。火性酒是气酒,也会使气发散。况且火性酒的阳气之味甚浓。阳气之味必然会上升到头部和面部,火热之毒就会因此而直接归于脑中。而脑中之精最害怕被发散,但也最容易被发散,得到了火性酒的辛热之气,就会随之进入而随之发散。在这种情况下,脑气就会散发在脑中,而瞳子则会相应地散大于外。而气血并未虚弱的人,其脑气还不会完全散发了,所以瞳子也没有出现散大之象。但是眼睛没有不昏蒙的。"

云师说:"好!"

陈士铎评论说:"瞳子的散大,不只是由火性酒造成的。一般来说,肾水的不足也会造成瞳子的散大。但是水的不足,则说明了火的有余。补益了阴,火就会下降。如果火下降了,瞳子的散大就会停止了。难道不可因此而感悟到火的肆虐吗?如果认为这完全是火性酒所导致,显然是不懂道理。"

reduce fire. [When] fire is reduced, [the pupils will] not dilate. [Such a measure certainly enables us] to understand why fire is rampant. To regard strong alcohol as the only [cause of dilation of pupils] is perhaps not the perfect axiom."

卷六

诊原篇第四十六

【原文】

雷公曰问于岐伯曰:"五脏六腑各有原穴,诊之可以知病,何也?"

岐伯曰:"诊脉不若诊原也。"

雷公曰:"何谓也?"

岐伯曰:"原者,脉气之所注也。切脉之法繁而难知,切腧之法约而易识。"

雷公曰:"请言切腧之法。"

岐伯曰:"切腧之法,不外阴阳。气来清者,阳也。气来浊者,阴也。气来浮者,阳也。气来沉者,阴也。浮而无者,阳将绝也。沉而无者,阴将绝也。浮而清者,阳气之生也。沉而清者,阴气之生也。浮而浊者,阴血之长也。浮而清者,阳血之长也。以此诊腧,则生死浅深如见矣。"

陈士铎曰:"诊原法不传久矣!天师之论,真得其要也。"

【今译】

雷公请问岐伯:"五脏六腑各有原穴,为什么通过诊断原穴就可以

Volume 6

【英译】

Chapter 46
Examination of Original [Acupoint]

Leigong asked Qibo, "There is original acupoint in each of the five Zang-organs and six Fu-organs. Why can examining original acupoint reveal [the condition of] disease?"

Qibo answered, "To examine meridian is not equal to to examine original [acupoint]."

Leigong asked,"What is the reason?"

Qibo answered, "Original [acupoint is the place that] meridian Qi penetrates through. [The method for] taking pulse is complicated and difficult to reveal [the condition of disease], [but the method for] taking acupoint is simple and easy to reveal [the condition of disease]."

Leigong asked,"Please explain [how] to take acupoint."

Qibo answered, "The method [for] taking acupoint is inseparable from Yin and Yang. Qi [that is] lucid [when] coming is Yang [while] Qi [that is] turbid [when] coming is Yin. Qi [that is] floating [when] coming is Yang [while] Qi [that is] deep [when] coming is Yin. [If Qi is] floating but [there is] no [way to find], [it indicates that] Yang will be isolated; [if Qi] is deep but [there is] no [way to find], [it indicates that] Yin will be isolated. [If Qi is] deep and lucid, [it indicates that] Yang Qi is produced; [if Qi

知道病情呢？"

岐伯说："诊脉其实不如诊原穴。"

雷公问："怎么理解呢？"

岐伯说："原穴是脉气的贯注之处。切脉的方法既繁琐又难解，切诊腧穴的方法简约易懂。"

雷公问："请说明切诊腧穴之法。"

岐伯说："切诊腧穴之法，不外乎阴和阳。气来而清的为阳，气来而浊的为阴。气来而浮的为阳，气来而沉的为阴。浮取无脉的，说明阳气将要绝了；沉取无脉的，说明阴气将要绝了。气浮而清的，说明阳气产生了；气沉而清的，说明阴气长成了。气浮而浊的，说明阴血生长了；气浮而清的，说明阳血生长了。以此法诊断腧穴，人的生死和病的深浅都会一目了然。"

陈士铎评论说："诊断原穴之法很久都没有再传承了。天师的论述，确实揭示了其要义。"

is⌉ floating and lucid, ⌈it indicates that⌉ Yin Qi is produced; ⌈if Qi is⌉ floating and turbid, ⌈it indicates that⌉ Yin blood is produced; ⌈if Qi is⌉ floating and lucid, ⌈it indicates that⌉ Yang blood is produced. To examine acupoint in such ⌈a way⌉, ⌈it is quite easy⌉ to find ⌈the time of⌉ life and death ⌈as well as⌉ mildness and severity ⌈of disease⌉."

Chen Shiduo's comment, "For a long time the method for examining original ⌈acupoint⌉ failed to inherit! The Celestial Master's discussion has revealed the gist."

精气引血篇第四十七

【原文】

力牧问于岐伯曰："九窍出血何也？"

岐伯曰："血不归经耳。"

力牧曰："病可疗乎？"

岐伯曰："疗非难也，引其血之归经，则瘳矣。"

力牧曰："九窍出血，脏腑之血皆出矣。难疗而曰易疗者，何也？"

岐伯曰："血失一经者重，血失众经者轻。失一经者，伤脏腑也。失众经者，伤经络也。"

力牧曰："血已出矣，何引而归之？"

岐伯曰："补气以引之，补精以引之也。"

力牧曰："气虚则血难摄，补气摄血则余已知之矣。补精引血余实未知也。"

岐伯曰："血之妄行，由肾火之乱动也。肾火乱动，由肾水之大衰也。血得肾火而有所归，亦必得肾水以济之也。夫肾水、肾火如夫妇之不可离也。肾水旺而肾火自归。肾火安，而各经之血自息。犹妇在家而招其夫，夫既归宅，外侮辄散。此补精之能引血也。"

力牧曰："兼治之乎，抑单治之乎？"

岐伯曰："先补气后补精，气虚不能摄血，血摄而精可生也。精虚

Volume 6

【英译】

Chapter 47
Guidance of the Blood with Essential Qi

Limu asked Qibo, "Why [is there] bleeding in the nine orifices?"

Qibo answered, "[Because] the blood does not enter the meridians."

Limu asked, "Can [such a] disease be treated?"

Qibo answered, "Treatment is not difficult. To guide the blood to return to the meridians will cure [the disease]."

Limu asked, "Bleeding in the nine orifices [indicates that] the same case also occurs in all the Zang-organs and Fu-organs. [This disease is originally] difficult to treat, [but you] have said [that it is] easy to treat. Why?"

Qibo answered, "[When] bleeding in one meridian is serious, bleeding in all the meridians is light. Loss [of blood in] one meridian damages the Zang-organs and Fu-organs [while] loss [of blood in] all the meridians damages meridians and collaterals."

Limu asked, "[When] the blood is already lost, how to guide [it] to return [to the meridians]?"

Qibo answered, "[It can be] guided by tonifying Qi. [It can also be] guided by tonifying essence."

Limu asked, "Qi deficiency [makes it] difficult to control the blood. I have already known [how] to control the blood by

不能藏血,血藏而气益旺也。故补气必须补精耳。"

力牧曰:"善。虽然血之妄出,疑火之祟耳。不清火而补气,毋乃助火乎?"

岐伯曰:"血至九窍之出,是火尽外泄矣!热变为寒,焉可再泄火乎? 清火则血愈多矣。"

力牧曰:"善。"

陈士铎曰:"失血补气,本是妙理。谁知补精即补气乎? 补气寓于补精之中,补精寓于补血之内,岂是泛然作论者? 寒变热,热变寒,参得个中趣,才是大罗仙。"

【今译】

力牧请问岐伯:"九窍出血,是什么原因呢?"

岐伯说:"是因血不归经。"

力牧问:"此病可以治疗吗?"

岐伯说:"治疗并不难,只要引导血液回归经脉,疾病就会痊愈。"

力牧问:"如果九窍出了血,脏腑也都会出血,难以治疗的反而说容易治疗,为什么呢?"

岐伯说:"如果血失于一经,病情就严重;如果血失于多经,病情就较轻。如果血失于一经,就会伤及脏腑;如果血失于多经,就会伤及经络。"

力牧问:"血液已经流出,怎么才能引导其归经呢?"

岐伯说:"通过补气来引导,通过补精来引导。"

tonifying Qi. ［But］ I don't know how to guide the blood by tonifying essence."

Qibo answered, "Wanton flow of the blood is caused by wanton movement of kidney-fire. Wanton movement of kidney-fire is due to serious debilitation of kidney-water. With ［the help of］ kidney-fire, the blood can return ［to the meridians］. ［Such a way of returning］ also depends on the support of kidney-water. Kidney-water and kidney-fire are just like husband and wife ［that］ cannot separate ［from each other］. ［If］ kidney-water is exuberant, kidney-fire will return spontaneously. ［When］ kidney-fire is harmonized, the blood in all the meridians will be in peace spontaneously. ［It is］ just like a wife at home calling her husband. ［When her］ husband has returned home, any insult ［made by others will be］ prevented. This ［is the reason why］ tonifying essence can guide the blood."

Limu asked, "Is it a concurrent treatment or an independent treatment?"

Qibo answered, "［If］ Qi is tonified first and then essence is tonified, Qi ［will be］ deficient and cannot control the blood. ［Only when］ the blood is controlled can essence be produced. ［If］ essence is deficient, ［it］ cannot store the blood; ［if］ the blood is stored, Qi ［will be］ promoted ［and become］ prosperous. Thus tonifying Qi must depend on tonifying essence."

Limu asked, "Excellent ［explanation］! However, wanton flowing of the blood ［from the meridians］ is perhaps caused by finagled movement of fire ［Qi］. ［If measure is taken］ not for clearing fire ［-Qi］ but for tonifying Qi, isn't it assisting fire ［-

力牧问："气虚则血难以调摄,补气摄血我已经知道了。但补精引血我还不知道。"

岐伯说："血的妄行,是肾火乱动所致。肾火的乱动,是肾水极度衰弱所致。血得到了肾火,就有所归了,同时也必须得到肾水的既济。肾水和肾火,正如夫妇一样,不可分离。如果肾水旺,肾火就能自然回归;如果肾火安,各经之血就能自然平息。这正如妻子在家召唤自己的丈夫一样,如果丈夫回家了,外来的欺侮就会马上消失,这就是为什么补精能引血。"

力牧问："应用兼治之法还是单治之法?"

岐伯说："先补气后补精,则气虚不能摄血,只有调摄了血,精才能产生,精虚不能藏血,只有血藏了,气才会日益旺盛。所以补气就必先补精。"

力牧问："好!血因妄行而出,可能是火气作祟所致,如果不清火而只补气,这怎么能助火呢?"

岐伯说："血之所以从九窍流出,是火完全外泄而导致的后果。如果热变为寒,怎么能再泄火呢?只有清肃了火,因血流失或血妄行所导致的各种疾病就会痊愈。"

力牧说："好!"

陈士铎评论说："失血了补气,这本来是奇妙的道理。但谁又懂得补精就是补气呢?补气蕴含于补精之中,补精蕴含于补血之内,这怎么可能是泛泛而论呢?寒变为热,热变为寒,彻悟了其中的意趣,才是真正的大罗仙。"

Qi] ?"

Qibo answered, "Bleeding from the nine orifices indicates complete leakage of fire. [If] heat changes into cold, how can fire [-Qi] leak? [Thus] clearing fire [-Qi] can cure [the disease marked by] bleeding."

Limu said, "Excellent [explanation]!"

Chen Shiduo's comment, "[To treat] serious bleeding [through] tonifying Qi originally is an excellent way. [But] who knows [that] tonifying essence is [actually] tonifying Qi? [In fact] tonifying Qi depends on tonifying essence and tonifying essence depends on tonifying the blood. How could it be a general discussion? [The idea about] cold changing into heat and heat changing into cold has well revealed the significance [in it]. The greatest god indeed!"

天人一气篇第四十八

【原文】

大挠问于岐伯曰:"天有转移,人气随天而转移,其故何也?"

岐伯曰:"天之转移,阴阳之气也。人之气亦阴阳之气也。安得不随天气为转移乎?"

大挠曰:"天之气分春夏秋冬,人之气恶能分四序哉? 天之气配日月支干,人之气恶能配两曜、一旬、十二时哉?"

岐伯曰:"公泥于甲子以论天也。天不可测,而可测。人亦不可测,而可测也。天之气有春、夏、秋、冬,人之气有喜、怒、哀、乐,未尝无四序也。天之气有日、月,人之气有水、火,未尝无两曜也。天之气,有甲、乙、丙、丁、戊、己、庚、辛、壬、癸。人之气,有阳跷、阴跷、带、冲、任、督、阳维、阴维、命门、胞络,未尝无一旬也。天之气有子、丑、寅、卯、辰、巳、午、未、申、酉、戌、亥。人之气有心、肝、脾、肺、肾、心包、胆、胃、膀胱、三焦、大小肠,未尝无十二时也。天有气,人即有气以应之。天人何殊乎?"

大挠曰:"天之气万古如斯,人之气何故多变动乎?"

岐伯曰:"人气之变动,因乎人,亦因乎天也。春宜温而寒,则春行冬令矣。春宜温而热,则春行夏令矣。春宜温而凉,则春行秋令矣。夏宜热而温,则夏行春令也。夏宜热而凉,则夏行秋令也。夏宜

Volume 6

【英译】

Chapter 48
The Sky and Man Sharing the Same Qi

Danao[1] asked Qibo, "The sky[2] occasionally changes and human Qi also changes with the sky. What is the reason?"

Qibo answered, "The changes of the sky [indicates the changes of] Qi in Yin and Yang. Qi [in] the human [body] is also Qi in Yin and Yang. How could it not change with [the changes of] weather?"

Danao asked, "Qi in the sky is divided into spring, summer, autumn and winter. How can Qi [in]the human [body] be divided into [such an] order [with] four [categories]? Qi in the sky coordinates with the sun, the mooth, the Earthly Branches and the Heavenly Stems. How can Qi [in] the human [body] match with the sun, the moon, a period [of ten days][3] and twelve hours[4]?"

Qibo answered, "You just rigidly adhere to description about the sky with Jiazi[5]. The sky is unmeasurable, but [sometimes] measurable. Human beings are also unmeasurable, but [sometimes] measurable. Qi in the sky is divided into spring, summer, autumn and winter [while] Qi in the human [body] is divided into pleasure, anger, sorrow and joy, certainly with the order of four [categories]. [Within] Qi from the sky, there are the sun and the moon; [within] Qi from the human [body] there are water and fire, certainly bearing two bright stars[6]. [In] Qi from the sky,

热而寒,则夏行冬令也。秋宜凉而热,非秋行夏令乎?秋宜凉而温,非秋行春令乎?秋宜凉而寒,非秋行冬令乎?冬宜寒而温,是冬行春令矣。冬宜寒而热,是冬行夏令矣。冬宜寒而凉,是冬行秋令矣。倒行逆施,在天既变动若此,欲人脏腑中不随天变动必不得之数矣。"

大挠曰:"天气变动,人气随天而转移,宜尽人皆如是矣。何以有变,有不变也?"

岐伯曰:"人气随天而变者,常也。人气不随天而变者,非常也。"

大挠曰:"人气不随天气而变,此正人守其常也。天师谓非常者,予不得其旨,请言其变。"

岐伯曰:"宜变而不变,常也。而余谓非常者,以其异于常人也。斯人也必平日固守元阳,未丧其真阴者也。阴阳不凋,随天气之变动,彼自行其阴阳之正令,故能不变耳。"

大挠曰:"彼变动者何以治之?"

岐伯曰:"有余者泻之,不足者补之,郁则达之,热则寒之,寒则温之,如此而已。"

陈士铎曰:"天人合一,安能变乎?说得合一之旨。"

【今译】

大挠请问岐伯:"天之气有转移的时候,人之气也随着天气而转

there are [ten stems, known as the Heavenly Stems[7], including] Jia, Yi, Bing, Ding, Wu, Ji, Geng, Xin, Ren and Kui. [In] Qi from the human [body], there are Yangqiao [vessel/meridian], Yinqiao [vessel/meridian], belt [vessel/meridian], thoroughfare [vessel/meridian], conception [vessel/meridian], governor [vessel/meridian], Yangwei [vessel/meridian], Yinwei [vessel/meridian], life gate and uterine collateral, certainly having a group [of ten categories]. [In] Qi from the sky, there are [twelve branches, known as the Earthly Branches[8], including] Zi, Chou, Yin, Mao, Chen, Si, Wu, Wei, Shen, You, Xu and Hai. [In] Qi from the human [body], there are heart, liver, spleen, lung, kidney, pericardium, gallbladder, stomach, bladder, triple energizer, large intestine and small intestine, certainly having [the system of] twelve hours. There is Qi in the sky and certainly there is Qi in the human [body] to correspond to it. How could there be difference bwtween the sky and man?"

Danao asked, "Qi from the sky remains the same forever. [But] why does Qi from the human [body] tend to change?"

Qibo answered, "Changes of Qi [in] the human [body] is due to human being and also the sky. [For instance,] spring should be warm but cold, [indicating that there is] winter climate in the spring; spring should be warm but hot, [indicating that there is] summer climate in the spring; spring should be warm but cool, [indicating that there is] autumn climate in the spring. Summer should be hot but warm, [indicating that there is] spring climate in the summer; summer should be warm but cool, [indicating that there is] autumn climate in the summer; summer should be hot but

移,这是什么原因呢?"

岐伯说:"天之气的转移,实际上是阴阳之气的转移。人之气也是阴阳之气,怎么能不随着天之气的转移而转移呢?"

大挠问:"天之气分为春、夏、秋、冬四类,人之气怎么能也按此顺序分为四种呢? 天之气与日月和支干相配,人之气又怎么能与日月、十天和十二时辰相配呢?"

岐伯说:"您只是拘泥于以甲子而论天。天不能测量,但也可以测量;人也不可测量,但也可以测量。天之气有春、夏、秋、冬之分,人之气有喜、怒、哀、乐之分,未尝没有四时的分序;天之气有日月,人之气有水火,并不是没有日月两曜之分;天之气有甲、乙、丙、丁、戊、己、庚、辛、壬、癸之分,人之气有阳跷、阴跷、带脉、冲脉、任脉、督脉、阳维、阴维、命门、胞络之分,并不是没有十个种类的划分;天之气有子、丑、寅、卯、辰、巳、午、未、申、酉、戌、亥之分,人之气有心、肝、脾、肺、肾、心包、胆、胃、膀胱、三焦、大肠和小肠之分,并不是没有十二时辰之分。天有气,人也有气与之相应,天与人又有何异呢?"

大挠问:"天之气万古如此而不变,人之气为什么会变化多端呢?"

岐伯说:"人之气的变动既是人自身的缘故,也与天有一定的关系。春天应当温暖,但有时反而寒冷,这是因为春天行使了冬令;春天应当温暖,但有时反而炎热,这是因为春天行使了夏令;春天应当温暖,但有时反而清凉,这是因为春天行使了秋令。夏天应当炎热,但有时反而温暖,这是因为夏天行使了春令;夏天应当炎热,但有时反而清凉,这是因为夏天行使了秋令;夏天应当炎热,有时反而寒冷,这是因

cold, [indicating that there is] winter climate in the summer. Autumn should be cool but hot, isn't it summer climate in the autumn? Autumn should be cool but warm, isn't it spring climate in the autumn? Autumn should be cool but cold, isn't it winter climate in the autumn? Winter should be cold but warm, [indicating that there] is spring climate in the winter; winter should be cold but hot, [indicating that there] is summer climate in the winter; winter should be cold but cool, [indicating that there] is autumn climate in the winter. [It is well proved that] retroaction [happens in the sky]. Now that the sky retroacts in such a way, it is impossible to prevent the Zang-organs and Fu-organs in the human [body] from following the changes of the sky."

Danao asked, "[When] Qi in the sky changes, Qi in the human [body] should follow the sky to change. [And such a change] should take place in everyone. [But] why is there change [in some people] but no change [in some others]?"

Qibo answered, "[It is] normal [that] Qi in the human [body] changes in correspondence to [that of] the sky. [It is] abnormal [if] Qi in the human [body] does not follow [that of] the sky to change."

Danao asked, "Qi in the human [body] does not follow [that of] the sky to change, [it shows that] people have followed the normal law. [But] Celestial Master have regarded [it as] abnormal, I cannot understand. Please explain such changes."

Qibo answered, "[What] should change but does not change [is actually] normal. [What] I have mentioned abnormal refers to the difference from the normal people. Such people often firmly defend

为夏天行使了冬令。秋天应当清凉,但有时反而炎热,这难道不是秋天行使了夏令吗? 秋天应当清凉,但有时反而温暖,这难道不是秋天行使了春令吗? 秋天应当清凉,但有时反而寒冷,这难道不是秋天行使了冬令吗? 冬天应当寒冷,但有时反而温暖,这是因为冬天行使了春令;冬天应当寒冷,但有时反而炎热,这是因为冬天行使了夏令;冬天应当寒冷,但有时反而清凉,这是因为冬天行使了秋令。可见天有时违反常理,倒行逆施。既然天如此变动,要使人的脏腑不随着天而变动,这怎么可能呢?"

大挠问:"天之气变化了,人之气也应当随着天之气而变化,应当人人都如此,但为什么有变也有不变的呢?"

岐伯说:"人之气随着天之气而变化,这是正常的;人之气不随天之气而变化,这是不正常的。"

大挠说:"人之气不随天之气而变化,这正是人对常理的遵守,但天师却说这是不正常的,我不明白其中的道理,请解释其变化之故。"

岐伯说:"应当变化的却没有变化,这是正常的。我之所以说这是不正常的,是因为这有异于正常之人。这类人平时必然要固守元阳,这样就不会丧失真阴,阴阳之气也不会凋零,他们就会随着天之气的变化而自行尊奉阴阳的常理,所以就能不变。"

大挠问:"变动了的人该怎么治疗呢?"

岐伯说:"如果有余,可以用泻下法;如果有不足,可以用补益法;如果木郁,可以用通达法;如果炎热,可以用寒凉法;如果寒冷,可以用

the original Yang and never lose any genuine Yin [in it]. [Qi in] Yin and Yang never forfeits, following the changes of Qi in the sky and spontaneously adhering to the normal order of Yin and Yang. That is why [it] never changes."

Danao asked, "How to treat those with changes?"

Qibo answered, "[For those with] excess, purgation [can be used to treat them]; [for those with] insufficiency, tonification [can be used to treat them]; [for those with] stagnation, unobstruction [can be used to treat them]; [for those with] heat, cold [therapy can be used to treat them]; [for those with] cold, warming [therapy can be used to treat them]. [The treatment can be done] just in such [a way]."

Chen Shiduo's comment, "[When] the sky and man are integrated, how could there be change? [This chapter is a thorough] description about the principle [of such an integration of the sky and man]."

Notes

[1] Danao (大挠)was the minister of Yellow Emperor.

[2] The sky here refers to weather. The changes of the sky refer to the changes of weather.

[3] Traditionally in China, one month is divided into three periods and each period is generally composed of ten days.

[4] Please see [3] in Chapter 11.

[5] Jiazi (甲子), a cycle of sixty years, is a traditional way to analyze and systematize the time of an hour, a day, a month, a year

温热法。治疗之法也不过如此而已。"

陈士铎评论说："天人合一,怎么会有变化呢？本文详述了天人合一的主旨精神。"

and sixty years. Please see [7] and [8].

[6] Bright stars refer to the sun and the moon.

[7] The Heavenly Stems (天干), including ten signs, and the Earthly Branches (地支), including twelve signs, are two sets of signs, with one being taken from each set to form 60 pairs, designating years, formerly also months, days, and hours.

[8] See the explanation mentioned above.

地气合人篇第四十九

【原文】

大挠问曰："天人同气，不识地气亦同于人乎？"

岐伯曰："地气之合于人气，《素问》《灵枢》已详哉言之。何公又问也？"

大挠曰："《内经》言地气统天气而并论也，未尝分言地气。"

岐伯曰："三才并立，天气即合于地气，地气即合于人气，原不必分言之也。"

大挠曰："地气有独合于人气之时，请言其所以合也？"

岐伯曰："言其合则合，言其分则分。"

大挠曰："请言人之独合于地气。"

岐伯曰："地有九州，人有九窍，此人之独合于地也。"

大挠曰："《内经》言之矣。"

岐伯曰："虽言之未尝分晰之也。"

大挠曰："请言其分。"

岐伯曰："左目合冀，右目合雍，鼻合豫，左耳合扬，右耳合兖，口合徐，脐合荆，前阴合营，后阴合幽也。"

大挠曰："其病何以应之？"

岐伯曰："冀之地气逆，而人之左目病焉。雍之地气逆，而人之右

Volume 6

【英译】

Chapter 49
Integration of Qi from the Earth and Man

Danao asked, "The sky and man share the same Qi. [I] don't know [whether] the earth also shares the same Qi with man."

Qibo answered, "[About] integration of Qi from the earth and man, there is detailed discussion in *Su Wen* (*Plain Conversation*) and *Ling Shu* (*Spiritual Pivot*). Why do you ask [such a question]?"

Danao said, "[In the *Yellow Emperor's*] *Internal Canon* [of *Medicine*], Qi in the earth is discussed together with Qi in the sky. [It] never talks about Qi in the earth independently."

Qibo said, "The three elements[1] exist side by side. [Since] Qi in the sky coordinates with Qi in the earth and Qi in the earth coordinates with Qi in the human [body]. Originally [there is] no need to discuss separately."

Danao asked, "Qi in the earth sometimes independently coordinates with Qi in the human [body]. Please explain the reason of [such a] coordination."

Qibo answered, "[When] talking about coordination, [there is] coordination; [when] talking about separation, [there is] separation."

Danao asked, "Please explain independent coordination of [Qi in] the human [body] with Qi in the earth."

Qibo answered, "There are nine states in the earth and nine

目病焉。豫之地气逆,而人之鼻病焉。扬之地气逆,而人之左耳病焉。兖之地气逆,而人之右耳病焉。徐之地气逆,而人之口病焉。荆之地气逆,而人之脐病焉。营之地气逆,而人之前阴病焉。幽之地气逆,而人之后阴病焉。此地气之合病气也。"

大挠曰:"有验,有不验何也?"

岐伯曰:"验者,人气之漓也。不验者,人气之固也。固者多,漓者少,故验者亦少。似地气之不尽合人气也,然而合者理也。"

大挠曰:"既有不验,恐非定理。"

岐伯曰:"医统天地人以言道,乌可缺而不全乎?宁言地气听其验不验也。"

大挠曰:"善。"

陈士铎曰:"地气实合于天,何分于人?地气有验不验者,非分于地气已。说其合,胡必求其合哉?"

【今译】

大挠请问岐伯:"天之气与人之气相同,不知地之气也与人之气是否也相同?"

岐伯说:"地之气与人之气是相合的,《素问》《灵枢》已经有详细的说明,您为什么又问呢?"

大挠说:"对于地之气,《内经》是与天之气一同论述的,并没有单独解说地之气。"

orifices in the human [body]. That is why [Qi in] the human [body] independently coordinates with [Qi in] the earth."

Danao said, "[This is already] mentioned in [*Yellow Emperor's*] *Internal Canon* [*of Medicine*]."

Qibo said, "Although [it is] mentioned, there is no [detailed] analysis."

Danao asked, "Please explain separative [coordination]."

Qibo answered, "The left eye coordinates with Ji[2], the right eye coordinates with Yong[3], the nose coordinates with Yu[4], the left ear coordinates with Yang[5], the right ear coordinates with Yan[6], the mouth coordinates with Xu[7], the navel coordinates with Jing[8], the genital coordinates with Ying[9] and the anus coordinates with You[10]."

Danao asked, "How does it correspond to [the concerned] disease?"

Qibo answered, " [When] Qi from the earth in Ji [area is] in counterflow, the left eye of a man [will be in] disorder; [when] Qi from the earth in Yong [area is] in counterflow, the right eye of man [will be in] disorder; [when] Qi from the earth in Yu [area is] in counterflow, the nose of a man [will be in] disorder; [when] Qi from the earth in Yang [area is] in counterflow, the left ear of a man [will be in] disorder; [when] Qi from the earth in Yan [area is] in counterflow, the right ear of a man [will be in] disorder; [when] Qi from the earth in Xu [area is] in counterflow, the mouth of a man [will be in] disorder; [when] Qi from the earth in Jing [area is] in counterflow, the navel of a man [will be in] disorder; [when] Qi from the earth in Ying [area is] in counterflow, the

岐伯说："天、地、人这三才是并立的,天之气即与地之气相合,地之气即与人之气相合,原本不必分别论述。"

大挠说："地之气有时会单独与人之气相合,请说明其合的原因。"

岐伯说："说其相合就会相合,说其分离就会分离。"

大挠说："请说明人独自与地之气的相合。"

岐伯说："地有九州,人有九窍,这就是人独自与地之气相合的原因。"

大挠说："这一点《内经》已经讲过了。"

岐伯说："虽然讲过了,但并没有进行分析。"

大挠说："请予以说明。"

岐伯说："人的左眼与冀州相合,右眼与雍州相合,鼻子与豫州相合,左耳扬州相合,右耳兖州相合,嘴巴与徐州相合,肚脐与荆州相合,前阴与营州相合,后阴与幽州相合。"

大挠问："人得的病又如何与之相应呢?"

岐伯说："如果冀州的地气逆行,人的左眼就会发病;如果雍州的地气逆行,人的右眼就会发病;如果豫州的地气逆行,人的鼻子就会发病;如果扬州的地气逆行,则人的左耳就会发病;如果兖州的地气逆行,人的右耳就会发病;如果徐州的地气逆行,人的口腔就会发病;如果荆州的地气逆行,人的肚脐就会发病;如果营州的地气逆行,人的前阴就会发病;如果幽州的地气逆行,人的后阴就会发病,这就是地气与病气的相应。"

大挠问："为什么有的应验有的却不应验呢?"

genital of a man [will be in] disorder; [when] Qi from the earth in You [area is] in counterflow, the anus of a man [will be in] disorder. This is the coordination of Qi in the earth with Qi in the disease."

Danao asked, "Why [sometimes] there is correspondence but [sometimes] there is no correspondence?"

Qibo answered, "Correspondence [indicates] permeation of Qi in the human [body with Qi in the earth]; no correspondence [indicates that] Qi in the human [body] fixes [in it and never changes]. [If] more [Qi in the human body] fixes [in it] and less permeates, there is certainly less correspondence. [It] seems [that] Qi in the earth cannot thoroughly coordinate with Qi in the human [body]. However [it is] normal [that Qi in the earth and human body should] coordinate [with each other]."

Danao asked, "Since there is no correspondence, perhaps [it is] not the reasonable law."

Qibo answered, "Discussion about the law [of medicine made by] doctors [certainly] involve the sky, earth and man. How could [such a discussion is] incomplete or partial? [We can] rather admit [that there is] correspondence [and there is also] no correspondence [between] Qi in the earth [and in the human body. But we must remember that it is a natural law that Qi in the earth and in the human body must correspond to and coordinate with each other]."

Danao said, "Excellent [explanation]!"

Chen Shiduo's comment, "Actually Qi in the earth coordinates with [Qi in] the sky. Why [it is necessary] to be assigned to man? [In] Qi from the earth, [sometimes] there is correspondence and

岐伯说:"应验的是人的气薄弱,不应验的是人的气坚固。如果人的气在经常都坚固,那么薄弱的就很少,所以应验的也很少。似乎地之气不能完全与人之气相合,但地之气与人之气的相合才是合情合理的。"

大挠问:"既然有的不应验,这恐怕不是常理吧?"

岐伯说:"医道应与天、地、人这三才综合而论,怎么能缺而周全呢? 我宁愿谈谈地之气,看看其与人之气究竟应验还是不应验。"

大挠说:"好!"

陈士铎评论说:"地之气实际上与天之气相合,为什么要将其与人之气分开呢? 地之气与人之气的应验与不应验,并非完全是地之气所致。谈到人之气与地之气的相合,何必一味地强调相合呢?"

[sometimes] there is no correspondence, [indicating that it is] not just assigned to Qi in the earth. [Although it is theoretically] said [that man and the earth should] coordinate [with each other], [in fact it is not absolutely necessary]. Why should there be coordination?"

Notes

[1] Three elements (三才), literally three talents, refer to the sky, earth and man which are traditionally regarded as the three basic components of the universe.

[2] Ji (冀) refers to Jizhou (冀州), one of the nine States in ancient China, now an area in Hebei (河北) Province.

[3] Yong (雍) refers to Yongzhou (雍州), one of the nine States in ancient China, now an area in Shaanxi (陕西) Province.

[4] Yu (豫) refers to Yuzhou (豫州), one of the nine States in ancient China, now an area in Henan (河南) Province.

[5] Yang (扬) refers to Yangzhou (扬州), one of the nine States in ancient China, now an area in Jiangsu (江苏) Province.

[6] Yan (兖) refers to Yanzhou (兖州), one of the nine States in ancient China, now an area in Shandong (山东) Province.

[7] Xu (徐) refers to Xuzhou (徐州), one of the nine States in ancient China, now an area in Anhui (安徽) Province.

[8] Jing (荆) refers to Jingzhou (荆州), one of the nine States in ancient China, now an area in Hubei (湖北) Province.

[9] Ying (营) refers to Yingzhou (营州), one of the nine States in ancient China, now an area in Liaoning (辽宁) Province.

[10] You (幽) refers to Youzhou (幽州), one of the nine States in ancient China, now an area in Hebei (河北) Province.

三才并论篇第五十

【原文】

鬼臾区问曰："五运之会,以司六气。六气之变,以害五脏。是五运之阴阳,即万物之纲纪,变化之父母,生杀之本始也。夫子何以教区乎?"

岐伯曰："子言是也。"

臾区退而作《天元纪》各论,以广五运六气之义。

岐伯曰："臾区之言大而肆乎! 虽然执臾区之论,概治五脏之病,是得一而失一也。"

臾区曰:"何谓乎?"

岐伯曰:"五运者,五行也。谈五运即阐五行也。然五行止有五,五运变成六,明者视六犹五也。昧者眩六为千矣。"

臾区曰:"弟子之言非欤?"

岐伯曰:"子言是也。"

臾区曰:"弟子言是,夫子有后言,请亟焚之。"

岐伯曰:"医道之大也,得子言大乃显然。而医道又微也,执子言微乃隐。余所以有后言也。虽然余之后言,正显子言之大也。"

臾区曰:"请悉言之。"

岐伯曰:"五运乘阴阳而变迁,五脏因阴阳而变动。执五运以治病未必有合也,舍五运以治病未必相离也。遗五运以立言,则医理缺其

Volume 6

【英译】

Chapter 50
Integrative Discussion about Three Elements[1]

Kui Yuqu[2] asked, "Meeting of the five motions[3] controls six [kinds of] Qi[4]. Changes of six [kinds of] Qi damage the five Zang-organs. Yin and Yang in the five motions are the laws and orders of all the things, the origin of all changes and the causes of life and death. How could you teach me?"

Qibo answered, "You can talk about it."

Kui Yuqu retreated and wrote an article [entitled] _Universal Law [of Motions and Changes]_ to explain the significance of five motions and six [kinds of] Qi.

Qibo said, "Kui Yuqu's discussion is great but wanton. However, guided by Kui Yuqu's discussion, treatment of diseases in the five Zang-organs [can] succeed [in] one [case] but fail [in] another [case]."

Kui Yuqu asked, "What is the reason?"

Qibo answered, "[The so-called] five motions are the five elements. To talk about the five motions is to explain the five elements. However the five elements are just five, [but] the five motions have transformed into six [kinds of Qi]. [Those who are] clear [about it usually] take six [kinds of Qi] as five [elements]. [Those who are] ignorant take six as thousand."

Kui Yuqu asked, "What I have said is incorrect?"

半。统五运以立言,则医道该其全。予故称子言之大而肆也。”

鬼臾区曰:“请言缺半之理。”

岐伯曰:“阴阳之气有盈有虚,男女之形有强有弱。盈者虚之兆,虚者盈之机,盖两相伏也。强者弱之媒,弱者强之福,盖两相倚也。合天地人以治邪,不可止执五运以治邪也;合天地人以扶正,不可止执五运以扶正也。”

鬼臾区曰:“医道合天地人者,始无弊乎?”

岐伯曰:“人之阴阳与天地相合也。阳极生阴,阴极生阳,未尝异也。世疑阴多于阳,阴有群阴,阳无二阳。谁知阳有二阳乎?有阳之阳,有阴之阳,君火为阳之阳,相火为阴之阳,人有君火、相火,而天地亦有之,始成其为天,成其为地也,使天地无君火,万物何以昭苏?天地无相火,万物何以震动?天地之君火,日之气也。天地之相火,雷之气也。雷出于地而轰于天,日临于天而照于地。盖上下相合,人亦何独不然?合天地人以治病则得其全,执五运以治病则缺其半矣。”

鬼臾区稽首而叹曰:“大哉!圣人之言乎,区无以测师矣。”

陈士铎曰:“六气即五行之论,知五行即知六气矣。世不知五运,即不知五行也;不知五行,即不知六气矣。”

【今译】

鬼臾区请问岐伯:“五运通过交会控制六气,而六气的变化则会损害五脏。所以五运的阴阳,是万物的纲纪,变化的根源,生杀的本源。天师如何就此予以指教呢?”

Qibo answered, "What you have said is right."

Kui Yuqu asked, "[Although what] I have said is right, your explanation later [is great]. Please burn up [what I have written]."

Qibo answered, "The law of medicine is great and your discussion can greatly reveal [it]. The law of medicine is also subtle, and guided by your discussion, [it will become] obscure. That is why I have analyzed [it] later. Nevertheless, what I have said later is to prove [what] you have said is great."

Kui Yuqu asked, "Please explain it in details."

Qibo answered, "The five motions follow Yin and Yang to change and transfer [while] the five Zang-organs are forced by Yin and Yang to change and move. Firmly holding the five motions in treating disease will not necessarily ensure coordination [while] abandonment of the five motions in treating disease will not necessarily cause separation. [If] the five motions are omitted in discussion, half of the principles of medicine will be absent; [if] the five motions are applied to discussion, the principles of medicine will be perfect. That is why I have said [that] your discussion is wanton."

Kui Yuqu asked, "Please explain the reason [why half of the principles are] absent."

Qibo answered, "Qi in Yin and Yang is sometimes exuberant and sometimes deficient. The body of a man or a woman is either strong or weak. Exuberance is the premonition of deficiency and deficiency is an advantage of exuberance, because they depend on each other. Strength is the media of weakness and weakness is the chance of strength, because they rely on each other. [It is

岐伯说："你可以说说。"

鬼臾区退下后写出了《天元纪》各论，以论述五运六气的意义。

岐伯说："鬼臾区的论述宏观而偏颇。如果按鬼臾区的论述治疗五脏之病，可能会得一而失一。"

鬼臾区问："为什么是这样的呢？"

岐伯说："五运就是五行，谈论五运既阐述五行。但是五行只有五，而五运则变成六，所以明智之人看到'六'正如看到'五'一样，而愚昧之人由于迷惑，看到'六'则以为看到了千千万万。"

鬼臾区问："学生我说的不对吗？"

岐伯说："你说的也对。"

鬼臾区问："虽然学生说的对，有老师后面讲的话，我讲的就焚烧了吧。"

岐伯说："医道博大精深，你的论述使得医道显得更加博大。然而医道又是精微的，按照你的论述而行，则医道的精微就会变得隐晦，这就是为什么我还有话要说。尽管如此，我要说的话，也是为了体现你对医道博大精深的论述。"

鬼臾区问："请予详解。"

岐伯说："五运随阴阳而变迁，五脏因阴阳而变动。依照五运而治病，未必会有彼此相合的效果；舍弃五运而治病，也未必会有彼此相离的结果。如果不依五运来统筹论述，则医理就会缺失一半；如果依据五运来总体论述，医道的阐释才会完善。这就是为什么我说你的论述宏观而偏颇。"

鬼臾区问："请说明医理为什么会缺失一半。"

岐伯说："阴阳之气有盈余的时候，也有虚亏的时候，这就是为什

appropriate] to coordinate with the sky, earth and man in treating disease [and] inappropriate to only adhere to the five motions in treating disease; [it is appropriate] to coordinate with the sky, earth and man in supporting healthy [Qi and] inappropriate only to adhere to the five motions in supporting healthy [Qi]. "

Kui Yuqu asked, "Is there any malpractice in coordination with the sky, earth and man [in terms of] the law of medicine?"

Qibo answered, "Yin and Yang in the human [body] coordinate with the sky and earth. [When] Yang [goes to] the extreme, Yin [is] promoted; [when] Yin [goes to] the extreme, Yang [is] promoted. There is no difference [in such a case]. [People in this] world doubt [that] Yin is more than Yang, [believing that] there is a crowd in Yin [but] even no double in Yang. Who knows [that] there is double Yang? [In fact] there is Yang within Yang and there is Yang within Yin. Monarch-fire is Yang within Yang and ministerial fire is Yang within Yin. [In] the human [body], there exist both monarch-fire and ministerial fire, and so do the sky and earth, [making it possible] to develop into the sky and earth. If there is no monarch-fire in the sky and earth, how could all things revive? [If] there is no ministerial fire in the sky and earth, how could all things be shaken? Monarch-fire in the sky and earth is Qi from the sun and ministerial fire in the sky and earth is Qi from thunder. Thunder originates from the earth and roars in the sky [while] the sun flies in the sky and lights up the earth because the upper and the lower coordinate with each other. How could human beings be not so? Coordination with the sky, earth and man in treating disease will ensure full recovery [but] adherence to

么男女的形体有强盛的时候,也有衰弱的时候。盈余是虚亏的前兆,虚亏是盈余的先机,两者相互依存;强盛是衰弱的表现,衰弱是强盛的体现,两者也相互依存。天、地、人要相合才能祛邪,不能只依靠五运来祛邪;天、地、人要相合才能扶正,不能只依靠五运来扶正。"

鬼臾区问:"医道只有与天、地、人相合,才能无弊吗?"

岐伯说:"人身之阴阳要与天地之阴阳相合。阳发展到了极致就会生阴,阴发展到了极致就会生阳,这是正常的,没有什么不同。世人总是怀疑阴多于阳,而且以为阴中有群阴,而阳中无阳,谁会知道阳中也有两个阳呢?实际上,阳中除了有阳中之阳,也有阴中之阳。君火就是阳中之阳,相火即为阴中之阳。人体中有君火和相火,而天地中也有君火和相火,这样上者才能成为天,下者才能成为地。如果天地中没有君火,万物又怎么会得以复苏呢?如果天地中没有相火,万物怎么会振兴呢?所以天地中的君火,就是太阳之气;天地中的相火,就是雷之气。雷从大地发出,而轰鸣于天上,太阳高悬于天空而普照于大地,这是上下相合的体现。人自身又怎么能不是如此的呢?只有天、地、人相合而治病,才能是全面的。如果只是依赖五运来治病,就会缺失一半。"

鬼臾区说:"天师的教导如圣人之教诲,博大而精深!我根本无法预知天师的思想啊!"

陈士铎评论说:"六气就是对五行的阐述,只有懂得了五行,才能懂得六气。如果世人不懂得五运,当然就不懂得五行了;如果不懂得五行,也就自然不懂得六气了。"

the five motions in treating disease will reduce half ⌈of the possibility to recover⌉."

Kui Yuqu kowtowed and sighed: "How great ⌈the explanation is⌉! ⌈This is⌉ sage's speech! ⌈I⌉ cannot explore ⌈what Celestial⌉ Master ⌈have said⌉!"

Chen Shiduo's comment, "⌈The so-called⌉ six ⌈kinds of⌉ Qi is a discussion about the five elements. Understanding the five elements means understanding the six ⌈kinds of⌉ Qi. ⌈If people in⌉ this world do not know the five motions, ⌈they⌉ certainly do not know the five elements; ⌈if they⌉ do not know the five elements, ⌈they⌉ certainly do not know the six ⌈kinds of⌉ Qi."

Notes

⌈1⌉ Please see ⌈1⌉ in Chapter 49.

⌈2⌉ Kui Yuqu（鬼臾区）was an important minister of Yellow Emperor.

⌈3⌉ Five motions（五运）refer to movements of wood, fire, earth, metal and water in the five elements. The five elements match with the five orientations. Thus the so-called five motions actually refer to the movement of Qi in these five orientations responsible for climatic changes.

⌈4⌉ Six ⌈kinds of⌉ Qi actually refer to the six normal climatic changes, i. e. wind, cold, summer-heat, dampness, dryness and fire.

五运六气离合篇第五十一

【原文】

鬼臾区问曰："五运与六气并讲，人以为异，奈何？"

岐伯曰："五运非六气，则阴阳难化。六气非五运，则疾病不成。二者合而不离也，夫寒、暑、湿、燥、风、火，此六气也。金、木、水、火、土，此五运也。六气分为六、五运分为五，何不可者？讵知六气可分，而五运不可分也。盖病成于六气，可指为寒、暑、湿、燥、风、火，病成于五运，不可指为金、木、水、火、土。以金病必兼水，水病必兼木，木病必兼火，火病必兼土，土病必兼金也。且有金病而木亦病，木病而土亦病，土病而水亦病，水病而火亦病，火病而金亦病也。故六气可分门以论证，五运终难拘岁以分门。诚以六气随五运以为转移，五脏因六气为变乱，此分之不可分也。"

鬼臾区曰："然则何以治六气乎？"

岐伯曰："五运之盛衰随五脏之盛衰为强弱，五脏盛而六气不能衰，五脏强而六气不能弱。逢司天、在泉之年，寒、暑、湿、燥、风、火有病、有不病者，正五脏强而不弱也。所以五脏盛者，何畏运气之侵哉？"

鬼臾区曰："善。"

陈士铎曰："六气之病，因五脏之不调也。五脏之不调，即五行之

【英译】

Chapter 51
Separation and Coordination of
the Five Motions and Six Qi

Kui Yuqu asked, "People feel [that there is] difference [if] the five motions[1] and six [kinds of] Qi[2] are discussed together. How [to explain it]?"

Qibo answered, "[If] the five motions are separated from the six [kinds of] Qi, Yin and Yang are difficult to change; [if] the six [kinds of] Qi are separated from the five motions, disease cannot be formed. They coordinate [with each other] and never separate [from each other]. Cold, summer-heat, dampness, dryness, wind and fire are the six [kinds of] Qi [while] metal, wood, water, fire and earth are the five motions. The six [kinds of] Qi are divided into six and the five motions are divided into five. Why [it is] impossible? Who knows [that] the six [kinds of] Qi can be separated but the five motions cannot be separated? Because diseases caused by the six [kinds of] Qi can be designated cold, summer-heat, dampness, dryness, wind and fire, [but] diseases caused by the five motions cannot be designated metal, wood, water, fire and earth. The reason [is that] metal-disease must be related to water, water-disease must be related to wood, wood-disease must be related to fire, fire-disease must be related to earth and earth-disease must be related to metal. Furthermore, [when] there is metal-disease,

不正也,调五行即调六气矣。"

【今译】

鬼臾区问:"五运与六气一并讲解时,人们认为有差别,这该怎么办呢?"

岐伯说:"五运如果偏离了六气,阴阳就难以转化;六气如果偏离了五运,疾病就不能形成。所以五运和六气总是相合,而不能分离。寒、暑、湿、燥、风、火,这是六气;金、木、水、火、土,这是五运。六气分为六,五运分为五,这有什么不可以呢?谁又懂得六气可以分而五运不可分呢?因为疾病是由六气所致,所以可以指定其属于寒、暑、湿、燥、风、火;而由五运所致之疾病,则不能指定其属于金、木、水、火、土。因为金病必然涉及水,水病则必然涉及木,木病则必然涉及火,火病则必然涉及土,土病则必然涉及金。而且如果金病出现了,木病也会产生;如果木病出现了,土病也会产生;如果土病出现了,水病也会产生;如果水病出现了,火病也会产生;如果火病出现了,金病也会产生。因此六气可以通过分门别类来论证疾病,而五运则终究难以根据年份来对疾病进行分门别类,这主要是因为六气总是随着五运而转变和移动,而五脏则总是随着六气而变化和动乱,这就是既可分又不可分的原由。"

鬼臾区问:"那么该如何治疗六气所致之病呢?"

岐伯说:"五运的盛衰将随着五脏的盛衰而变化,或强或弱。如果五脏盛,六气就不会衰;如果五脏强,则六气就不会弱。遇到司天和在泉之年,寒、暑、湿、燥、风、火有的会引发疾病,有的则不会引发疾病,这

there is also wood-disease; [when] there is wood-disease, there is also earth-disease; [when] there is earth-disease, there is also water-disease; [when] there is water-disease, there is also fire-disease; [when] there is fire-disease, there is also metal-disease. That is why the six [kinds of] Qi can be classified to analyze disease, [but] the five motions are difficult to classify just [according to the time of] a year. The fact [is that] the six [kinds of] Qi follow the five motions to transfer and the five Zang-organs, due to the six [kinds of] Qi, change into disorders. This [is the reason why there are] separability and inseparability."

Kui Yuqu asked, "Then how to treat the six [kinds of] Qi?"

Qibo answered, "Exuberance and debilitation of the five motions, accompanied by exuberance and debilitation of the five Zang-organs, [will eventually develop into] strength and weakness. [When] the five Zang-organs are exuberant, the six [kinds of] Qi cannot be debilitated; [when] the five Zang-organs are strong, the six [kinds of] Qi cannot be weak. In the years of Sitian (governing the sky) and Zaiquan (in the spring[3]), [among] cold, summer-heat, dampness, dryness, wind and fire, some have disease, some do not have, [indicating that] the five Zang-organs are strong, not weak. So [if] the five Zang-organs are exuberant, how could it fear invasion of [the five] motions [and six kinds of] Qi?"

Kui Yuqu said, "Excellent [explanation]!"

Chen Shiduo's comment, "Disease caused by the six [kinds of] Qi is due to inability of the five Zang-organs in regulation. Inability of the five Zang-organs in regulation indicates [that] the five

正是五脏强而不弱的缘故。所以五脏强盛者,怎么会畏惧六运之气的侵袭呢?"

鬼臾区说:"好!"

陈士铎评论说:"六气之所以引发疾病,是因为五脏不调的缘故。五脏之所以不调,则是五行不正所致。所以调理五行就是调理六气。"

elements are abnormal . [Thus] regulation of the five elements means
regulation of the six [kinds of] Qi ."

Notes

[1] Please see [3] in Chapter 50.

[2] Please see [4] in Chapter 50.

[3] Spring here refers to a place where water comes up
naturally from the ground.

六气分门篇第五十二

【原文】

雷公问于岐伯曰："五运六气合而不离,统言之可也。何鬼臾区分言之,多乎?"

岐伯曰："五运不可分,六气不可合。"

雷公曰："其不可合者,何也?"

岐伯曰："六气之中有暑火之异也。"

雷公曰："暑火皆火也,何分乎?"

岐伯曰:"火,不一也。暑外火,火内火也。"

雷公曰:"等火耳。火与火相合,而相应也。奈何异视之?"

岐伯曰:"内火之动,必得外火之引。外火之侵,必得内火之召也。似可合以立论,而终不可合以分门者,内火与外火异也。盖外火,君火也;内火,相火也。君火即暑,相火即火,暑乃阳火,火乃阴火。火性不同,乌可不区而别乎? 六气分阴阳,分三阴三阳也,三阴三阳中分阳火阴火者,分君相之二火也。五行概言火而不分君相。六气分言火而各配支干。二火分配,而暑与火各司其权,各成其病矣。故必宜分言之也。臾区之说,非私言也。实闻予论,而推广之。"

雷公曰:"予昧矣,请示世之不知二火者。"

【英译】

Chapter 52
Separation of Six Qi

Leigong asked Qibo, "The five motions[1] and the six [kinds of] Qi[2] are coordinated [with each other] and cannot separate [from each other]. [This can be] analyzed in general. [But] why did Kui Yuqu analyze separately? [Is it] unnecessary?"

Qibo answered, "The five motions cannot separate [from each other while] the six [kinds of] Qi cannot coordinate [with each other]."

Leigong asked, "Why can it not coordinate [with each other]?"

Qibo answered, "[Because there is] difference between summer [-heat] and fire."

Leigong asked, "Summer [-heat] and fire are all fire. How to differentiate?"

Qibo answered, "Fire is not all the same. Summer[-heat] is external fire [while] fire is internal fire."

Leigong asked, "Fire is the same. Fire and fire coordinate with each other and correspond to each other. [But] why to analyze it in different ways?"

Qibo answered, "Movement of internal fire must be guided by external fire [and] invasion of external fire must be summoned by internal fire. [It] seems reasonable to discuss [internal fire and external fire] comprehensively, but in fact [it] is unreasonable to

陈士铎曰："五行止有一火,六气乃有二火,有二火乃分配支干矣。支干虽分,而君相二火实因六气而异。言之于不可异而异者,异之于阴阳之二火也。"

【今译】

雷公请问岐伯："五运六气合而不离,总体来说当然是可以的。为什么鬼臾区要分开来说呢? 太偏颇了吧?"

岐伯说："五运不可分开,六气不可相合。"

雷公问："为什么不能相合呢?"

岐伯说："因为六气之中,暑与火是有差异的。"

雷公问："暑与火都是火,怎么才能区分呢?"

岐伯说："火不都是一样的,暑是外火,而火则是内火。"

雷公问："暑与火同样都是火吧。火与火彼此相合而相应,为什么认为其中有差异的呢?"

岐伯说："只有得到外火的引导,内火才能运动;只有得到内火的召唤;外火才能侵入。这似乎可以合而论之,但终究不能为了分门别类而使之相合,因为内火与外火之间存在着差异。外火是君火,内火是相火。君火即暑,相火即火。暑属于阳火,火则属于阴火。既然火性不同,为什么不能对其加以区别呢? 六气分为阴阳,即可以分为三阴和三阳,而三阴和三阳中又可分为阳火和阴火,可以分为君火和相火这两类。五行则是总体地论述火,而不分君火和相火。六气则分别论述火,并与地支和天干相配。两类火分开时,暑与火则各有权限,且各自引发

do so in a separate way [because] internal fire and external fire are different. External fire is monarch-fire and internal fire is ministerial fire. Monarch-fire is summer [-heat] and ministerial fire is fire. Summer [-heat] is Yang-fire and fire is Yin-fire. The nature of fire differs. Why can it not be differentiated? The six [kinds of] Qi are divided into Yin and Yang, i. e. three Yin and three Yang. [In] three Yin and three Yang, [fire is] divided into Yang fire and Yin fire, respectively called monarch-fire and ministerial fire. The [concept of] the five elements is a general analysis of fire without classification of monarch [-fire] and ministerial [fire]. The six [kinds of] Qi analyze fire separately, matching respectively to the Heavenly Stems[3] and Earthly Branches[4]. [In terms of] assignment of double fire, summer [-heat] and fire [have their] duty respectively and are responsible for different diseases. That is why [it is] appropriate to discuss separately. What Kui Yuqu said is not private talk. In fact [he was trying] to carry forward [what] I discussed before. "

Leigong said, "I am really ignorant! Please show [this idea to those who are] unclear about double fire in this world. "

Chen Shiduo's comment, " There is just one fire in the five elements. [But] there are two [kinds of] fire in the six [kinds of] Qi. [Only when] there are two [kinds of] fire can [it] match with the Heavenly Stems and Earthly Branches. [Although these two kinds of fire can] match with the Heavenly Stems and Earthly Branches, monarch-fire and ministerial fire are different because the six [kinds of] Qi [are diverse]. Discussion about difference in [what] should

不同的疾病。所以必须对其进行分别论述。因此鬼臾区所论述的，不是自说自话，实际上是听了我的论述，然后又推而广之。"

雷公说："我太愚昧了！请以此指导不懂君火和相火的世人。"

陈士铎评论说："五行中只有一种火，六气中则有两种火，有两种火就可以与地支和天干相合。地支和天干虽然可分，君火与相火则因六气的不同而存在差异。之所以谈到其无差异而实际上却有差异的问题，是因为阴阳二火之间存在差异的缘故。"

be the same depends on diversity of double fire ⌈*related to*⌋ *Yin and Yang.*"

Notes

⌈1⌋ Please see ⌈3⌋ in Chapter 50.

⌈2⌋ please see ⌈4⌋ in Chapter 50.

⌈3⌋ Please see ⌈7⌋ in Chapter 48.

⌈4⌋ Please see ⌈7⌋ in Chapter 48.

六气独胜篇第五十三

【原文】

雍父问曰："天地之气，阴阳尽之乎？"

岐伯曰："阴阳足以包天地之气也。虽然阴阳之中，变化错杂，未可以一言尽也。"

雍父曰："请言其变。"

岐伯曰："六气尽之矣。"

雍父曰："六气是公之已言也，请言所未言。"

岐伯曰："六气之中有余不足，胜复去留，奥区言之矣。尚有一端未言也。遇司天在泉之年，不随天地之气转移，实有其故，不可不论也。"

雍父曰："请悉论之。"

岐伯曰："辰戌之岁，太阳司天，而天柱不能窒抑之，此肝气之胜也。巳亥之岁，厥阴司天，而天蓬不能窒抑之，此心气之胜也。丑未之岁，太阴司天，而天蓬不能窒抑之，此包络之气胜也。子午之岁，少阴司天而天冲不能窒抑之，此脾气之胜也。寅申之岁，少阳司天，而天英不能窒抑之，此肺气之胜也。卯酉之岁，阳明司天，而天芮不能窒抑之，此肾气之胜也。"

雍父曰："司天之胜，予知之矣。请言在泉之胜。"

Volume 6

【英译】

Chapter 53
Domination of Six Qi

Yongfu[1] asked, "Can Qi in the sky and earth be clearly explained [with] Yin and Yang?"

Qibo answered, "Yin and Yang fully include Qi in the sky and earth. However changes in Yin and Yang are complicated and cannot be thoroughly explained in one sentence."

Yongfu asked, "Please explain the changes."

Qibo answered, "[I have already] thoroughly explained six [kinds of] Qi[2]."

Yongfu asked, "You have already talked about the six [kinds of] Qi. Please talk [about what you have] not mentioned."

Qibo answered, "There is surplus and insufficiency in the six [kinds of] Qi. About domination, restoration, leaving and remaining, Kui Yuqu has already mentioned. [However,] there is still one part necessary to analyze. In the years of Sitian[3] and Zaiquan[4], [it] does not follow Qi in the sky and earth to transfer because of certain reasons. [So it is] quite necessary to discuss."

Yongfu asked, "Please explain in details."

Qibo answered, "[In] the year of Chenxu, Taiyang dominates the sky and Tianzhu[5] cannot inhibit it, indicating domination of liver-Qi. [In] the year of Sihai, Jueyin dominates the sky and Tianpeng[6] cannot inhibit it, indicating domination of heart-Qi.

岐伯曰:"丑未之岁,太阳在泉,而地晶不能窒抑之,此肝胆之气胜也。寅申之岁,厥阴在泉,而地玄不能窒抑之,此心与小肠之气胜也。辰戌之岁,太阴在泉,而地玄不能窒抑之,此包络三焦之气胜也。卯酉之岁,少阴在泉,而地苍不能窒抑之,此脾胃之气胜也。巳亥之岁,少阳在泉,而地彤不能窒抑之,此肺与大肠之气胜也。子午之岁,阳明在泉,而地阜不能窒抑之,此肾与膀胱之气胜也。"

雍父曰:"子闻顺天地之气者昌,逆天地之气者亡。今不为天地所窒抑,是逆天地矣,不夭而独存何也?"

岐伯曰:"顺之昌者,顺天地之正气也。逆之亡者,逆天地之邪气也。顺可逆而逆可顺乎?"

雍父曰:"同是人也,何以能独胜乎?"

岐伯曰:"人之强弱不同,纵欲与节欲异也。"

雍父曰:"善。"

陈士铎曰:"天蓬、地玄独有二者,正分其阴阳也。阴阳同而神亦同者,正显其顺逆也,可见宜顺不宜逆矣!"

【今译】

雍父问道:"天地之气,可以用阴阳阐释清楚吗?"

岐伯说:"阴阳足以包括天地之气。但由于阴阳之中的变化错综复杂,一两句话是很难说清楚的。"

雍父问:"请解释其中的变化。"

Volume 6

[In] the year of Chouwei, Taiyin dominates the sky and Tianpeng cannot inhibit it, indicating domination of the pericardium. [In] the year of Ziwu, Shaoyin dominates the sky and Tianchong[7] cannot inhibit it, indicating domination of spleen-Qi. [In] the year of Yinshen, Shaoyang dominates the sky and Tianying[8] cannot inhibit it, indicating domination of lung-Qi. [In] the year of Maoyou, Yangming dominates the sky and Tianrui[9] cannot inhibit it, indicating domination of kidney-Qi."

Yongfu asked, "I have known domination of the sky. Please explain domination [of being] in the spring[10]."

Qibo answered, "[In] the year of Chouwei, Taiyang is in the spring and Dijing[11] cannot inhibit it, indicating domination of Qi in the liver and gallbladder. [In] the year of Yinshen, Jueyin is in the spring and Dixuan[12] cannot inhibit it, indicating domination of Qi in the heart and small intestine. [In] the year of Chenxu, Taiyin is in the spring and Dixuan cannot inhibit it, indicating domination of Qi in the pericardium and triple energizer. [In] the year of Maoyou, Shaoyin is in the spring and Dicang[13] cannot inhibit it, indicating domination of Qi in the spleen and stomach. [In] the year of Sihai, Shaoyang is in the spring and Ditong[14] cannot inhibit it, indicating domination of Qi in the lung and large intestine. [In] the year of Ziwu, Yangming is in the spring and Difu[15] cannot inhibit it, indicating domination of Qi in the kidney and bladder."

Yongfu asked, "I have heard [that] following the sky and earth ensures prosperity [while] violating the sky and earth causes death. Now [it] cannot be inhibited by the sky and earth. [This] is violation of the sky and earth. Why [it] does not die but just exist?"

岐伯说:"六气此前已经解释清楚了。"

雍父问:"六气您确实已经解释清楚了,请说说您还没有谈到过的。"

岐伯说:"六气之中存在着有余和不足以及胜复与去留。对此,鬼臾区已经说过了。但还有一点他没有谈到。遇到司天、在泉之年,之所以不随天地之气而转变和移动,其实是有原因的,这一点不能不予以论述。"

雍父问:"请予以详细说明。"

岐伯说:"辰戌之年,太阳主管天,而天柱星却不能加以抑制,此时的肝气就会强盛;巳亥之年,厥阴主管天,而天蓬星却不能加以抑制,此时的心气就会强盛;丑未之年,太阴主管天,而天蓬星却不能加以抑制,此时的包络之气就会强盛;子午之年,少阴主管天,而天冲星却不能加以抑制,此时的脾气就会强盛;寅申之年,少阳主管天,而天英星却不能抑制,此时的肺气就会强盛;卯酉之年,阳明主管天,而天芮星却不能抑制,此时的肾气就会强盛。"

雍父问:"司天的强盛,我知道了,请解释在泉的强盛。"

岐伯说:"丑未之年,太阳在泉,而地晶却不能加以抑制,此时的肝胆之气就会强盛;寅申之年,厥阴在泉,而地玄却不能加以抑制,此时的心与小肠之气就会强盛;辰戌之年,太阴在泉,而地玄却不能加以抑制,此时的包络与三焦之气就会强盛;卯酉之年,少阴在泉,而地苍却不能加以抑制,此时的脾胃之气就会强盛;巳亥之年,少阳在泉,而地彤却不能加以抑制,此时的肺与大肠之气就会强盛;子午之年,阳明在泉,而地

Qibo answered, "[The idea that] following [the sky and earth ensures] prosperity [means] to follow healthy Qi in the sky and earth [and that] violating [the sky and earth causes] death [means] to violate evil-Qi in the sky and earth. [Isn't it not proved that] following can [change into] violating while violating can [change into] following?"

Yongfu asked, "[We] are all human beings. [But] why can some succeed independently?"

Qibo answered, "[Because] people are either strong or weak [in constitution], [and also] different in sexual proclivities and abstinence."

Yongfu said, "Excellent [explanation]!"

Chen Shiduo's comment, "*To classify Tianpeng and Dixuan into two [different categories is for the purpose of] differentiating Yin and Yang in them. Yin and Yang are the same, and so are gods, demonstrating [their characteristics in] following and violating [activities]. [It is] obvious [that] following is appropriate [while] violating is inappropriate.*"

Notes

[1] Yongfu (雍父) was a minister of Yellow Emperor.

[2] Please see [7] in Chapter 48.

[3] Please see [3] in Chapter 51.

[4] please see [4] in Chapter 51.

[5] According to the book entitled *Tu Yi* (《图翼》), "The five stars have different names in the sky and the earth. The Jupiter (木

阜却不能加以抑制,此时的肾与膀胱之气就会强盛。"

雍父问:"我听说顺应天地之气的就会昌盛,悖逆天地之气的就会衰亡。如今不能被天地所节制的,这就是对天地的悖逆,而悖逆者不但没有衰亡,反而还能独自存活,这是为什么原因呢?"

岐伯说:"所谓顺之者昌,指的是顺应天地的正气;所谓逆之者亡,指的是悖逆天地的邪气。这样顺不就可以变为逆,而逆不就可以变为顺了吗?"

雍父问:"同样都是人,为什么有的却能独自强盛呢?"

岐伯说:"这是因为人有强弱的不同,正如纵欲与节欲的差异一样。"

雍父说:"好!"

陈士铎评论说:"天蓬与地玄之所以特意分开,就是为了区分其中的阴阳。阴阳相同而神也相同,这正好揭示了其顺逆的问题。可见应当顺应而不应当悖逆。"

星）is called Tianchong（天冲）in the sky and Dicang（地苍）on the earth; the Mars（火星）is called Tianying（天英）in the sky and Ditong（地彤）on the earth; the Saturn（土星）is called Tianrui（天芮）in the sky and Difu（地阜）on the earth; the Venus（金星）is called Tianzhu（天柱）in the sky and Dijing（地晶）on the earth; the Mercury（水星）is called Tianpeng（天蓬）in the sky and Dixuan（地玄）on the earth."

［6］Please see［5］in this chapter.

［7］Please see［5］in this chapter.

［8］Please see［5］in this chapter.

［9］Please see［5］in this chapter.

［10］Please see［3］in Chapter 51.

［11］Dijing（地晶）refers to metal in the west, representing metal-Qi on the earth.

［12］Dixuan（地玄）refers to water in the north, representing water-Qi on the earth.

［13］Dicang（地苍）refers to wood in the east, representing wood-Qi on the earth.

［14］Ditong（地彤）refers to fire in the south, representing fire-Qi on the earth.

［15］Difu（地阜）refers to earth in the center, representing earth-Qi on the earth.

三合篇第五十四

【原文】

雷公问曰:"寒暑燥湿风火,此六气也。天地之运化何合于人而生病?"

岐伯曰:"五行之生化也。"

雷公曰:"人之五脏,分金木水火土,彼此有胜负。而人病,此脏腑之自病也,何关于六气乎?"

岐伯曰:"脏腑之五行,即天之五行,地之五行也。天地人三合而生化出矣。"

雷公曰:"请问三合之生化。"

岐伯曰:"东方生风,风生木,木生酸,酸生肝,肝生筋,筋生心,在天为风,在地为木,在体为筋,在气为柔,在脏为肝,其性为暄,其德为和,其用为动,其色为苍,其化为荣,其虫毛,其政为散,其令宣发,其变摧拉,其眚陨落,其味为酸,其志为怒,怒伤肝,悲胜怒,风伤肝,燥胜风,酸伤筋,辛胜酸,此天地之合人肝也。

南方生热,热生火,火生苦,苦生心,心生血,血生脾,在天为热,在地为火,在体为脉,在气为炎,在脏为心,其性为暑,其德为显,其用为燥,其色为赤,其化为茂,其虫羽,其政为明,其令郁蒸,其变炎烁,其眚燔炳,其味为苦,其志为喜,喜伤心,恐胜喜,热伤气,寒胜热,苦伤气,咸

Volume 6

【英译】

Chapter 54
Three Coordinations

Leigong asked, "Cold, summer [-heat], dryness, dampness, wind and fire are six [kinds of] Qi. Why may the motion and transformation of the sky and earth coordinate with man cause disease?"

Qibo answered, "[This is due to] production and transformation of the five elements."

Leigong asked, "The five Zang-organs in the human [body] are classified into metal, wood, water, fire and earth, [among which] there are mutual promotion and restriction. Disease in the human [body is actually] disease [occurring] spontaneously in the Zang-organs and Fu-organs. Why is it related to the six [kinds of] Qi?"

Qibo answered, "The five elements in the Zang-organs and Fu-organs are also the five elements in the sky and the earth. [Only when] the sky, earth and man are integrated [with each other] can there be production and transformation."

Leigong asked, "Please explain integration of the three [as well as] production and transformation."

Qibo answered, "The east produces wind, the wind produces wood, the wood produces sour [taste], the sour [taste] produces the liver, the liver produces sinews and the sinews produce the heart[1]. [It is demonstrated by] wind in the sky, wood in the earth, sinews

胜苦,此天地之合人心也。

中央生湿,湿生土,土生甘,甘生脾,脾生肉,肉生肺,在天为湿,在地为土,在体为肉,在气为克,在脏为脾,其性静坚,其德为濡,其用为化,其色为黄,其化为盈,其虫倮,其政为谧,其令云雨,其变动注,其眚淫溃,其味为甘,其志为思,思伤脾,怒胜思,湿伤肉,风胜湿,甘伤脾,酸胜甘,此天地之合人脾也。

西方生燥,燥主金,金生辛,辛生肺,肺生皮毛,在天为燥,在地为金,在体为皮毛,在气为成,在脏为肺,其性为凉,其德为清,其用为固,其色为白,其化为敛,其虫介,其政为劲,其令雾露,其变肃杀,其眚苍落,其味为辛,其志为忧,忧伤肺,喜胜忧,热伤皮毛,寒胜热,辛伤皮毛,苦胜辛,此天地之合人肺也。

北方生寒,寒生水,水生咸,咸生肾,肾生骨髓,髓生肝,在天为寒,在地为水,在体为骨,在气为坚,在脏为肾,其性为凛,其德为寒,其用为藏,其色为黑,其化为肃,其虫鳞,其政为静,其令为寒,其变凝冽,其眚冰雹,其味为咸,其志为恐;恐伤肾,思胜恐,寒伤血,燥胜寒,咸伤血,甘胜咸,此天地之合人肾也,五脏合金木水火土,斯化生之所以出也。天地不外五行,安得不合哉。"

雷公曰:"五行止五,不应与六气合也。"

岐伯曰:"六气即五行也。"

雷公曰:"五行五而六气六,何以相合乎?"

岐伯曰:"使五行止五,则五行不奇矣。五行得六气,则五行之变化无穷。余所以授六气之论,而奥区乃肆言之也。"

in the human body, softness in Qi and the liver in the Zang-organs. [It is characterized] by warmth in property, harmony in nature[1], movement in function, blue in color, prosperity in transformation, caterpillar in animals, dispersion in function, dissemination in seasonal activity, destruction in changes, falling in disasters, sourness in tastes and anger in emotions. [Excessive] anger damages the liver [while] sorrow dominates over anger; wind damages the liver [while] dryness dominates over wind; sourness damages the sinews [while] pungency dominates over sourness. This is the coordination of the sky and earth with the human liver.

The south produces heat, the heat produces fire, the fire produces bitterness, the bitterness produces the heart, the heart produces the blood and the blood produces the spleen. [It is demonstrated as] heat in the sky, fire in the earth, the meridians in the human body, growth in Qi and the heart in the Zang-organs. [It is characterized by] summer [-heat] in property, reflection in nature, dryness in function and redness in color, flourishing in transformation, bird in animals, brightness in action, hotness in seasonal activity, scorching in changes, burning in disasters, bitterness in tastes and joy in emotions. Excessive joy damages the heart [while] fear dominates over joy; heat damages Qi [while] cold dominates over heat; bitterness damages Qi [while] saltiness dominates over bitterness. This is the coordination of the sky and earth with the human heart.

The center (the central region) produces dampness, the dampness produces earth, the earth produces sweet [flavor], the sweet [flavor] produces the spleen, the spleen produces muscles and

雷公曰:"六气之中,各配五行,独火有二,此又何故?"

岐伯曰:"火有君相之分耳。人身火多于水,五脏之中无脏非火也,是以天地之火亦多于金木水土也,正显天地之合于人耳。"

雷公曰;"大哉言乎! 释蒙解惑,非天师之谓欤? 请载登《六气》之篇。"

陈士铎曰:"五行不外五脏,五脏即六气之论也。因五行止有五,惟火为二,故六气合二火而论之,其实合五脏而言之也。"

【今译】

雷公问:"寒、暑、燥、湿、风、火,这是六气。为什么天地之运化与人相合会引发疾病呢?"

岐伯说:"这是五行生化的缘故。"

雷公问:"人的五脏分为金、木、水、火、土,彼此之间还存在着强盛和衰弱的问题。而人之所以得病,是因为脏腑自行发病所致,这为什么会关乎到六气呢?"

岐伯说:"脏腑的五行就是天的五行和地的五行,这就是天、地、人这三才相合而生化出来的。"

雷公问:"请问天、地、人这三才相合而生化的是什么呢?"

岐伯说:"当东方生起了风,风就会生起了木,木就会产生了酸,酸就会滋生了肝,肝就会滋生了筋,筋就会滋生了心;其在天的体现是风,其在地的体现是木,其在人体的体现是筋,其在气的体现是柔和,其在

the muscles produce the lung. [It is demonstrated as] dampness in the sky, soil in the earth, muscles in the human body, sufficiency in Qi, the spleen in the Zang-organs, tranquility in property, moisture in nature, transformation in function, yellow in color, fullness in transformation, naked insect in animals, quietness in action, cloud and rain in seasonal activity, permeation in changes, collapse in disasters, sweetness in tastes and contemplation in emotions. Excessive contemplation damages the spleen [while] anger dominates over contemplation; excessive dampness damages the spleen [while] wind dominates over dampness; excessive sweetness damages the spleen [while] sourness dominates over sweetness. This is the coordination of the sky and earth with the human spleen.

The west produces dryness, the dryness produces metal, the metal produces pungency, the pungency produces the lung and the lung produces the skin and hair. [It is demonstrated as] dryness in the sky, metal in the earth, skin and hair in the human body, reaping in Qi, the lung in the Zang-organs, coolness in property, clearness in nature, firmness in action, white in color, astringency in transformation, scale insect in animals, hardness in function, fog and dew in seasonal activity, destruction in changes, drop in disasters, pungency in tastes and grief in emotions. Excessive grief damages the lung [while] joy dominates over grief; excessive heat damages the skin and hair [while] cold dominates over heat; excessive pungency damages the skin and hair [while] bitterness dominates over pungency. This is the coordination of the sky and earth with the human lung.

The north produces cold, the cold produces water, the water

五脏的体现是肝;其本性的体现为温暖,其德性的体现为和合,其功用的体现是运动,其色彩的体现是苍色,其传化的体现是营血,其虫类的体现是毛虫,其政制的体现是发散,其号令的体现是宣发,其变化的体现是摧拉,其过失的体现是陨落,其滋味的体现是酸味,其情志的体现是愤怒;怒会伤害肝,悲会胜过怒;风会伤害肝,燥会胜过风;酸会伤害筋,辛会胜过酸,这就是天地与人体之肝的相合。"

岐伯说:"当南方生起了热,热就会生起了火,火就会产生苦,苦就会滋生心,心就会滋生血,血就会滋生脾;其在天的体现为热,其在地的体现为火,其在人体的体现为脉,其在气的体现为炎热,其在五脏的体现为心;其本性的体现是暑热,其德性的体现是彰显,其作用的体现是干燥,其色彩的体现是红色,其传化的体现是繁茂,其虫类的体现是羽虫,其政制的体现是宣明,其号令的体现是郁蒸,它的变化的体现是炎热,其过失的体现是闷热,其滋味的体现是苦味,其情志的体现是喜悦;喜会伤害心,恐能胜过喜;热会伤害气,寒能胜过热;苦会损伤气,咸能胜过苦。这就是天地与人体之心的相合。"

岐伯说:"当中央生起湿气,湿气就会滋生土,土就会滋生甘,甘就会滋生脾,脾就会滋生肉,肉就会滋生肺;其在气的体现为湿,其在地的体现为土,其在人体的体现为肉,其在气的体现为充,其在五脏的体现为脾;其本性的体现是坚实,其德性的体现是濡养,其作用的体现是传化,其色彩的体现是黄色,其化生的体现是充盈,其虫类的体现是倮虫,其政制的体现是平静,其号令的体现是云雨,其变动的体现是注入,其过失的体现是淫溃,其滋味的体现是甘,其情志的体现是思;思会伤害

produces saltiness, the saltiness produces the kidney, the kidney produces bone marrow and the marrow produces the liver. [It is demonstrated as] cold in the sky, water in the earth, bones in the human body, solidity in Qi and the kidney in the Zang-organs. [It is characterized by] sharpness in property, cold in nature, storage in action, black in color, depuration in transformation, scaled insect in animals, quietness in function, snow in seasonal activity, icy cold in changes, hailstone in disasters, saltiness in tastes and fear in emotions. Excessive fear damages the kidney [while] contemplation dominates over fear; excessive cold damages the blood [while] dryness dominates over cold; excessive saltiness damages the blood [while] sweetness dominates over saltiness. [3] This is the coordination of the sky and earth with the human kidney. The five Zang-organs coordinate with metal, wood, water, fire and earth respectively. This is the cause of transformation and production. [In] the sky and earth, [there is] nothing more than the five elements. How could there be no coordination?"

Leigong asked, "The five elements just have five [kinds of Qi] and are inappropriate to coordinate with the six [kinds of] Qi. "

Qibo answered, "The six [kinds of] Qi are actually the five elements. "

Leigong asked, "The five elements [only have] five [kinds of Qi] but the six [kinds of] Qi [have] six [categories]. How could [they] coordinate [with each other]?"

Qibo answered, "If the five elements just have five [kinds of Qi], it is not strange at all. [When] coordinated with the six [kinds of] Qi, the five elements are changeable all the way. That is why I

脾,怒能胜过思;湿会伤害肉,风能胜过湿;甘会损伤脾,酸能胜过甘。这就是天地与人体之脾的相合。"

岐伯说:"当西方生起了燥气,燥就会生成金,金就会滋生辛,辛就会滋生肺,肺就会滋生皮毛;其在天的体现为燥,其在地的体现为金,其在人体的体现为皮毛,其在气的体现为成形,其在五脏的体现为肺;其本性的体现是清凉,其德性的体现是清新,其作用的体现是坚固,其色彩的体现是白色,其化生的体现是收敛,其虫类的体现是介虫,其政制的体现是强劲,其号令的体现是雾露,其变化的体现是肃杀,其过失的体现是苍落,其滋味的体现是辛,其情志的体现是忧;忧会伤害肺,喜能胜过忧;热会伤害皮毛,寒能胜过热;辛会损伤皮毛,苦能胜过辛。这就是天地与人体之肺脏的相合。"

岐伯说:"当北方生起了寒,寒就会滋生水,水就会滋生咸,咸就会滋生肾,肾就会滋生骨髓,髓就会滋生肝;其在天的体现为寒,其在地的体现为水,其在人体的体现为骨,其在气的体现为坚固,其在五脏的体现为肾;其本性的体现是凛冽,其德性的体现是寒冷,其作用的体现是收藏,其色彩的体现是黑色,其转化的体现是肃静,其虫类的体现是鳞虫,其政制的体现是宁静,其号令的体现是寒冷,其变化的体现是凝冽,其过失的体现是冰雹,其滋味的体现是咸,其情志的体现是恐;恐会伤害肾,思能胜过恐;寒会伤害血,燥会胜过寒;咸会损伤血,甘能胜过咸。这就是天地与人体之肾的相合。五脏与金木水火土分别相合,这是化生得以形成的原由。天地运行的体现,不外乎五行而已,怎么能不相合呢?"

have mentioned the six [kinds of] Qi. Kui Yuqu's discussion [about it] is wanton. "

Leigong asked, "Among the six [kinds of] Qi, each [one] matches with [another one in] the five elements. But why does fire [in the five elements coordinate with] two [of the six kinds of Qi]?"

Qibo answered, "[Because] fire is divided into monarch-fire and ministerial fire. [In] the human body, fire is more than water. [Among] the five Zang-organs, no one does not have fire. Thus fire in the sky and earth is also more than that in metal, wood, water and earth [in the five elements], demonstrating [the fact that] the sky and earth coordinate with man. "

Leigong said, "How great [your] analysis is! [Nobody can] explain such questions and resolve such doubts except Celestial Master! Please record [this analysis in] the Chapter of Six [Kinds of] Qi. "

Chen Shiduo's comment, " The five elements are just the five Zang-organs and the five Zang-orgtans are the six [kinds of] Qi. Since [there are] just five [kinds of Qi in] the five elements, fire thus [bears] two [kinds]. That is why the six [kinds of] Qi coordinate with two [kinds of] fire in discussion. In fact [this is] the coordination [of the six kinds of Qi] with the five Zang-organs in discussion. "

Notes

[1] The sentence "The east produces wind, the wind produces

雷公问："五行只有五气,不应与六气相合吧?"

岐伯说："六气实际上就是五行。"

雷公问："五行为五,而六气则为六,这怎么能相合呢?"

岐伯说："如果五行只有五,那么五行也就没有什么奇特之处了。五行只有得到了六气,其变化才能无穷。这就是我要传授六气之理的原由,而鬼臾区的论述则宏观而偏颇。"

雷公问："六气分别与五行相合,唯独火有两种,这又是什么原因呢?"

岐伯说："火有君火和相火之别,而人身体中的火又多于水,五脏之中无一缺火,所以天地之火就比金木水土要多,这正体现了天地与人相合的事实。"

雷公说："天师讲的真好啊! 彻底消解了我的迷茫和疑惑,除了天师还有谁能达到这样的境界呢? 请将这一论述登载在《六气》篇中。"

陈士铎评论说："五行不外乎五脏而已,五脏也就是对六气的论述。五行只有五类,惟独火有两类,所以六气与两类火结合起来论述,其实就是与五脏结合起来论述。"

wood, the wood produces sour [taste], the sour [taste] produces the liver, the liver produces sinews and the sinews produces the heart" is a literally translation of the original sentence "东方生风,风生木,木生酸,酸生肝,肝生筋,筋生心". In this original Chinese sentence, the verb "生", literally "production", is used for six times, but the meaning is not all the same. It sometimes means to produce, sometimes means to promote, sometimes means to nourish, sometimes means to strengthen. Thus this original Chinese sentence can be freely translated as "The east produces wind, the wind promotes [the growth of] wood, the wood produces sour [taste], the sour [taste] nourishes the liver, the liver replenishes sinews and the sinews strengthen the heart". The following description about the south, the center, the west and the north are the same.

[2] The original Chinese character is De (德) which literally means morality, but actually means the nature of natural things. The following description about the south, the center, the west and the north are the same.

[3] This passage about the east, south, center, west and north is also mentioned in Chapter 5 in *Su Wen* (《素问》, *Plain Conversation*), the first fascicle of *Huang Di Nei Jing* (《黄帝内经》, *Yellow Emperor's Internal Canon of Medicine*). To understand this passage, please see the notes from [25] to [43] in Chapter 5 in the English version of *Su Wen* (《素问》, *Plain Conversation*). The English version was published by World Book Publishing Company in 2005.

卷七

四时六气异同篇第五十五

【原文】

天老问曰："五脏合五时,六经应六气,然《诊要经终》以六气应五脏而终于六经,《四时刺逆从论》以六经应四时而终于五脏,《诊要篇》以经脉之生于五脏而外合于六经,《四时刺逆从论》以经脉本于六气而外连于五脏,何也?"

岐伯曰："人身之脉气,上通天,下合地,未可一言尽也,故彼此错言之耳。"

天老曰："章句同而意旨异,不善读之,吾恐执而不通也。"

岐伯曰："医统天地人以立论。不知天,何知地? 不知地,何知人? 脉气循于皮肉筋骨之间,内合五行,外合六气,安得一言而尽乎? 不得不分之以归于一也。"

天老曰："请问归一之旨。"

岐伯曰："五时之合五脏也,即六气之合五脏也。六气之应六经也,即五时之应六经也。知其同,何难知异哉!"

天老曰："善。"

陈士铎曰："何尝异,何必求同;何尝同,不妨言异。人惟善求之可耳!"

Volume 7

【英译】

Chapter 55
Four Seasons and Six Qi

Tianlao asked, "The five Zang-organs coordinate with the five seasons and the six meridians correspond to the six [kinds of] Qi. However [in] *Discussion on the Essentials of Diagnosis and Destination of Meridians*[1], the six [kinds of] Qi correspond to the five Zang-organs and terminate at the six meridians; [in] *Discussion on Following and Against [the Changes in] the Four Seasons*[2], the six [kinds of] Qi correspond to the four seaons and terminate at the five Zang-organs. [In] *Essentials of Diagnosis*[3], the meridians originate from the five Zang-organs and externally coordinate with the six meridians; [in] *Discussion on Following and Against [the Changes in] the Four Seasons* the meridians originate from the six [kinds of] Qi and externally connected with the five Zang-organs. What is the reason?"

Qibo answered, "Meridian Qi in the human body communicates with the sky in the upper and coordinates with the earth in the lower, [which is] hard to describe in one sentence. That is why there is confused description."

Tianlao said, "The massages and sentences are the same but the order is different. I am afraid [that those who are] not good at reading will be stubborn [in thinking and therefore] cannot understand."

Qibo answered, "[The theory and practice of] medicine depend on [coordination of] the sky, earth and man. [If one is] unclear about the sky, how [can he] know the earth? [If one is] unclear

【今译】

天老问道:"五脏与五时相合,六经与六气相应。但在《素问·诊要经终论篇》中,却认为六气对应于五脏,最终则结于六经。在《素问·四时刺逆从论篇》中,则认为六经对应于四时,最终则结于五脏。在《素问·诊要经终论篇》中,则认为经脉生于五脏,但在外又与六经相合。在《素问·四时刺逆从论篇》中,则认为经脉之本在于六气,但在外则与五脏相连。这是什么原因呢?"

岐伯说:"人身的脉气,在上与天相通,在下与地相合,一句话是难以说清楚的。所以彼此之间总是相互交错而论。"

天老说:"《黄帝内经》虽然章句相同,但旨意却有一定的差异,不善于阅读的人,我担心一定会固执僵化,很难融会贯通的。"

岐伯说:"医道以天、地、人为基础统一立论。不懂得天的人怎么能懂得地呢?不懂得地的人怎么可能懂得人呢?经脉之气循行在皮肉筋骨之中,在内合于五行,在外合于六气,怎么能一句话就说完了呢?所以不得先对其加以区分,然后再将其合而为一。"

天老问:"请问合而为一是什么意思呢?"

岐伯说:"五时与五脏的相合,就是六气与五脏的相合;六气与六经的对应,也就是五时与六经的对应。如果懂得其相同性,又怎么能不懂其差异呢?"

天老说:"好!"

陈士铎评论说:"何尝会有差异,何必求其同一;何尝会有相同,何妨论其差异。人只要善于求索,没有实现不了目标的。"

about the earth, how [can he] understand man? Qi in the meridians circulates in between the skin and fleshes [as well as] sinews and bones, internally coordinating with the five elements and externally coordinating with the six [kinds of] Qi. How can [it be] described in one sentence? [For this reason, they] must be described separately [and finally] integrated into one."

Tianlao asked, "Please explain the principle for integrating into one."

Qibo answered, "The coordination of the five seasons with the five Zang-organs is also the coordination of the six [kinds of] Qi with the five Zang-organs. The correspondence of the six [kinds of] Qi to the six meridians is also the correspondence of the five seasons to the six meridians. [If one] knows their sameness, [it will be very] easy to know [their] difference."

Tianlao said, "Excellent [explanation]!"

Chen Shiduo's comment, "[If] there is no difference, how could there be sameness? [If] there is no sameness, [it is certainly] appropriate to talk about difference. [All this depends on] people's trials to find the truth."

Notes

[1] This is the title of Chapter 16 in *Su Wen* (《素问》, *Plain Conversation*), the first fascicle of *Huang Di Nei Jing* (《黄帝内经》, *Yellow Emperor's Internal Canon of Medicine*).

[2] This is the title of Chapter 64 in *Su Wen* (《素问》, *Plain Conversation*), the first fascicle of *Yellow Emperor's Internal Canon of Medicine*.

[3] This title is not included in *Su Wen* (《素问》, *Plain Conversation*), the first fascicle of *Yellow Emperor's Internal Canon of Medicine*, and *Ling Shu* (《灵枢》, *Spiritual Pivot*), the second fascicle of *Yellow Emperor's Internal Canon of Medicine*. It is not clear where this title comes from.

司天在泉分合篇第五十六

【原文】

问曰："司天在泉,二气相合,主岁何分?"

岐伯曰："岁半以上,天气主之。岁半以下,地气主之。"

天老曰："司天之气主上半岁乎? 在泉之气主下半岁乎?"

岐伯曰："然。"

天老曰："司天之气何以主上半岁也?"

岐伯曰："春夏者,天之阴阳也,阳生阴长,天之气也,故上半岁主之。"

天老曰："在泉之气何以主下岁也?"

岐伯曰："秋冬者,地之阴阳也。阴杀阳藏,地之气也,故下半岁主之。"

天老曰："一岁之中,天地之气截然分乎?"

岐伯曰："天地之气,无日不交。司天之气始于地之左,在泉之气本乎天之右。一岁之中,互相感召,虽分而实不分也。"

天老曰："然则司天在泉,何必分之乎?"

岐伯曰："不分言之,则阴阳不明,奚以得阴中有阳,阳中有阴之义乎? 司天之气始于地而终于天,在泉之气始于天而终于地。天地升降,环转不息,实有如此,所以可合而亦可分之也。"

Volume 7

【英译】

Chapter 56
Coordination of Sitian and Zaiquan

Tianlao asked, "Qi from Sitian (dominating the sky) and Qi from Zaiquan (in the spring[1]) coordinate with each other and dominate for one year. How to differentiate?"

Qibo answered, "[In] the first half of the year, Qi from the sky is in domination; [in] the second half of the year, Qi from the earth is in domination."

Tianlao asked, "Is it Qi from Sitian (dominating the sky) [that] dominates over the first half of the year? Is it Qi from Zaiquan (in the spring) [that] dominates over the second half of the year?"

Qibo answered, "Right."

Tianlao asked, "Why can Qi from Sitian (dominating the sky) dominate over the first half of the year?"

Qibo answered, "The spring and summer are Yin and Yang in the sky. Yang grows and Yin develops, [demonstrating the property of] Qi from the sky. That is why [it] dominates over the first half of the year."

Tianlao asked, "Why can Qi from Zaiquan (in the spring) dominate over the second half of the year?"

Qibo answered, "Autumn and winter are Yin and Yang in the earth. Yin kills and Yang stores, [demonstrating the property of]

天老曰："司天之气何以始于地？在泉之气何以始于天乎？"

岐伯曰："司天之气始于地之左，地中有天也；在泉之气始于天之右，天中有地也。"

天老曰："善。"

陈士铎曰："司天在泉，合天地以论之，才是善言天地者。"

【今译】

天老问："司天与在泉二气相合，所主管的一年该如何区分呢？"

岐伯说："上半年由天气主之，下半年由地气主之。"

天老问："意思是说上半年由司天之气主管？下半年由在泉之气主管？"

岐伯说："对的。"

天老问："为什么司天之气能主管上半年呢？"

岐伯说："春和夏代表天之阴阳。阳生阴长所体现的，就是天之气，这就是为什么司天之气能主管上半年。"

天老问："为什么在泉之气能主管下半年呢？"

岐伯说："秋和冬代表地之阴阳。阴杀阳藏所体现的，就是地之气，这就是为什么在泉之气能主管下半年。"

天老问："一年之中，天地之气会截然分开吗？"

岐伯说："天地之气，无时无刻不相交。司天之气始于地之左侧，在泉之气源自天之右侧，一年之中互相感应和召唤，虽然形式上分开，

Qi from the earth. That is why [it] dominates over the second half of the year."

Tianlao asked, "Is Qi from the sky and the earth absolutely separated from each other in a year?"

Qibo answered, "Qi from the sky and earth communicates with each other every day. Qi from Sitian (dominating the sky) originates from the left [side] of the earth and Qi from Zaiquan (in the spring) starts from the right [side] of the sky. In the whole year [they] impel and inspire each other. Although [they are physically] separate [from each other], in fact [they] never separate [from each other]."

Tianlao asked, "But why do Sitian (dominating the sky) and Zaiquan (in the spring) separate [from each other]?"

Qibo answered, "[If it is] not discussed separately, Yin and Yang will be unclear. [If so,] how [could one] know [that] there is Yang in Yin and there is Yin in Yang? Qi from Sitian (dominating the sky) starts from the earth but terminates at the sky; Qi from Zaiquan (in the spring) starts from the sky but terminates at the earth. [Qi from] the sky and earth ascends and descends cyclically and constantly. Just for this reason, [they] not only can coordinate [with each other], but also separate [from each other]."

Tianlao asked, "Why does Qi from Sitian (dominating the sky) start from the earth? Why does Qi from Zaiquan (in the spring) start from the sky?"

Qibo answered, "[The reason why] Qi from Sitian (dominating the sky) starts from the left [side] of the earth [is that] there is sky

但实际上却并未分开。"

天老问："那么司天和在泉又何必分开呢?"

岐伯说："如果不分开来论述,阴阳就不明确,怎么能使人理解阴中有阳、阳中有阴的含义呢? 司天之气起始于地而终止于天,在泉之气起始于天而终止于地,天地之气始终不息地上升、下降、环绕和转移,事实也确实如此。正因为如此,司天和在泉才可以相合,也可以分开。"

天老问："为什么司天之气起始于地呢? 为什么在泉之气会起始于天呢?"

岐伯说："司天之气起始于地之左侧,这是地中有天的体现;在泉之气起始于天之右侧,这是天中有地的体现。"

天老说："好!"

陈士铎评论说："只有将司天和在泉与天地结合起来论述,才是完善地论述天与地。"

in the earth; [the reason why] Qi from Zaiquan (in the spring) starts from the right [side] of the sky [is that] there is earth in the sky."

Tianlao said, "Excellent [explanation]!"

Chen Shiduo's comment, *"Discussion of Sitian (dominating the sky) and Zaiquan (in the spring) together with the sky and earth [indicates that it] is an excellent analysis of the sky and earth."*

[1] Please see [3] in Chapter 51.

从化篇第五十七

【原文】

天老问曰："燥从热发,风从燥起,埃从风生,雨从湿注,热从寒来,其故何欤?"

岐伯曰："五行各有胜,亦各有制也。制之太过,则受制者应之,反从其化也。所以热之极者,燥必随之,此金之从火也;燥之极者,风必随之,此木之从金也;风之极者,尘霾随之,此土之从木也;湿蒸之极者,霖雨随之,此水之从土也;阴寒之极者,雷电随之,此火之从水也。乃承制相从之理,何足异乎?"

天老曰："何道而使之不从乎?"

岐伯曰："从火者润其金乎,从金者抒其木乎,从木者培其土乎,从土者导其水乎,从水者助其火乎,毋不足、毋有余,得其平而不从矣!"

天老曰："润其金而金仍从火,抒其木而木仍从金,培其土而土仍从木,导其水而水仍从土,助其火而火仍从水,奈何?"

岐伯曰："此阴阳之己变,水火之已漓,非药石针灸之可疗也。"

陈士铎曰："言浅而论深。"

Volume 7

【英译】

Chapter 57
Following Transformation

Tianlao asked, "Dryness stems from heat, wind from dryness, dust from wind, rain from dampness permeation, heat from cold. What is the reason?"

Qibo answered, "[Among] the five elements, there is superiority and also constraint respectively. [If] constraint is excessive, [the one that is] constrained [will eventually] adapt to it [and], on the contrary, change [itself according to the constraint]. Thus [if] there is extreme heat, there must be dryness, this [is the change of] metal according to [that of] fire; [if] there is extreme dryness, there must be wind, this [is the change of] wood according to [that of] metal; [if] there is extreme wind, there must be dust, this [is the change of] earth according to [that of] wood; [if] there is extreme steaming of dampness [-heat], there must be great rain, this [is the change of] water according to [that of] earth; [if] there is extreme Yin cold, there must be thunder, this [is the change of] fire according to [that of] water. This is the principle of coordination and constraint. How [could there be anything] strange?"

Tianlao asked, "Is there any way to prevent any follower?"

Qibo answered, "[The one that] follows fire moistens [Qi] in metal; [the one that] follows metal promotes [Qi] in wood; [the

【今译】

天老问："燥从热发，风从燥起，埃从风生，雨从湿注，热从寒来，这是什么原因呢？"

岐伯说："五行各有其优胜之处，也各有其制约的因素。如果制约太过，则被制约者就会适应，否则就会制约者就会产生变化。因此，热势发展到了极点，燥气就必然相随，这是金随着火而变化的缘故；干燥发展到了极点，风气就必然相随，这是木随着金而变化的缘故；狂风发展到了极点，尘埃就必然会随之产生，这是土随着木而变化的缘故；湿热熏蒸发展到了极点，大雨就必然相随，这是水随着土而变化的缘故；阴寒发展到了极点，雷电必然相随，这是火随着水而变化的缘故。这是承接与制约相互跟随的原理，有什么值得奇异的呢？"

天老问："有什么方法可以使之不跟随呢？"

岐伯说："随火的滋润其金气，随金的抒发其木气，随木的培植其土气，随土的疏导其水气，随水的助长其火气，不要不足，不要有余，得到平顺就不会再有跟随了。"

天老问："滋润金气而金仍然跟随着火，抒发木气而木仍然跟随着金，培植土气而土仍然跟随着木，疏导水气而水仍然跟随着土，助长火气而火仍然跟随着水，这该怎么办呢？"

岐伯说："这说明阴阳已经产生了变化，水火已经分离了，这种情况并非可以用药物、砭石、针灸治疗了。"

陈士铎评论说："虽然论述简朴，但道理却非常深奥。"

one that] follows wood cultivates [Qi] in earth; [the one that] follows earth dredges [Qi] in water; [the one that] follows water assists [Qi] in fire. [There should be] neither insufficiency nor excess. [When] there is peace [in circulation of Qi], there will be no follower [in movement]."

Tianlao asked, "[When] metal is moistened, it still follows fire; [when] wood is promoted, it still follows metal; [when] earth is cultivated, it still follows wood; [when] water is dredged, it still follows earth; [when] fire is assisted, it still follows water. How to solve [it]?"

Qibo answered, "This [indicates that] Yin and Yang have already changed [and that] water and fire have already separated [from each other], [which is] impossible to be treated by medicinals, stone needle, acupuncture and moxibustion."

Chen Shiduo's comment, "*The explanation is simple but the analysis is profound.*"

冬夏火热篇第五十八

【原文】

胡孔甲问于岐伯曰："冬令严冷凛洌之气逼人肌肤,人宜畏寒,反生热证,何也?"

岐伯曰："外寒则内益热也。"

胡孔甲曰："外寒内热,人宜同病,何故独热?"

岐伯曰："肾中水虚,不能制火,因外寒相激而火发也。人身无脏非火,无腑非火也,无不藉肾水相养。肾水盛则火藏,肾水涸则火动。内无水养则内热已极,又得外寒束之,则火之郁气一发,多不可救。"

胡孔甲曰："火必有所助而后盛,火发于外,外无火助,宜火之少衰,乃热病发于夏转轻,发于冬反重,何也?"

岐伯曰："此正显火郁之气也。暑日气散而火难居,冬日气藏而火难泄。难泄而泄之,则郁怒之气所以难犯而转重也。"

胡孔甲曰："可以治夏者治冬乎?"

岐伯曰："辨其火热之真假耳,毋论冬夏也。"

胡孔甲曰："善。"

陈士铎曰："治郁无他治之法,人亦治郁而已矣。"

Volume 7

【英译】

Chapter 58
Heat and Fire in Winter and Summer

Hu Kongjia asked Qibo, "[In] winter, extreme cold threatens human skin and man should fear cold. But why are there heat symptoms and signs?"

Qibo answered, "[If there is] external cold, [there will be] internal heat."

Hu Kongjia asked, "[If there is] external cold and internal heat, people should suffer from the same disease. But why do [a few people suffer from] heat [disease]?"

Qibo answered, "Water in the kidney is deficient and unable to control fire. When stimulated by external cold, fire [inside the body will] outbreak. [In] the human body, all the Zang-organs belong to fire, and so do all the Fu-organs. [Among the Zang-organs and Fu-organs,] no one does not [depend on] water in the kidney to nourish. [When] water in the kidney is exuberant, fire will conceal [itself in the body]; [when] water in the kidney is dry, fire will act [rashly]. [If] there is no internal water to nourish, internal heat will go to the extreme. [When] fettered by external cold, stagnated Qi from fire will outbreak. [When such an accident happens,] many [people suffering from it] cannot be saved."

Hu Kongjia asked, "[Only when] assisted can fire become exuberant. [In fact,] fire outbreaks in the external and in the

【今译】

胡孔甲问岐伯："冬天严寒凛冽之气侵袭威逼人体的肌肤,人体应当出现畏惧寒冷的症状,如今反而出现发热的症状,这是为什么呢?"

岐伯说："外面天气寒冷,人体内部热气就会更加严重。"

胡孔甲问："体外寒冷,体内发热。在这种情况下,人们应当都同时发病,但为什么只有一些人发热,而不是全体都发热呢?"

岐伯说："这是因为肾水虚弱,不能制伏火气,又因为外来寒气的刺激,从而导致内热发生。人身的没有哪个脏器不是火的,没有哪个腑器也不是火的,没有哪个脏腑不是凭藉肾水来滋养的。如果肾水旺盛,火气就隐藏在体中;如果肾水干涸,火气就会妄动。如果体内没有水的滋养,且内热已达到极点,同时又遇到外寒束缚,那么火的郁气一旦发生,大多情况下就无法挽救了。"

胡孔甲问："火必然因有所助才会旺盛。火发生在外,如果外无火助,火就应当是衰少了。但内热病发生在夏天时则比较轻,而发生在冬天时反而严重,这是为什么呢?"

岐伯说："这实际上正是显示火的郁气。在暑热的夏季,真气容易发散,火气难以滞留在身内。在寒冷的冬天,真气内藏,火气就难以发泄。如果难以发泄但却勉强发泄了,那么郁怒之气因为难以制伏而加重。"

胡孔甲问："可以用治疗夏天火热之法来治疗冬天的火热吗?"

岐伯说："治疗时只须辨别火热的真假即可,不必论述冬天和夏天的季节问题。"

胡孔甲说："好!"

陈士铎评论说："治疗郁热并无其他方法,只是努力根治郁热而已。"

external there is no water to assist. [For this reason,] fire should be faint. However, heat disease occurring in summer is light but occurring in winter is severe. What is the reason?"

Qibo answered, "This demonstrates stagnated Qi in fire. [In] summer, Qi [tends] to dissipate but fire is difficult to remain [inside the body]. [In] winter, Qi conceals [inside the body] but fire is difficult to disperse. [If it tries] to disperse [when there is] difficulty to disperse, severely stagnated Qi becomes more serious [because it is] hard to subdue."

Hu Kongjia asked, "Can [the therapeutic method used] to treat [heat disease in] summer [be applied to] treatment [of heat disease occurring in] winter?"

Qibo answered, "[What should be cared is] to differentiate [whether] fire and heat are true or false, not just to discuss winter or summer."

Hu Kongjia said, "Excellent [explanation]!"

Chen Shiduo's comment, "[*There is*] *no other* [*special*] *method for treating stagnated* [*heat disease*]. [*What*] *man* [*should do is*] *also to treat stagnated* [*heat disease*]."

暑火二气篇第五十九

【原文】

祝融问于岐伯曰："暑与火皆热证也,何六气分为二乎?"

岐伯曰："暑病成于夏,火病四时皆有,故分为二也。"

祝融问曰："火病虽四时有之,然多成于夏,热蕴于夏而发于四时,宜暑包之矣。"

岐伯曰："火不止成于夏,四时可成也。火宜藏不宜发,火发于夏日者,火以引火也。其在四时虽无火之可发,而火蕴结于脏腑之中,每能自发,其酷烈之势较外火引之者更横,安可谈暑而不谈火乎?"

祝融曰："火不可发也,发则多不可救,与暑热之相犯有异乎?"

岐伯曰："暑与火热同而实异也。惟其不同,故夏日之火,不可与春秋冬之火共论;惟其各异,即夏日之暑,不可与夏日之火并举也。盖火病乃脏腑自生之热,非夏令暑热所成之火,故火证生于夏,仍是火证,不可谓火是暑,暑即是火也。"

祝融曰："暑、火非一也,分二气宜矣。"

陈士铎曰："暑与火不可并论,独吐至理。"

Volume 7

【英译】

Chapter 59
Double Qi from Summer [-Heat] and Fire

Zhurong asked Qibo, "Summer [-heat] and fire are all heat syndrome/pattern. Why [is it] divided into two in the six [kinds of] Qi?"

Qibo answered, "Summer [-heat] disease occurs in summer [while] fire disease occurs in all seasons. That is why [it is] divided into two."

Zhurong asked, "Although there is fire disease in the four seasons, [it] mainly occurs in summer . [Since] heat accumulates in summer but appears in the four seasons, [it] should include summer [-heat]."

Qibo answered, "Fire not only occurs in summer, [but also] occurs in the four seasons[1]. [It is] appropriate for fire to conceal, not to outbreak. [The reason why] fire outbreaks in summer [is that] fire induces fire. Although there is no outbreak of fire in the four seasons, fire accumulates and binds in the Zang-organs and Fu-organs, frequently outbreaking spontaneously. Its fierce tendency is more violent than that of external fire. Why does the discussion only focus on summer [-heat], not on fire?"

Zhurong asked, "Fire cannot outbreak. [If it] outbreaks, many [sufferers] cannot be saved. [In] what [way is it] different from summer-heat?"

【今译】

祝融问岐伯："暑热与火热都是热症,为何在六气中反而分为二种呢?"

岐伯说："暑热之病只发生在夏天,而火热之病一年四季都有发生,所以将其分为二种。"

祝融问："火热之病虽然一年四季都有,但多数还是发生在夏季。火热因为蕴藏在夏天,而发生在四季,这当然应包括暑热了。"

岐伯说："火热之病并不只是发生在夏天,可以发生在一年四季之中。火应当蕴藏而不应当发泄。火热发生在夏天,是因为有火引火的缘故。在四季中虽然没有火来引发,但火热蕴结于脏腑之中,每每可以自动发生,其酷烈之势与外来之火引发的情势相比,情况更为猛烈,怎么可以只谈暑热而不谈火热呢?"

祝融问："火热不能发作,发作后多数患者不能救治。这与暑热的侵袭有何差异?"

岐伯说："暑热与火热表面上似乎相同,但实际上却是有差异的。正因为存在差异,所以夏天之火不能与春、秋、冬之火共论。正因为存在差异,夏天的暑热就不能与夏天的火热同论。这是因为火热病是脏腑自生的热气,并非夏天的暑热所形成的火气,因此火证发生在夏天仍然是火证,不能认为火就是暑,也不能认为暑就是火。"

祝融说："暑与火确实不是一种,应当分为二种。"

陈士铎评论说："暑热与火热不可相提并论,但关键的道理则在这里得到了独特的阐述。"

Volume 7

Qibo answered, "Summer [-heat] and fire-heat [seem to be] the same but actually different. Because [they are] different, fire in summer cannot be discussed together with fire in spring, autumn and winter; because [they are] different, summer [-heat] in summer cannot be analyzed together with fire in summer. [This is] due to [the fact that] fire disease [is caused by] heat produced spontaneously by the Zang-organs and Fu-organs, not [caused by] fire produced by summer-heat in summer. That is why fire syndrome/pattern caused in summer is still fire syndrome/pattern. [For this reason,] fire cannot be called summer [-heat] and summer [-heat cannot be called] fire."

Zhurong said, "Summer [-heat] and fire are not the same [and it is] appropriate to divide [it into] two [kinds of] Qi."

Chen Shiduo's comment, "Summer [-heat] and fire cannot be mentioned in the same way. The unique discussion [in this Chapter is the analysis of] the great principle."

Notes

[1] Traditionally in China, the time of a year is divided into five seasons, i. e. spring, summer, late summer, autumn and winter.

阴阳上下篇第六十

【原文】

常伯问于岐伯曰："阳在上,阴在下,阳气亦下行乎?"

岐伯曰："阴阳之气上下相同,阳之气未尝不行于下也。"

常伯曰："寒厥到膝不到巅,头痛到巅不到膝,非阴气在下,阳气在上之明验乎?"

岐伯曰："阴气生于阳,阳气生于阴,盖上下相通,无彼此之离也。阳气从阴出于经脉之外,阴气从阳入于经脉之中,始得气血贯通,而五脏七腑无不周遍也。寒厥到膝,阳不能达也,非阳气专在上而不在下也;头痛到巅,阴不能降也,非阴气专在下而不在上也。天地不外阴阳,天地之阴阳不交,则寒暑往来,生长收藏咸无准实,人何独异哉?"

陈士铎曰："阳宜达,阴宜降也。二者相反,则达者不达,降者不降矣。论理阳之达有降之势,阴之降有达之机,总贵阴阳之不可反也。"

【今译】

常伯请问岐伯："阳气在上,阴气在下,阳气也能行于下吗?"

岐伯说："阴阳之气上下相同,阳气并不是不能行于下的。"

常伯问："寒厥之证发展到膝盖但没有到头顶,头痛发生在头顶而

Volume 7

【英译】

Chapter 60
Yin and Yang, Upper and Lower

Changbo asked Qibo, "Yang is in the upper and Yin is in the lower. Does Yang Qi also flow downwards?"

Qibo answered, "Qi from both Yin and Yang all flows upwards and downwards in the same way. [It does] not mean [that] Qi from Yang never flows downwards."

Changbo asked, "Reveral cold only extends to the knee and never to the top of the head; headache only maintains on the top of the head and never extends to the knee. Is it proved [that] Yin Qi is in the lower and Yang Qi is in the upper?"

Qibo answered, "Yin Qi originates from Yang and Yang Qi originates from Yin. [As a result,] the upper and the lower are connected with each other and never separated from each other. Yang Qi, following Yin Qi, flows to the external of meridians; Yin Qi, following Yang Qi, enters the meridians, consequently ensuring connection of Qi and blood in all the five Zang-organs and seven Fu-organs. [The reason that] reversal cold [just] extends to the knee [is that] Yang [Qi] cannot reach [it], not [indicating that] Yang Qi is only in the upper and not in the lower; [the reason that] headache just maintains on the top of the head [is that] Yin [Qi] cannot descend, not [indicating that] Yin Qi is just in the lower and not in the upper. [In] the sky and earth, [there are] no more than

不发展到膝盖,这难道不是阴气在下、阳气在上的明证吗?"

岐伯说:"阴气生于阳,阳气生于阴,因为上下相通,所以彼此不相分离。阳气随着阴气运行到经脉之外,阴气随着阳气进入到经脉之中,这样才能气血贯通,从而使五脏七腑没有不通畅的。寒厥之症之所以只发展到膝盖,是因为阳气不能到达的缘故,并非是阳气只在上而不在下的原因;头痛发生在头顶,这是阴气不能下降的缘故,并不是阴气只在下而不在上的原因。天地之中所存在的不外乎阴阳二气,如果天地之中的阴阳之气不交,那么寒暑的往来以及收藏生长都没有准则和实际了,人又怎么会独自存有差异呢?"

陈士铎评论说:"阳气应当上达,阴气应当下降。假若二者相反,则上达的不能上达,下降的不能下降。就道理而言,阳气虽然上达,也有下降的趋势,阴气虽然下降,但也有上达的机遇。总之,重要的是阴阳的运行不能完全相反。"

Volume 7

Yin and Yang. [If] Yin and Yang in the sky and earth are unable to connect [with each other], alternate attack of cold and heat [will make it] impossible [for all things] to sprout, grow, [transform], retrain [or collect] and store. How could there be difference in human beings?"

Chen Shiduo's comment, " *Yang* [*Qi*] *should ascend* [*while*] *Yin* [*Qi*] *should descend.* [*If*] *they are opposite,* [*the one that should*] *ascend cannot ascend and* [*the one that*] *should descend cannot descend. According to the law, Yang* [*Qi*] *ascends but also tends to descend and Yin* [*Qi*] *descends but also has the chance to ascend. Anyway Yin and Yang cannot* [*move in*] *the opposite* [*way*].*"*

营卫交重篇第六十一

【原文】

雷公曰："阳气出于卫气,阴气出于营气。阴主死,阳主生。阳气重于阴气,宜卫气重于营气矣。"

岐伯曰："营卫交重也。"

雷公曰："请问交重之旨。"

岐伯曰："宗气积于上焦,营气出于中焦,卫气出于下焦。盖有天地,有阳气,有阴气。人禀天地之二气,亦有阴阳。卫气即阳也,由下焦至中焦,以升于上焦,从阴出阳也;营气即阴也,由中焦至上焦,以降于下焦,从阳入阴也。二气并重,交相上下,交相出入,交相升降,而后能生气于无穷也。"

雷公曰："阴阳不可离,予既已知之矣,但阴气难升者谓何?"

岐伯曰："阴气精专,必随宗气以同行于经隧之中。始于手太阴肺经太渊穴,而行于手阳明大肠经、足阳明胃经、足太阴脾经、手少阴心经、手太阳小肠经、足太阳膀胱经、足少阴肾经、手厥阴心包经、手少阳三焦经、足少阳胆经、足厥阴肝经,而又始于手太阴肺经。盖阴在内不在外,阴主守内不主卫外,纡折而若难升,实无暑之不升也。故营卫二气,人身并重,未可重卫轻营也。"

雷公曰："善。"

陈士铎曰："营卫原并重也。世重卫而轻营者,不知营卫也。"

【英译】

Chapter 61
Overlapping of Nutrient [Qi] and Defense [Qi]

Leigong said, "Yang Qi manifests as defense Qi and Yin Qi manifests as nutrient Qi. Yin [Qi is] responsible for death [while] Yang [Qi is] responsible for life. [When] Yang Qi overlaps with Yin Qi, defense Qi should overlap with nutrient Qi."

Qibo answered, "[This is] overlapping of defense [Qi] with nutrient [Qi]."

Leigong said, "Please explain the meaning of overlapping."

Qibo answered, "Pectoral Qi accumulates in the upper energizer, nutrient Qi starts from the middle energizer and defense Qi starts from the lower energizer, because there exist the sky, the earth, Yang Qi and Yin Qi. Human beings receive Qi from the sky and earth and therefore bear Yin and Yang. Defense Qi is Yang [Qi], [flowing] from the lower energizer to the middle energizer, [and finally] rising up to the upper energizer, [indicating] Yang emerging from Yin; nutrient Qi is Yin [Qi], [flowing] from the middle energizer to the upper energizer, [and finally] descending to the lower energizer, [indicating] Yang entering Yin. [These] two [kinds of] Qi overlap [with each other], communicating with each other upwards and downwards, going out and coming in together, ascending and descending together. Only in this way can [they] produce infinite vital Qi."

【今译】

雷公说:"阳气表现为卫气,阴气表现为营气。阴气主管死亡,阳气主管生存。阳气重于阴气,卫气也应重于营气。"

岐伯说:"这是营气与卫气之间的相互重叠。"

雷公说:"请问相互重叠的含义是什么。"

岐伯说:"宗气积聚在上焦,营气从中焦发出,卫气从下焦发出。因为有天地,有阳气,有阴气,而人禀受天地之二气,所以也有阴阳二气。卫气就是阳气,由下焦发出后到达中焦,又上升到上焦,这就是从阴出阳。营气则是阴气,由中焦发出后到达上焦,再从上焦下降到下焦,这就是从阳入阴。二气相互重叠,相互上下,相互出入,相互升降,然后才能产生无穷的气。"

雷公问:"阴阳不能分离,这我已经知道了,但为什么阴气难以上升呢?"

岐伯说:"阴气精致专一,必须随着宗气一同运行于经络之中,从手太阴肺经的太渊穴开始,循行于手阳明大肠经、足阳明胃经、足太阴脾经、手少阴心经、手太阳小肠经、足太阳膀胱经、足少阴肾经、手厥阴心包经、手少阳三焦经、足少阳胆经、足厥阴肝经,然后再从手太阴肺经开始循行。因为阴气在内不在外,所以阴气主管固守于里,不负责防卫表,其运行曲折,好像难以上升,但实际上却无时无刻不在上升。因此对于人身而言,营气和卫气都是非常重要的,不能只重视卫气而忽视营气啊!"

雷公说:"好!"

陈士铎评论说:"营气和卫气原本是同等重要的。但在人世间,有的人重视卫气而轻视营气,因为没有认识到营气和卫气重要性啊!"

Leigong asked, "Yin and Yang cannot separate [from each other], I have already known. But why is Yin Qi difficult to rise up?"

Qibo answered, "Yin Qi is exquisite and special, certainly flowing in the meridians and collaterals with pectoral Qi. [It] starts from Taiyuan (LU 9) in the lung meridian of hand-Taiyin, flowing in the large intestine meridian of hand-Yangming, the stomach meridian of foot-Yangming, the spleen meridian of foot-Taiyin, the heart meridian of hand-Shaoyin, the small intestine meridian of hand-Taiyang, the bladder meridian of foot-Taiyang, the kidney meridian of foot-Shaoyin, the pericardium meridian of hand-Jueyin, the triple energizer meridian of hand-Shaoyang, the gallbladder meridian of foot-Shaoyang and the liver meridian of foot-Jueyin, and finally restarting from the lung meridian of hand-Taiyin. [This is] because [that] Yin [Qi] is in the internal, not in the external; [and that] Yin [Qi] governs the internal, not defending the external. [It seems that Yin Qi flows] tortuously and is difficult to rise up. In fact [it] never stops rising up. Hence defense [Qi] and nutrient [Qi] are all very important in the human body. [So it is] incorrect just to pay more attention to defense [Qi and less to nutrient [Qi]."

Leigong said, "Excellent [explanation]!"

Chen Shiduo's comment, "Nutrient [Qi] and defense [Qi] are all very important. [In this] world [those who] pay more attention to defense [Qi] and less to nutrient [Qi] do not understand nutrient [Qi] and defense [Qi]."

五脏互根篇第六十二

【原文】

雷公问于岐伯曰："阳中有阴，阴中有阳，余既知之矣。然论阴阳之变迁也，未知阴中有阳，阳中有阴，亦有定位乎？"

岐伯曰："阴阳互根也，原无定位，然求其位亦有定也。肺开窍于鼻，心开窍于舌，脾开窍于口，肝开窍于目，肾开窍于耳，厥阴与督脉会于巅，此阳中有阴，阴居阳位也；肝与胆为表里，心与小肠为表里，肾与膀胱为表里，脾与胃为表里，肺与大肠为表里，包络与三焦为表里，此阴中有阳，阳居阴位也。"

雷公曰："请言互根之位。"

岐伯曰："耳属肾而听声，声属金，是耳中有肺之阴也。鼻属肺而闻臭，臭属火，是鼻中有心之阴也。舌属心而知味，味属土，是舌中有脾之阴也。目有五轮，通贯五脏，脑属肾，各会诸体，是耳与脑有五脏之阴也。大肠俞在脊十六椎旁，胃俞在脊十二椎旁，小肠俞在背第十八椎，胆俞在脊十椎旁，膀胱俞在中膂第二十椎，三焦俞在肾俞之上，脊第十三椎之旁，包络无俞，寄于膈俞，在上七椎之旁，是七腑阳中有阴之位也。惟各有位，故其根生生不息也，否则虚器耳，何根之有哉？"

雷公曰："善。"

Volume 7

【英译】

Chapter 62
Interdependence of the Five Zang-organs

Leigong asked Qibo, "There is Yin in Yang and there is Yang in Yin. [This fact] I have already known. But in discussing changes of Yin and Yang, [I] do not know [whether] there is Yang in Yin and Yin in Yang. Is there any position?"

Qibo answered, "Yin and Yang are interdependent and originally there is no fixed position. But [if you] look for the position, the position is certainly fixed. The lung opens [its] orifice[1] in the nose, the heart opens [its] orifice in the tongue, the spleen opens [its] orifice in the mouth, the liver opens [its] orifice in the eyes, the kidney opens [its] orifice in the ears. Jueyin and the governor vessel meet at the top of the head, [indicating that] there is Yin in Yang [and that] Yin is located in Yang position. [Besides,] the liver and the gallbladder are externally and internally [related to each other], the heart and the small intestine are externally and internally [related to each other], the kidney and the bladder are externally and internally [related to each other], the spleen and the stomach are externally and internally [related to each other], the lung and the large intestine are externally and internally [related to each other], and the pericardium and the triple energizer are externally and internally [related to each other], [indicating that] there is Yang in Yin [and that] Yang is located in

陈士铎曰:"阴中有阳,阳中有阴,无位而有位者,以阴阳之有根也。"

【今译】

雷公请问岐伯:"阳中有阴,阴中有阳,这我已经知道了。但论述阴阳的变迁,却不知阴中有阳,阳中有阴,这也有定位吗?"

岐伯说:"阴阳互根,本来就没有固定的位置。但如果一定要寻求它们的位置,也是可以定位的。肺开窍于鼻,心开窍于舌,脾开窍于口,肝开窍于目,肾开窍于耳,厥阴与督脉会聚于头顶,这是阳中有阴,也是阴气居于阳位的体现。肝与胆相表里,心与小肠相表里,肾与膀胱相表里,脾与胃相表里,肺与大肠相表里,包络与三焦相表里,这是阴中有阳,也是阳气居于阴位的体现。"

雷公说:"请说明五脏互根的位置。"

岐伯说:"耳属于肾而主管听声,声则属于金,这是耳中有肺之阴气的体现。鼻属于肺而主管闻香臭,香臭属于火,这是鼻中有心之阴气的体现。舌属于心而主管味道,味道属于土,这是舌中有脾之阴气的体现。眼睛中有五轮,通贯五脏,而脑则属于肾,会合身体的各个部位,这是耳与脑中有五脏之阴气的体现。大肠俞位于脊柱的第十六椎旁,胃俞位于脊柱的第十二椎旁,小肠俞位于脊柱的第十八椎旁,胆俞位于脊柱的第十椎旁,膀胱俞位于中膂的第二十椎,三焦俞位于肾俞之上、脊柱的第十三椎旁,包络没有俞,寄居于膈俞,位于脊柱的第七椎的旁,这是七腑阳中有阴的位置。只有七腑各居其位,才能生生不息,否则就会

Yin position."

Leigong asked,"Please explain the position of interdependence."

Qibo answered, "The ears belong to the kidney and [are responsible for] listening to sound which belongs to metal, indicating [that] there is Yin from the lung in the ears; the nose belongs to the lung and [is responsible for] smelling flavor [which] belongs to fire, indicating [that] there is Yin from the heart in the nose; the tongue belongs to the heart and [is responsible for] testing taste [which] belongs to earth, indicating [that] there is Yin from the spleen in the tongue. There are five wheels in the eyes [that] are connected with the five Zang-organs. The brain belongs to the kidney and coordinates with all parts of the body, indicating [that] there is Yin from the five Zang-organs in the ears and brain. Dachangshu (BL 25) [is located] at the side of the sixteenth spinal vertebra, Weishu (BL 21) [is located] at the side of the twelfth spinal vertebra, Xiaochangshu (BL 27) [is located] at the side of the eighteenth spinal vertebra, Danshu (BL 19) [is located] at the side of the tenth spinal vertebra, Pangguangshu (BL 28) [is located] at the side of the twentieth hip vertebra, Sanjiaoshu (BL 22) [is located] above Shenshu (BL 23) at the side of the thirteenth spinal vertebra. [In] the pericardium there is no acupoint, [so it is] located in Geshu (BL 17) above the side of the seventh spinal vertebra, indicating [that] there is Yin position in Yang from the seven Fu-organs. Only when everyone has its own position can [it] exist forever. Otherwise [it is] an organ of nihility. How [could it] have the root[2]?"

Leigong said,"Excellent [explanation]!"

变成虚无的脏器,怎么可能互根呢?"

雷公说:"好!"

陈士铎评论说:"阴中有阳,阳中有阴,彼此之间形式上没有位置,但实际上却是有位置的,因为阴阳皆有其根。"

Volume 7

Chen Shiduo's comment, "There is Yang in Yin and Yin in Yang, [indicating that actually] there is position [when there appears] no position because both Yin and Yang are interdependent."

Notes

[1] The original Chinese characters for "open into" are Kaiqiao (开窍) which means to open orifices. Traditional Chinese medicine uses this term to describe the close relationship between two organs. It does not necessarily mean that there is a canal that links the two interrelated organs. For example, when we say that the liver opens into the eyes, we just emphasize the close relationship between the liver and the eyes and we certainly do not think that there is a canal that links the liver and the eyes. However, the concept of "open into" can well be explained according to the theory of Jingluo (经络 meridians and collaterals).

[2] Root here refers to the foundation of existence.

八风固本篇第六十三

【原文】

雷公问于岐伯曰:"八风出于天乎? 出于地乎? 抑出于人乎?"

岐伯曰:"八风出于天地,人身之五风合而成病。人无五风,天地之风不能犯也。"

雷公曰:"请问八风之分天地也。"

岐伯曰:"八风者,春夏秋冬东西南北之风也。春夏秋冬之风,时令之风也,属于天;东西南北之风,方隅之风也,属于地。然而地得天之气,风乃长;天得地之气,风乃大。是八风属于天地,可合而不可分也。"

雷公曰:"人之五风,何以合天地乎?"

岐伯曰:"五风者,心肝脾肺肾之风也,五脏虚而风生矣。以内风召外风,天地之风始翕然相合。五脏不虚,内既无风,外风何能入乎?"

雷公曰:"风既入矣,祛外风乎? 抑消内风乎?"

岐伯曰:"风由内召,不治内将何治乎?"

雷公曰:"治内风而外风不散奈何?"

岐伯曰:"内风不治,外风益入,安得散乎? 治脏固其本,治风卫其标,善治八风者也。"

雷公曰:"何言之善乎! 请志之,传示来者。"

Volume 7

【英译】

Chapter 63
Eight [Kinds of] Wind[1]Consolidating the Root[2]

Leigong asked Qibo, "Where do the eight [kinds of] wind come from? From the sky, earth or man?"

Qibo answered, "The eight [kinds of] wind come from the sky and earth and, [when] combining with the five [kinds of] wind in the human body, will cause disease. [If there are] no five [kinds of] wind in the human [body], wind from the sky and earth cannot invade [the body]."

Leigong asked, "Please explain how to allocate the eight [kinds of] wind to the sky and earth."

Qibo answered, "The eight [kinds of] wind [refer to] wind [blowing] in the spring, summer, autumn and winter [as well as] in the east, south, west and north. Wind [blowing] in spring, summer, autumn and winter is seasonal wind and belongs to the sky; wind [blowing] in the east, south, west and north is oriental wind and belongs to the earth. However, [when] the earth has received Qi from the sky, wind can grow; [when] the sky has received Qi from the earth, wind can increase. Hence the eight [kinds of] wind belong to the sky and earth, [physically] separable but [actually] inseparable."

Leigong asked, "How can the five [kinds of] wind in the human [body] combine with the sky and earth?"

陈士铎曰："小风之来,皆外感也,外感因于内召。故单治内不能也,单治外亦不可也。要在分之中宜合,合之中宜分也。"

【今译】

雷公请问岐伯:"八风究竟源自于天,还是源自于地,抑或源自于人?"

岐伯说:"八风源自于天地,与人身的五风相合就会引发疾病。如果人体没有五风,则源自天地之风就不能侵犯。"

雷公问:"请问八风如何分之于天地?"

岐伯说:"八风指的是春、夏、秋、冬、东、西、南、北之风。春、夏、秋、冬之风,是时令之风,属于在天之风;东、西、南、北之风,是方位之风,属于在地之风。然而,地只有得到了天之气,其风才能增长;天只有得到地之气,风才能壮大。所以八风虽然分别属于天地,其形式上可分,但实际上是不可分的。"

雷公问:"人体的五风,如何与天地的八风相合呢?"

岐伯说:"五风指的是心、肝、脾、肺、肾之风,只有五脏虚弱的时候内风才会产生。当人体的内风召感外风时,天地之风才会开始与之相合。如果五脏不虚弱,身内就不会有风,外风又怎么能够进入人体呢?"

雷公问:"外风既然进入人体了,到底是该祛除外风呢? 还是要抑制和消除内风呢?"

岐伯说:"外风是由人身之内风召感而来的,如果不治内风,又怎么能治外风呢?"

Qibo answered, "The five [kinds of] wind [refer to] wind from the heart, liver, spleen, lung and kidney. [When] the five Zang-organs are weak, wind [begins] to appear. Only [when] internal wind calls for external wind can wind from the sky and earth combine with [it]. [When] the five Zang-organs are not weak, there will be no internal wind. How can external wind enter [the body]?"

Leigong asked, "[When external] wind has entered [the body], [should] external wind be eliminated [or] internal wind be resolved?"

Qibo answered, "[It is] the internal [wind that has] beckoned [the external] wind. [If] the internal [wind is] not resolved, how can [invasion of external wind be] eliminated?"

Leigong asked, "[When] the internal wind is resolved, but the external wind is not eliminated. How [to deal with it]?"

Qibo answered, "[If] the internal wind is not resolved, invasion of the external wind [will be] more serious. How can [it be] eliminated? To treat the Zang-organs can consolidate the root and to treat wind can defend the tip[3]. [This is] the right [way] to deal with the eight [kinds of] wind."

Leigong said, "Excellent explanation! Please record [this explanation] and pass on to the next generation."

Chen Shiduo's comment, "[External] breeze is all external contraction beckoned by the internal [wind]. That is why the internal [wind] alone is impossible to be resolved and the external [wind] alone is unable to be eliminated. [One must be clear that it

雷公问："治疗内风,但是外风不消散又该怎么办呢?"

岐伯说："如果内风得不到治疗,外风的入侵就会更加严重,怎么能将其消散呢? 治疗五脏就可坚固其本,治疗风气就可防卫其标,这才是善于治疗八风的表现!"

雷公说："分析得真好啊! 请记载下来,传给后来人。"

陈士铎评论说："外来的小风都是外感的体现。外感是内风召感所致。所以单纯治疗体内症候是不可的,单纯治疗体外的症候也是不可的。所以要在分离之中关注结合,要在结合之中注意分离。"

is] *appropriate to combine in separation and to separate in combination.* "

Notes

[1] Eight [kinds of] wind refer to wind blowing in spring, summer, autumn and winter as well as in the east, south, west and north. Wind blowing in spring, summer, autumn and winter is seasonal wind; wind blowing in the east, south, west and north is oriental wind.

[2] Root （本）, an important concept in traditional Chinese culture, refers to foundation or origin of anything.

[3] Tip （标）, an important concept in traditional Chinese culture, refers to the secondary aspect or superficial aspect of anything.

卷八

八风命名篇第六十四

【原文】

少俞问于岐伯曰："八风分春夏秋冬、东西南北乎？"

岐伯曰："然。"

少俞曰："东西南北不止四风，合之四时，则八风不足以概之也。"

岐伯曰："风不止八，而八风实足概之。"

少俞曰："何谓也？"

岐伯曰："风从东方来，得春气也；风从东南来，得春气而兼夏气矣；风从南方来，得夏气也；风从西南来，得夏气而兼秋气矣；风从西方来，得秋气也；风从西北来，得秋气而兼冬气矣；风从北方来，得冬气也；风从东北来，得冬气而兼春气矣。此方隅、时令合而成八也。"

少俞曰："八风有名乎？"

岐伯曰："东风名和风也，东南风名薰风也，南风名热风也，西南风名温风也，西风名商风也，西北风名凉风也，北风名寒风也，东北风名阴风也，又方隅时令合而名之也。"

少俞曰："其应病何如乎？"

岐伯曰："和风伤在肝也，外病在筋；薰风伤在胃也，外病在肌；热风伤在心也，外病在脉；温风伤在脾也，外病在腹；商风伤在肺也，外病

Volume 8

【英译】

Chapter 64
Nomenclature of the Eight [Kinds of] Wind

Shaoshu asked Qibo, "[Are] the eight [kinds of] wind classified into spring, summer, autumn and winter [as well as] the east, west, south and north?"

Qibo answered, "Right."

Shaoshu said, "[The categories of] wind [in] the east, west, south and north are not just four. [When] combined with the four seasons, the eight [kinds of] wind are unable to generalize [all that concerned]."

Qibo answered, "[It is true that] wind is more than eight [kinds]. But the eight [kinds of] wind are enough to generalize [all that concerned]."

Shaoshu asked, "How to explain it?"

Qibo answered, "[What] wind from the east gets is spring-Qi; [what] wind from the southeast gets is spring-Qi and also summer-Qi; [what] wind from the south gets is summer-Qi; [what] wind from southwest gets is summer-Qi and also autumn-Qi; [what] wind from the west gets is autumn-Qi; [what] wind from the northwest gets is autumn-Qi and also winter-Qi; [what] wind from the north gets is winter-Qi; [what] wind from the northeast gets is winter-Qi and also spring-Qi. That [is how] the orientations and the seasons

在皮;凉风伤在膀胱也,外病在营卫;寒风伤在肾也,外病在骨;阴风伤在大肠也,外病在胸胁。此方隅时令与脏腑相合而相感也。然而脏腑内虚,八风因得而中之,邪之所凑,其气必虚,非空言也。"

少俞曰:"人有脏腑不虚而八风中之者,又是何谓?"

岐伯曰:"此暴风猝中,不治而自愈也。"

陈士铎曰:"八风之来皆外感也,外感因于内召。故治内而外邪自散。若自外病者,不必治之。"

【今译】

少俞请问岐伯说:"八风分为春、夏、秋、冬、东、西、南、北吗?"

岐伯说:"是的。"

少俞问:"东、西、南、北不只是四风,与四时配合后,八风不足以对其加以概括了。"

岐伯说:"虽然不只是八风,但实际上八风还是可以概括的。"

少俞问:"原因呢?"

岐伯说:"从东方来的风,得到的是春天之气;从东南来的风,得到的是春天之气并兼有夏天之气;从南方来的风,得到的是夏天之气;从西南来的风,得到的是夏天之气并兼有秋天之气;从西方来的风,得到的是秋天之气;从西北来的风,得到的是秋天之气并兼有冬天之气;从北方来的风,得到的是冬天之气;从东北来的风,得到的是冬天之气并兼有春天之气。这是方位与时令相配合而形成的八风。"

are combined to form the eight [kinds of] wind. "

Shaoshu asked, "How to name the eight [kinds of] wind?"

Qibo answered, "The east wind is named harmony wind, the southeast wind is named fragrant wind, the south wind is named heat wind, the southwest wind is named warm wind, the west wind is named autumnal wind, the northwest wind is named cool wind, the north wind is named cold wind and the northeast wind is named cloudy wind. This nomenclature is [based on] combination of the orientations and seasons. "

Shaoshu asked, "How about the diseases related to them?"

Qibo answered, "Harmony wind damages the liver [and causes] disease externally in the sinews; fragrant wind damages the stomach [and causes] disease externally in the muscles; heat wind damages the heart [and causes] disease externally in the vessels/meridians; warm wind damages the spleen [and causes] disease externally in the abdomen; autumnal wind damages the lung [and causes] disease externally in the skin; cool wind damages the bladder [and causes] disease externally in the nutrient and defense [aspects]; cold wind damages the kidney [and causes] disease externally in the bones; cloudy wind damages the large intestine [and causes] disease externally in the chest and rib-side. Such [causes and locations of diseases demonstrate] the result of the combination of the orientations, seasons and Zang-organs and Fu-organs. However, [only when] the Zang-organs and Fu-organs are weakened can the eight [kinds of] wind invade [the body]. [Hence in the place where] evil accumulates, Qi must be deficient. [This is certainly] not idle talk. "

少俞问："这八种风有名称吗？"

岐伯说："东风名为和风，东南风名为薰风，南风名为热风，西南风名为温风，西风名为商风，西北风名为凉风，北风名为寒风，东北风名为阴风。这也是方向与时令相配合而命名的名称。"

少俞问："其对应的病又是怎么样的呢？"

岐伯说："和风在体内伤害肝脏，在外病在筋；薰风在体内伤害胃脏，在外病在肌肉；热风在体内伤害心脏，在外病在脉；温风在体内伤害脾脏，在外病在腹；商风在体内伤害肺脏，在外病在皮肤；凉风在体内伤害膀胱，在外病在营卫；寒风在体内伤害肾脏，在外病在骨；阴风在体内伤害大肠，在外病在胸胁。这是方位、时令与脏腑相互配合而彼此感应的。但是只有脏腑内在的虚弱存在，八风才会因此而侵入人体。所以邪气所凑集之处，正气必然虚弱，这当然不是空虚的泛泛之论。"

少俞问："有的人脏腑并不虚弱，但是还是受到了八风的伤害，这是什么原因呢？"

岐伯说："这是暴风突然伤害的缘故，即便不治疗也会自然痊愈。"

陈士铎评论说："八风的入侵都是外感所致，外感则是体内五风感召所致。所以治疗体内症候会使外邪自然消散。如果是因外病所致，则不必治疗。"

Volume 8

Shaoshu asked, "[In] some people, Zang-organs and Fu-organs are not weakened, but the eight [kinds of] wind still attack them. What is the reason?"

Qibo answered, "This [is] sudden attack of violent storm. [If] not treated, [it still can] heal spontaneously."

Chen Shiduo's comment, " Invasion of the eight [kinds of] wind is all external contraction. [And] external contraction is caused by internal [wind that] beckons [external wind]. Thus [when] the internal is treated, external evil [will] disperse spontaneously. If [it] originates from external disease, [there is] no need to treat it."

太乙篇第六十五

【原文】

风后问于岐伯曰："八风可以占疾病之吉凶乎？"

岐伯曰："天人一理也，可预占以断之。"

风后曰："占之不验何也？"

岐伯曰："有验有不验者，人事之不同耳，天未尝不可占也。"

风后曰："请悉言之。"

岐伯曰："八风休咎，无日无时不可占也。如风从东方来，寅卯辰时则顺，否则逆矣，逆则病；风从西方来，申酉戌时则顺，否则逆矣，逆则病；风从南方来，巳午未时则顺，否则逆矣，逆则病；风从北方来，亥子丑时则顺，否则逆矣，逆则病。"

风后曰："予闻古之占风也，多以太乙之日为主。"

岐伯曰："无日无时不可占也，恐不可为训乎？占风以太乙日决病，所以验不验也。"

风后曰："舍太乙以占吉凶，恐不验更多耳。"

岐伯曰："公何以信太乙之深也？"

风后曰："太乙移日，天必应之风雨，风雨和则民安而病少，风雨暴则民劳而病多。太乙在冬至日有变，占在君；太乙在春分日有变，占在相；太乙在中宫日有变，占在相吏；太乙在秋分日有变，占在将；太乙在

Volume 8

【英译】

Chapter 65
Taiyi[1]

Fenghou asked Qibo, "Can the eight [kinds of] wind [be used] to analyze favourable and unfavourable [conditions of] disease?"

Qibo answered, "The sky and man are integrated. [Hence it is] possible to decide through prognosis."

Fenghou asked, "Why does augury not come true?"

Qibo answered, "[The reason that] sometimes [augury] comes true but sometimes comes false [is that there is] difference in human affairs. [So it does] not mean [that] the sky cannot be divined."

Fenghou asked, "Please explain in details."

Qibo answered, "The eight [kinds of] wind [should] not be blamed. [In fact] augury can be done every day and every hour. For instance, wind from the east is normal [at the time of] Yin (3:00 - 5:00), Mao (5:00 - 7:00) and Chen (7:00 - 9:00), otherwise [it is] adverse and causes disease; wind from the west is normal [at the time of] Shen (15:00 - 17:00), You (17:00 - 19:00) and Xu (19:00 - 21:00), otherwise [it is] adverse and causes disease; wind from the south is normal [at the time of] Si (9:00 - 11:00), Wu (11:00 - 13:00) and Wei (13:00 - 15:00), otherwise [it is] adverse and causes disease; wind from the north is normal [at the time of] Hai (21:00 - 23:00), Zi (23:00 - 1:00) and Chou (1:00 - 3:00), otherwise [it is] adverse and causes disease."

夏至日有变,占在民。所谓有变者,太乙居五宫之日,得非常之风也。各以其所主占之,生吉克凶,多不爽也。"

岐伯曰:"请言风雨之暴。"

风后曰:"暴风南方来,其伤人也,内舍于心,外在脉,其气主热。暴风西南方来,其伤人也,内舍于脾,外在肌,其气主弱。暴风西方来,其伤人也,内舍于肺,外在皮肤,其气主燥。暴风西北方来,其伤人也,内舍于小肠,外在手太阳脉,脉绝则溢,脉闭则结不通,善暴死,其气主清。暴风从北方来,其伤人也,内舍于肾,外在骨与肩背之膂筋,其气主寒。暴风东北方来,其伤人也,内舍于大肠,外在两胁腋骨下及肢节,其气主温。暴风东方来,其伤人也,内舍于肝,外在筋经,其气主湿。暴风东南方来,其伤人也,内舍于胃,外在肌肉,其气主重着。言风而雨概之矣。"

岐伯曰:"人见风辄病者,岂皆太乙之移日乎?执太乙以占风,执八风以治病,是泥于论风也。夫百病皆始于风,人之气血虚馁,风乘虚辄入矣,何待太乙居宫哉?"

陈士铎曰:"人病全不在太乙,说得澹而有味。"

【今译】

风后请问岐伯:"可以用八风占卜疾病的吉凶吗?"

岐伯说:"天与人是一样的道理,可以通过预测来诊断。"

风后问:"占卜却不应验,这是为什么呢?"

Volume 8

Fenghou said, "I have heard [that] augury in ancient times was mainly done on the day of Taiyi."

Qibo said, "[In fact] augury can be done at every day and every hour. [What you have mentioned is] perhaps not the instruction. To diagnose disease [by means of] augury on the day of Taiyi may come true or may come false."

Fenghou said, "[If] augury is not done on the day of Taiyi for [examining] favourable and unfavourable [condition of disease], [it may] frequently come false."

Qibo asked, "Why do you so believe Taiyi?"

Fenghou said, "[On] the day [when] Taiyi transfers, there must be wind and rain from the sky to correspond to it. [If] wind and rain are gentle, people [will live a] peaceful [life] and seldom [suffer from] disease; [if] wind and rain are violent, people [will live a] hard [life] and frequently [suffer from] disease. [When] Taiyi changes on the day of the winter solstice, augury corresponds to the monarch; [when] Taiyi changes on the day of the spring equinox, augury corresponds to the ministers; [when] Taiyi changes on the day of the central palace, augury corresponds to officials; [when] Taiyi changes on the day of the autumn equinox, augury corresponds to the military generals; [when] Taiyi changes on the day of the summer solstice, augury corresponds to the people. The so-called change refers to the day [that] Taiyi is located in the five palaces and meets abnormal wind. [Usually] augury is done on the day controlled by it. [Under such a condition,] promotion [indicates] favourable [while] restriction [indicates] unfavourable. [For this reason,] most [cases of augury] come true."

岐伯说："有的应验，也有的不应验，这是因为人事的差异所致，并非天时不可占卜。"

风后说："请详细说明。"

岐伯说："八风引起疾病的问题，并没有哪一天哪一个时辰不能占卜的。例如，风从东方来，寅卯辰时为顺，否则就是逆了，而逆就一定会生病。风从西方来，申酉戌时为顺，否则就是逆了，而逆就一定会生病。风从南方来，巳午未时为顺，否则就是逆了，而逆就一定会生病。风从北方来，亥子丑时为顺，否则就是逆了，而逆就一定会生病。"

风后说："我听说古代对于风的占卜，大多数情况下都是用太乙之日为主。"

岐伯说："实际上没有哪一天哪一个时辰不能占卜的，所以这一说法恐怕不全为实。通过太乙日占卜风向以诊断疾病，有些情况是应验的，也有些情况是不应验的。"

风后问："舍弃太乙日占卜吉凶，不应验的情况恐怕会更多吧?"

岐伯说："你为什么会如此深信太乙之日的占卜呢?"

风后说："太乙每日迁移，天必然出现相应的风雨，如果风雨和顺，民众则平安而少病，如果风雨狂暴，民众则辛劳而多病。太乙在冬至之日有变化，占卜将应验于君;太乙在春分之日有变化，占卜将应验于相;太乙在中宫之日有变，占卜将应验于吏;太乙在秋分之日有变化，占卜将应验于将;太乙在夏至之日有变化，占卜将应验于民。所谓有变化，指的是太乙位于五宫之日，将会遇到不正常之风。若分别以其所主宰之日占卜，相生则为吉，相克则为凶，大多数情况下都会应验的。"

Volume 8

Qibo asked, "Please explain violent wind and rain."

Fenghou answered, "Violent wind from the south damages human beings internally in the heart and externally in the vessels/meridians with heat controlled by its Qi[3]; violent wind from the southwest damages human beings internally in the spleen and externally in the fleshes with weakness controlled by its Qi; violent wind from the west damages human beings internally in the lung and externally in the skin with dryness controlled by its Qi; violent wind from the northwest damages human beings internally in the small intestine and externally in [the small intestine] meridian of hand-Taiyang with lucidity controlled by its Qi, [during which there is] overflow [if] vessels/meridians are broken [and] obstruction [if] vessels/meridians are blocked, frequently leading to sudden death; violent wind from the north damages human beings internally in the kidney and externally in the bones and the major sinews in the shoulder and back with cold controlled by its Qi; violent wind from the northeast damages human beings internally in the large intestine and externally in [the regions] below the rib-sides and armpits [as well as] joints of the limbs with warmth controlled by its Qi; violent wind from the east damages human beings internally in the liver and externally in the sinews and meridians with dampness controlled by its Qi; violent wind from the southeast damages human beings internally in the stomach and externally in the fleshes with heaviness controlled by its Qi. [Such a] description about wind also includes rain."

Qibo said, "People tend to contract disease [when] attacked by wind. How could it all [be caused by] transference on the day of

岐伯说："请说明风雨的狂暴。"

风后说："暴风从南方来,其对人的伤害,在内位于心,在外位于脉,其气为热气。暴风从西南方来,其对人的伤害,在内位于脾,在外位于肌肉,其气为弱气。暴风从西方来,其对人的伤害,在内位于肺,在外位于皮肤,其气为燥气。暴风从西北方来,其对人的伤害体,在内位于小肠,在外位于手太阳经,脉象绝则溢满,脉象闭则不通,常常会导致暴死,它的气是清气。暴风从北方来,它伤害人,在内位于肾,在外位于骨与肩背的大筋,其气为寒气。暴风从东北方来,其对人的伤害,在内位于大肠,在外位于两胁腋骨下和四肢关节,其气为温气。暴风从东方来,其对人的伤害体,在内位于肝,在外位于筋节,其气为湿气。暴风从东南方来,其对人的伤害,在内位于胃,在外位于肌肉,其气为重着之气。谈论风的时候,雨其实也包括其中。"

岐伯说："人遇到风常常就会生病,这岂能皆是太乙之日的迁移呢? 占卜风仅仅局限于太乙之日,诊治疾病仅仅局限于八风,这显然是拘泥性的论风。百病都起始于风,人的气血虚衰了,风就会乘虚而入,为何一定要要等待太乙位于某宫之后才开始占卜诊断呢?"

陈士铎评论说："人之患病与太乙之变迁没有任何关系,说得浅淡而有意味。"

Taiyi? Simply depending on Taiyi to forcast wind and the eight [kinds of] wind to treat disease is rigidly adhering to discussion of wind. All diseases result from wind. [When] Qi and blood in the human [body] are weakened, wind will take the chance to invade [the body]. Why [do you just] wait for [the time when] Taiyi is located in a certain palace?"

Chen Shiduo's comment, "[Occurrence of] disease [in] the human [body] has nothing to do with Taiyi. [Such an instruction is] simple but significant."

Notes

[1] Taiyi（太乙）, also called 太一 in traditional Chinese culture, refers to the original Qi（元气）that already exists before the separation of the sky and earth. So Taiyi（太乙）is the root of all sorts of Qi and all kinds of things in the universe. In the well known classic entitled *Lüshi Chunqiu*（《吕氏春秋》）, it says, "All the things in this universe are produced by Taiyi（太乙）and transformed by Yin and Yang."

[2] Fenghou（风后）was an official in the times of Yellow Emperor and responsible for augury.

[3] The description about something "controlled by its Qi" actually refers to the property of its Qi. For instance, "heat controlled by its Qi" means heat-Qi and "dryness controlled by its Qi" means dryness-Qi. The description about wind from different orientations in this chapter is the same.

亲阳亲阴篇第六十六

【原文】

风后问于岐伯曰："风与寒异乎？"

岐伯曰："异也。"

风后曰："何异乎？"

岐伯曰："风者，八风也；寒者，寒气也。虽风未有不寒者，要之风寒各异也。"

风后曰："风与寒有异，入人脏腑，亦有异乎？"

岐伯曰："风入风府，寒不入风府也。"

风后曰："其义何居？"

岐伯曰："风阳邪，寒阴邪。阳邪主降，阴邪主升。主降者由风府之穴而入，自上而下也；主升者不由风府，由脐之穴而入，自下而上也。"

风后曰："阴邪不从风府入，从何穴而入乎？"

岐伯曰："风府之穴，阳经之穴也；脐之穴，阴经之穴也。阳邪从阳而入，故风入风门也；阴邪从阴而入，故寒入脐也。阳亲阳，阴亲阴，此天地自然之道也。"

风后曰："风穴招风，寒穴招寒。风门，风穴也，宜风之入矣。脐非寒穴也，何寒从脐入乎？"

岐伯曰："脐非寒穴，通于命门，命门火旺则寒不能入，命门火衰则

Volume 8

【英译】

Chapter 66
Intimate Yang and Intimate Yin

Fenghou asked Qibo, "Are wind and cold different?"

Qibo answered, "Different."

Fenghou asked, "What is the difference?"

Qibo answered, "Wind [refers to] the eight [kinds of] wind; cold [refers to] cold Qi. Although no wind is not cold, the importance [is that there is] difference between wind and cold."

Fenghou asked, "There is difference between wind and cold. [When] entering the Zang-organs and Fu-organs, is there still difference [between them]?"

Qibo answered, "Wind enters wind palace[1], [but] cold does not enter wind palace."

Fenghou asked, "What does it mean?"

Qibo answered, "Wind [is] Yang evil [and] cold [is] Yin evil. Yang evil is responsible for descent [while] Yin evil is responsible for ascent. [The one] responsible for descent invades [the body] through Fengfu (GV 16), descending from the upper to the lower; [the one] responsible for ascent invades [the body] not through Fengfu (GV 16) but through Shenque (CV 8) [located] in the navel, ascending from the lower to the upper."

Fenghou asked, "Yin evil does not invade [the body] through Fengfu (GV 16). Through which acupoint [does it] invade [the

腹内阴寒,脐有不寒者乎? 阴寒之邪遂乘虚寒之隙,夺脐而入矣,奚论寒穴哉?"

风后曰:"善。"

陈士铎曰:"阳邪入风府,阴邪入脐,各有道路也。"

【今译】

风后请问岐伯:"风与寒有何差异吗?"

岐伯说:"有差异。"

风后问:"有什么差异呢?"

岐伯说:"风,指的是八风;寒,指的是寒气。虽然风没有不寒冷的,但关键是风与寒有差异的。"

风后问:"风与寒有差异,但当其侵入人体脏腑后,是否还有差异呢?"

岐伯说:"风气侵入风府,寒气则不能侵入风府。"

风后问:"这是什么意思呢?"

岐伯说:"风为阳邪,寒为阴邪。阳邪主下降,阴邪主上升。主下降的由风府穴侵入,自上而向下行;主上升的不从风府穴侵入,而从肚脐的穴位侵入,自下而向上行。"

风后问:"阴邪不能从风府穴侵入,该从什么穴位侵入呢?"

岐伯说:"风府之穴,是阳经的穴位;肚脐之穴,是阴经的穴位。阳邪从阳位侵入,所以风气从风门侵入;阴邪从阴位侵入,所以寒气从肚

body]?"

Qibo answered, "Fengfu (GV 16) [is an] acupoint [located in] the Yang meridian and Shenque (CV 8) [is an] acupoint [located in] the Yin meridian. Yang evil invades [the body] from Yang [position], that is why wind invades [the body] through wind gate[2]; Yin evil invades [the body] from Yin [position], that is why cold invades [the body] through the navel. Yang is intimate with Yang and Yin is intimate with Yin. This is the natural law of the sky and earth."

Fenghou asked, "Wind acupoint beckons wind and cold acupoint beckons cold. Wind gate [is] wind acupoint and wind can enter it. The navel is not cold acupoint. Why can cold enter the navel?"

Qibo answered, "The navel is not cold acupoint, [but it is] connected with Mingmen (GV 4). [When] fire in Mingmen (GV 4) is effulgent, cold cannot enter it; [when] fire in Mingmen (GV 4) is debilitated, [there will be] Yin cold in the abdomen. How could there be no cold in the navel? [In fact,] evil in Yin cold makes use of the navel, [which is] the canal of deficiency-cold, to invade [the body]. What is the need to discuss cold acupoint?"

Fenghou said, "Excellent [explanation]!"

Chen Shiduo's comment, " Yang evil enters Fengfu (GV 16) and Yin evil enters the navel, each [of which] has [its own] way [to invade the body]."

脐侵入。阳气与阳气相亲,阴气与阴气相亲,这是天地之间的自然之道。"

风后问:"风穴招来风气,寒穴招来寒气。风门是风穴,风气应当从中侵入;肚脐并不是寒穴,为什么寒气会从肚脐侵入人体呢?"

岐伯说:"肚脐虽然不是寒穴,但可连通于命门,命门火旺时寒气则不能侵入,命门火衰时腹内则会有阴寒,肚脐里怎么会没有寒气呢?于是阴寒之邪便乘肚脐虚寒之隙而从肚脐侵入,又如何需要论述寒穴呢?"

风后说:"好!"

陈士铎评论说:"阳邪侵入风府,阴邪侵入肚脐,各有侵入的通道。"

Volume 8

Notes

[1] Palace （府） here refers to the place where wind usually stays in it.

[2] Wind gate （风门） refers to the point 1. 5 *Cun* below and lateral to the spinous process of the second thoracic vertebra.

异传篇第六十七

【原文】

雷公问曰："各脏腑之病皆有死期,有一日即死者,有二三日死者,有四五日死者,有五六日至十余日死者,可晰言之乎?"

岐伯曰："病有传经不传经之异,故死有先后也。"

雷公曰："请问传经。"

岐伯曰："邪自外来,内入脏腑,必传经也。"

雷公曰："请问不传经。"

岐伯曰："正气虚自病,则不传经也。"

雷公曰："移寒移热,即传经之谓乎?"

岐伯曰："移即传之义,然移缓传急。"

雷公曰："何谓乎?"

岐伯曰："移者,脏腑自移;传者,邪不欲在此腑而传之彼脏也。故移之势缓而凶,传之势急而暴,其能杀人则一也。"

雷公曰："其传经杀人若何?"

岐伯曰："邪入于心,一日死。邪入于肺,三日传于肝,四日传于脾,五日传于胃,十日死。邪入于肝,三日传于脾,五日传于胃,十日传于肾,又三日邪散而愈,否则死。邪入于脾,一日传于胃,二日传于肾,三日传于膀胱,十四日邪散而愈,否则死。邪入于胃,五日传于肾,八日

Volume 8

【英译】

Chapter 67
Different Transmission

Leigong asked, "There is a time of death [in] the disease of every Zang-organ and Fu-organ. [The time of] death may be one day, or two to three days, or four to five days, or five to six days, or even over ten days. Could [you] explain it in detail?"

Qibo answered, "Disease transmits either in meridians or not in meridians. That is why [the time of] death is early or late."

Leigong asked, "Please explain transmission in the meridians."

Qibo answered, "[When] evil from the external enters into the Zang-organs and Fu-organs, [it] must transmit in the meridians."

Leigong asked, "Please explain no transmission in the meridians."

Qibo answered, "[When] healthy Qi is deficient [and the patient contracts] disease spontaneously, [the evil] will not transmit [in] the meridians."

Leigong asked, "Is transference of cold and heat also transmission [in] the meridians?"

Qibo answered, "Transference also means transmission. But transference is slow [while] transmission is rapid."

Leigong asked, "What it the reason?"

Qibo answered, "Transference [means] transference [of evil] spontaneously [in] the Zang-organs and Fu-organs; transmission

传于膀胱,又五日传于小肠,又二日传于心则死。邪入于肾,三日传于膀胱,又三日传于小肠,又三日传于心则死。

邪入于膀胱,五日传于肾,又一日传于小肠,又一日传于心则死。邪入于胆,五日传于肺,又五日传于肾,又五日传于心则死。邪入于三焦,一日传于肝,三日传于心则死。邪入于胞络,一日传于胃,二日传于胆,三日传于脾,四日传于肾,五日传于肝,不愈则再传,再传不愈则死。邪入于小肠,一日传于膀胱,二日传于肾,三日传于包络,四日传于胃,五日传于脾,六日传于肺,七日传于肝,八日传于胆,九日传于三焦,十日传于大肠,十一日复传于肾,如此再传,不已则死。邪入于大肠,一日传于小肠,二日传于三焦,三日传于肺,四日传于脾,五日传于肝,六日传于肾,七日传于心则死。不传心仍传小肠,则生也。邪入于胆,往往不传,故无死期可定。然邪入于胆,往往如见鬼神,有三四日即死者,此热极自焚也。"

雷公曰:"善。"

陈士铎曰:"移缓传急,确有死期可定,最说得妙。"

【今译】

雷公问:"各脏腑的病都有死期,有的一天就死亡,有的二三天死亡,有的四五天死亡,有的五六天甚至十多天死亡,可否予以详细解析呢?"

岐伯说:"疾病有传经和不传经的差异,所以导致的死亡日期有先

[means that] evil does not want to stay in one Zang-organ and thus transmits to another one. That is why transference is slow but dangerous [and] transmission is rapid but fierce, [the result of which in] killing people[1] is the same."

Leigong asked,"How does it transmit in the meridians and kill people?"

Qibo answered, "[When] evil enters into the heart, death [will be caused in] one day. [When] evil enters into the lung, [it will] transmit to the liver [in] three days, to the spleen [in] four days and to the stomach [in] five days, [causing] death [in] ten days. [When] evil enters into the liver, [it will] transmit to the spleen [in] three days, to the stomach [in] five days and to the kidney [in] ten days, dissipating [after] another three days. [Dissipation of evil after another three days ensures] cure [of disease], otherwise death [will be caused]. [When] evil enters into the spleen, [it will] transmit to the stomach [in] one day, to the kidney [in] two days, to the bladder [in] three days, dissipating after fourteen days. [Dissipation of evil after fourteen days ensures] cure [of disease], otherwise death [will be caused]. [When] evil enters into the stomach, [it will] transmit to the kidney [in] five days, to the bladder [in] eight days, to the small intestine [in] another five days and to the heart [in] another two days, causing death [when transmitting to the heart]. [When] evil enters into the kidney, [it will] transmit to the bladder [in] three days, to the small intestine [in] another three days and to the heart [in] another more three days, causing death [when transmitting to the heart].

[When] evil enters into the bladder, [it will] transmit to the

后的差异。"

雷公问："请问如何传经？"

岐伯说："邪气从外而侵入脏腑，必然会传经的。"

雷公问："请问如何不传经？"

岐伯说："若人的正气虚弱，就自然会发病，这种情况下就不会传经了。"

雷公问："寒气的迁移和热气的迁移，就是所谓的'传经'吗？"

岐伯说："迁移有传变之意，但转移缓慢，传变迅速。"

雷公问："什么道理呢？"

岐伯说："转移指的是病气在脏腑中的自行迁移；传变指的是邪气从某一腑传到另一脏。所以转移之势缓慢而凶险，传变之势迅速而暴烈，所以其导致人死亡的后果则是相同的。"

雷公问："传经是如何导致人死亡的呢？"

岐伯说："邪气侵入心，一天就会导致死亡。邪气侵入肺，三天后就会传到肝，四天后就会传到脾，五天后就会传到胃，十天后就会导致死亡。邪气侵入肝，三天后就会传到脾，五天后就会传到胃，十天后就会传到肾，又经过三天，邪气消散疾病就会痊愈，否则就会导致死亡。邪气侵入脾，一天就会传到胃，二天后就会传到肾，三天后就会传到膀胱，十四天后邪气消散疾病就会痊愈，否则就会导致死亡。邪气侵入胃，五天后传到肾，八天后传到膀胱，又经过五天后传到小肠，又经过二天后传到心就会导致死亡。邪气侵入肾，三天后传到膀胱，又经过三天后传到小肠，又经过三天后传到心就会导致死亡。邪气侵入膀胱，五天

kidney [in] five days, to the small intestine [in] one day and to the heart [in] another day, causing death [when transmitting to the heart]. [When] evil enters into the gallbladder, [it will] transmit to the lung [in] five days, to the kidney [in] another five days and to the heart [in] another more five days, causing death [when transmitting to the heart]. [When] evil enters into the triple energizer, [it will] transmit to the liver [in] one day, to the heart [in] three days, causing death [when transmitting to the heart]. [When] evil enters into the pericardium, [it will] transmit to the stomach [in] one day, to the gallbladder [in] two days, to the spleen [in] three days, to the kidney [in] four days and to the liver [in] five days. [If the disease is] not cured, [it will] transmit again. [When the disease is still] not cured [after] transmission again, [it will cause] death. [When] evil enters into the small intestine, [it will] transmit to the bladder [in] one day, to the kidney [in] two days, to the pericardium [in] three days, to the stomach [in] four days, to the spleen [in] five days, to the lung [in] six days, to the liver [in] seven days, to the gallbladder [in] eight days, to the triple energizer [in] nine days, to the large intestine [in] ten days and again to the kidney [in] eleven days. [If the disease is] not cured [when] such transmission continues, death [will be caused]. [When] evil enters into the large intestine, [it will] transmit to the small intestine [in] one day, to the triple energizer [in] two days, to the lung [in] three days, to the spleen [in] four days, to the liver [in] five days, to the kidney [in] six days and to the heart [in] seven days, causing death [when transmitting to the heart]. [If it does] not transmit to the heart but

后传到肾,又经过一天传到小肠,又经过一天传到心就会导致死亡。邪气侵入胆中,五天后传到肺,又经过五天则传到肾,又经过五天则传到心就会导致死亡。邪气侵入三焦,一天后传到肝,三天后传到心就会导致死亡。邪气侵入心包络,一天后传到胃,二天后传到胆中,三天后传到脾,四天后传到肾,五天后传到肝,如果不痊愈就会再次发生传变,再次发生传变而不痊愈就会导致死亡。邪气侵入小肠,一天后传到膀胱,二天后传到肾,三天后传到包络,四天后传到胃,五天后传到脾,六天后传到肺,七天后传到肝,八天后传到胆中,九天后传到三焦,十天后传到大肠,十一天后又传到肾,如果再次传变而不痊愈就会导致死亡。邪气侵入大肠,一天后传到小肠,二天后传到三焦,三天后传到肺,四天后传到脾,五天后传到肝,六天后传到肾,七天后传到心脏就会导致死亡。如果不传到心而依然传到小肠,人就可以存活。邪气侵入胆中后,往往不会传到其他脏腑之中,因此没有死期可以预测。但是当邪气侵入胆中,则往往就像遇到鬼神一样,有些情况下三四天就会导致死亡,这是热到极点而导致自焚的原因。"

雷公说:"好!"

陈士铎评论说:"转移缓慢而传变急速,的确有死期可以预测。这一解说妙极了!"

transmits to the small intestine, life [will be ensured]. [When] evil enters into the gallbladder, [it] usually never transmits. That is why the time of death cannot be forecasted. But [when] evil enters into the gallbladder, [it] usually appears like [meeting a] ghost [and may cause] death [in] three or five days due to extreme heat [that] burns spontaneously. "

Leigong said, "Excellent [explanation]!"

Chen Shiduo's comment, "[In terms of] slow transference and rapid transmission, the time of death surely can be forecasted. Excellent explanation!"

Notes

[1] Killing people means death caused by disease.

伤寒知变篇第六十八

【原文】

雷公问曰："伤寒一日，巨阳受之，何以头项痛，腰脊强也？"

岐伯曰："巨阳者，足太阳也。其脉起于目内眦，上额交巅，入络脑，还出别下项，循肩髆内，挟脊抵腰中。寒邪必先入于足太阳之经，邪入足太阳，则太阳之经脉不通，为寒邪所据，故头项痛，腰脊强也。"

雷公曰："二日阳明受之，宜身热、目疼、鼻干、不得卧矣；而头项痛、腰脊强，又何故欤？"

岐伯曰："此巨阳之余邪未散也。"

雷公曰："太阳之邪未散，宜不入阳明矣。"

岐伯曰："二日则阳明受之矣。因邪留恋太阳，未全入阳明，故头项尚痛，腰脊尚强，非二日阳明之邪全不受也。"

雷公曰："三日少阳受之，宜胸胁痛、耳聋矣，邪宜出阳明矣。既不入少阳，而头项腰脊之痛与强，仍未除者，又何故欤？"

岐伯曰："此邪不欲传少阳，转回于太阳也。"

雷公曰："邪传少阳矣，宜传入于三阴之经，何以三日之后太阳之证仍未除也？"

岐伯曰："阳经善变，且太阳之邪与各经之邪不同，各经之邪循经而入，太阳之邪出入自如，有入有不尽入也。惟不尽入，故虽六七日，而

Volume 8

【英译】

Chapter 68
Explanation of Change in Cold Damage

Leigong asked,"[In] the first day of cold damage, great Yang is attacked. [But] why [there appear] headache, nape pain and stiffness of the waist and spine?"

Qibo answered, "Great Yang is [the bladder meridian of foot-] Taiyang. This meridian starts from the inner canthus, running upwards to the forehead to connect [with the governor vessel at] the top [of the head], the collateral [of which] enters the brains, returning out and descending to the nape, circulating at the medial side of the shoulder and arriving at the middle of the back from both sides of the spine. Cold evil inevitably invades [the bladder] meridian of foot-Taiyang first. [When] evil has invaded [the bladder meridian of] foot-Taiyang, this meridian is certainly obstructed, and restricted by cold evil. That is why [there appear] headache, nape pain and stiffness of the waist and spine."

Leigong asked,"[In] the second day, Yangming [meridian] is attacked. There should be fever, pain of eyes, dryness of nose and inability to sleep. But [there still appear] headache, nape pain and stiffness of the waist and spine. What is the reason?"

Qibo answered, "Because the remaining evil [in] the great Yang [meridian] is not dissipated."

Leigong asked,"[When] the remaining evil [in] the Taiyang

其证未除耳。甚至七日之后,犹然头项痛,腰脊强,此太阳之邪乃原留之邪,非从厥阴复出而传之足太阳也。"

雷公曰:"四日太阴受之,腹满嗌干;五日少阴受之,口干舌燥;六日厥阴受之,烦满囊缩。亦有不尽验者,何也?"

岐伯曰:"阴经不变,不变而变者,邪过盛也。"

雷公曰:"然则三阳三阴之经皆善变也,变则不可以日数拘矣。"

岐伯曰:"日数者,言其常也;公问者,言其变也。变而不失其常,变则可生,否则死矣。"

雷公曰:"两感于寒者变乎?"

岐伯曰:"两感者,越经之传也,非变也。"

陈士铎曰:"伤寒之文,世人不知。读此论,人能悟否?无奈治伤寒者不能悟也。"

【今译】

雷公问:"伤寒第一天,太阳受侵,为何会出现头项痛和腰脊强呢?"

岐伯说:"太阳指的是足太阳膀胱经。其经脉起源于目内眦,上行交会于头顶,络脉进入脑中,回转下行到项部,循行到肩膊内,挟脊两旁而抵达腰中。寒邪必然先侵入足太阳经中。当邪气侵入足太阳经中,太阳经就会不通,这是被寒邪所拘束的缘故,所以才出现头项痛和腰脊强的症状。"

[meridian] is not dissipated, [it] should not invade the Yangming [meridian]."

Qibo answered, "[In] the second day, Yangming [meridian] is invaded. Since evil tends to linger in the Taiyang [meridian], [it has] not completely entered the Yangming [meridian]. That is why [there appear] headache, nape pain and stiffness of the waist and spine. [It does not mean that] no part of Yangming [meridian] is invaded by evil."

Leigong asked, "[In] the third day, Shaoyang [meridian] is invaded. [Consequently,] there should be pain in the chest and rib-side and deafness and evil should emerge from Yangming [meridian]. [Evil does] not enter Shaoyang [meridian], but [the symptoms and signs of] headache, nape pain and stiffness of the waist and spine are still not resolved. What is the reason?"

Qibo answered, "This [is because that] evil does not transmit to Shaoyang [meridian], [but] return to Taiyang [meridian]."

Leigong asked, "[When] evil transmits to Shaoyang [meridian], [it] should transmit to the three Yin meridians. Why after three days syndrome/pattern of Taiyang [meridian] is still not resolved?"

Qibo answered, "[Because] Yang meridian tends to change and evil in the Taiyang [meridian] is different from that in other meridians. Evil in other meridians enter along the meridians, [but] evil in Taiyang [meridian] comes out and enters into spontaneously, sometimes compeletely entering and sometimes incompletely entering. Only [when it] enters incompletely can the syndrome/pattern [of Taiyang meridian] not be resolved after six or seven

雷公问:"第二天阳明受侵后,应当出现身热、目疼、鼻干、不得卧等症状,但反而出现头项痛和腰脊强,这又是什么原因呢?"

岐伯说:"这是太阳的余邪没有散去的缘故。"

雷公问:"太阳的余邪没有散去,应当不传入阳明吧?"

岐伯说:"第二天就是阳明受侵了。因为邪气留滞于太阳,所以没有全部侵入阳明,因而才导致了头项仍然疼痛,腰脊仍然强硬,并非是第二天阳明全部不受邪侵的原因。"

雷公问:"第三天少阳受侵,应当引起胸胁痛和耳聋的症状,邪气应当从阳明出来。既然邪气没有侵入少阳,而头项疼痛和腰脊强硬的症状依然没有解除,这又是什么原因呢?"

岐伯说:"这是邪气没有侵入少阳,反而转回到太阳的缘故。"

雷公问:"邪气传入少阳经,应该继续传入三阴之经,但为什么三天之后太阳经的症状仍然没有消除呢?"

岐伯说:"阳经善于变化,并且太阳经中的邪气与其他各经中的邪气不同。其他各经中的邪气沿着经脉而入,而太阳经中的邪气则出入自如,有的完全进入而有的并不完全进入。正因为有的邪气并不完全进入,所以虽然过了六七天,太阳经的症状仍然没有消除。甚至过了七天之后,仍然会有头项疼痛和腰脊强硬的症状,这是因为太阳经中的邪气仍然是原来滞留的邪气,不是从厥阴经中出来后再传到足太阳经中的。"

雷公问:"第四天太阴经受侵,出现腹部胀满和咽喉干燥的症状;第五天少阴受侵,出现口干舌燥的症状;第六天厥阴受侵,出现少腹硬

days. Even after seven days, there still appear headache, nape pain and stiffness of the waist and spine because evil in the Taiyang [meridian] is the original one, not [the one] transmitting from the Jueyin [meridian] to [the bladder meridian of] foot-Taiyang."

Leigong asked, "[In] the fourth day, Taiyin [meridian] is attacked, [resulting in] abdominal fullness and dryness of the throat. [In] the fifth day, Shaoyin [meridian] is attacked, [resulting in] dryness of the mouth and tongue. [In] the sixth day, Jueyin [meridian] is attacked, [resulting in] vexation, fullness and contraction of scrotum. [But] there are still [some cases that do] not come true. What is the reason?"

Qibo answered, "Yin meridians [usually] do not change. [The one that originally should] not change but has changed [is caused by] exuberance of evil."

Leigong asked, "However the three Yang and three Yin meridians are all changeable. [But after] changes, [they should] not be confined to the number of days."

Qibo answered, "The number of days indicates the general rule. Your question indicates [the situation of] change. [In fact, such a] change does not violate the rule. [And only when there is] change can life [be ensured], otherwise death [will be caused]."

Leigong asked, "[When] two [meridians] are attacked by cold, [could there be] change?"

Qibo answered, "[Cold that has] attacked the two [meridians is] transmission over the meridians, not change."

Chen Shiduo's comment, "[*About*] *the article of cold damage*,

满和阴囊收缩的症状。但依然有不全部应验的,这是为什么呢?"

岐伯说:"正常情况下阴经不传变。但不应传变而又传变的现象,是邪气过于旺盛的缘故。"

雷公问:"但是三阳三阴的经脉都善于传变,传变后就不能强制天数了吧?"

岐伯说:"天数,指的是传变的规律;你所问的,是有关传变的情况。传变但又不违背规律的,这样的传变就有益于生存,否则就会导致死亡。"

雷公问:"如果两条经脉同时遭受了寒气的侵袭,会发生什么传变吗?"

岐伯说:"两条经络同时遭受了寒气的侵袭,这是越过两经的传变,并不是变化。"

陈士铎评论说:"有关伤寒的文章,世人是不清楚的。读了这篇文章的人,能领悟到其真谛吗?无奈治疗伤寒的人不能领悟啊!"

Volume 8

people in this world cannot understand. Can people understand [after] reading this discussion? Unfortunately [those who] treat cold damage cannot understand [it]."

伤寒异同篇第六十九

【原文】

雷公问于岐伯曰："伤寒之病多矣，可悉言之乎？"

岐伯曰："伤寒有六，非冬伤于寒者，举不得谓伤寒也。"

雷公曰："请言其异。"

岐伯曰："有中风，有中暑，有中热，有中寒，有中湿，有中疫，其病皆与伤寒异。伤寒者，冬月感寒邪，入营卫，由腑而传于脏也。"

雷公曰："暑热之证感于夏，不感于三时，似非伤寒矣，风寒湿疫多感于冬日也，何以非伤寒乎？"

岐伯曰："百病皆起于风。四时之风，每直中于脏腑，非若传经之寒，由浅而深入也。寒之中人，自在严寒，不由营卫直入脏腑，是不从皮肤渐进，非传经之伤寒也。水旺于冬，而冬日之湿反不深入，以冬令收藏也，他时则易感矣。疫来无方，四时均能中疫，而冬疫常少。二证俱不传经，皆非伤寒也。"

雷公曰："寒热之不同也，何热病亦谓之伤寒乎？"

岐伯曰："寒感于冬，则寒必变热；热变于冬，则热即为寒。故三时之热病不可谓寒，冬日之热病不可谓热，是以三时之热病不传经，冬日之热病必传经也。"

雷公曰："热病传经，乃伤寒之类也，非正伤寒也。何天师著《素

Volume 8

【英译】

Chapter 69
Difference and Sameness in Cold Damage

Leigong asked Qibo, "[There are] various diseases in cold damage. Could [you] explain in detail?"

Qibo answered, "There are six [kinds of] cold damage. [Only those that are] damaged by cold in winter can be called cold damage."

Leigong asked, "Please explain the difference."

Qibo answered, "Diseases [due to] wind attack, summer-heat attack, heat attack, cold attack, dampness attack and pestilence attack are all different from cold damage. Cold damage [refers to] attack of cold evil in winter [that] enters defense [Qi] and nutrient [Qi] and transmits to the Zang-organs through Fu-organs."

Leigong asked, "Syndrome/pattern of summer-heat occurs in summer, not in the other three seasons, [and therefore is] not similar to cold damage. Wind [attack], cold [attack], dampness [attack] and pestilence [attack] usually happen in winter. Why [are they] not cold damage?"

Qibo answered, "All diseases are caused by wind. Wind in the four seasons usually attacks the Zang-organs and Fu-organs directly, unlike cold transmitting in the meridians [that moves] from the shallow [level] to the deep [region]. Cold attack of people happens naturally in severe cold [season]. [Such cold] never moves directly

问》有热病传经之文,而伤寒反无之,何也?"

岐伯曰:"类宜辩而正不必辩也,知类即知正矣。"

雷公曰:"善。"

陈士铎曰:"伤寒必传经,断在严寒之时,非冬日伤寒,举不可谓伤寒也。辨得明说得出。"

【今译】

雷公请问岐伯:"伤寒病症很多,可详细予以论述吗?"

岐伯说:"伤寒有六种,除了冬天受到寒气的伤害之外,都不能称为伤寒。"

雷公问:"请解释其中的差异。"

岐伯说:"这些差异有中风,有中暑,有中热,有中寒,有中湿,有中疫,这些都与伤寒有差异。伤寒,指的是冬三月所感受的寒邪,该寒邪侵入营卫,由腑传到脏。"

雷公问:"暑热的病证发生于夏天,其他三个季节不会发生,似乎就不是伤寒了。风、寒、湿、疫多发生在冬天,但为什么就不是伤寒呢?"

岐伯说:"百病都起因于风。四时之风,每次都直接侵入脏腑,不像传经的寒气,由浅而深入。寒气对人体的伤害,自然发生在寒冬季节,不是由营卫直接侵入脏腑的。也不是从皮肤逐渐进入人体的,所以就不是传经的伤寒。水旺于冬季,但冬天的湿气反而不会深入人体,因为冬季是收藏的季节,但其他季节则容易感染了。疫病不受地方限制,

Volume 8

from nutrient [Qi] and defense [Qi] into the Zang-organs and Fu-organs. [Cold that does] not gradually enter [into the body] through the skin is not cold damage [that] transmits along the meridians. [In] winter, water is exuberant. [But in] winter dampness is not deep because winter [is the season for] storage. [In] other seasons, [it is very] easy to be infected. Pestilence is not [confined to any] areas and infects [people in all] the four seasons. However in winter, [infection of] pestilence is seldom. [These two] syndromes/patterns do not transmit in the meridians, and thus are not cold damage. "

Leigong asked, "Cold and heat are different. [But] why is heat disease also called cold damage?"

Qibo answered, "Cold is contracted in winter and must change into heat; heat is transformed in winter and certainly changes into cold. That is why heat disease in the other three seasons cannot be called cold, [but] heat disease in winter can be called heat. Hence heat disease in the other three seasons do not transmit in the meridians, [but] heat disease in winter must transmit in the meridians. "

Leigong asked, "Heat disease [that] transmits in the meridians belongs to the category of cold damage, [but is] not orthodoxical cold damage. [In] *Su Wen* (*Plain Conversation*) written by Celestial Master, there is a chapter about heat disease transmitting in the meridians, but there is no [discussion about] cold damage. Why?"

Qibo answered, "[The one that is] similar to [cold damage] should be differentiated, [but the one that is] orthodoxical [cold damage] is unnecessary to differentiate. [If one] understands [the

一年四季都可能被感染,但冬季疫病的感染却常常较少。这两种病证都不传经,所以都不是伤寒。"

雷公问:"寒热性质不同,为什么热病也称为伤寒呢?"

岐伯说:"寒气感染在冬天,所以寒气必然会变成热证;热病发生在冬天,那么热病也是寒气所致。因此,春、夏、秋三时的热病不能称为寒,冬天的热病也不能称为热,所以春、夏、秋三时的热病不传经,而冬天的热病则必然传经。"

雷公问:"热病传经属于伤寒之类,但却不是正伤寒。但天师在撰写《素问》时,有热病传经之文,反而没有伤寒之文,为什么呢?"

岐伯说:"类伤寒应当分辨清楚,而正伤寒则不必加以分辨,懂得了类伤寒,也就懂得了正伤寒。"

雷公说:"好!"

陈士铎评论说:"伤寒必然传于经,且必然发生在严寒时期。不是发生在冬季的伤寒,都不可称为伤寒。辨别得很明确,表达得很清楚。"

disease] similar to [cold damage], [he certainly] understands orthodoxical [cold damage]."

Leigong said,"Excellent [explanation]!"

Chen Shiduo's comment, "Cold damage must transmit in the meridians, especially in the severe cold [season]. Cold damage [that does] not occur in winter cannot be called cold damage. The analysis is clear and the explanation is thorough."

风寒殊异篇第七十

风后问于岐伯曰："冬伤于寒与春伤于寒，有异乎？"

岐伯曰："春伤于寒者，风也，非寒也。"

风后曰："风即寒也，何异乎？"

岐伯曰："冬日之风则寒，春日之风则温。寒伤深，温伤浅。伤深者入少阳而传里，伤浅者入少阳而出表，故异也。"

风后曰："传经乎？"

岐伯曰："伤冬日之风则传，伤春日之风则不传也。"

风后曰："其不传何也？"

岐伯曰："伤浅者，伤在皮毛也。皮毛属肺，故肺受之。不若伤深者，入于营卫也。"

风后曰："春伤于风，头痛鼻塞，身亦发热，与冬伤于寒者，何无异也？"

岐伯曰："风入于肺，鼻为之不利，以鼻主肺也。肺既受邪，肺气不宣，失清肃之令，必移邪而入于太阳矣。膀胱畏邪，坚闭其经，水道失行，水不下泄，火乃炎上，头即痛矣。夫头乃阳之首也，既为邪火所据，则一身之真气皆与邪争，而身乃热矣。"

风后曰："肺为胃之子，肺受邪，宜胃来援，何以邪入肺而恶热、口渴之证生，岂生肺者转来刑肺乎？"

Volume 8

【英译】

Chapter 70
Unique Difference in Wind and Cold

Fenghou asked Qibo, "Is there any difference between damage by cold in winter and damage by cold in spring?"

Qibo answered, "Damage by cold in spring [is due to] wind, not cold."

Fenghou asked, "Wind is cold. What is the difference?"

Qibo answered, "Wind in winter is cold [but] wind in spring is warm. Damage by cold [wind] is deep [while] damage by warm [wind] is shallow. Deep damage permeates into the Shaoyang [meridian] and transmits to the internal [while] shallow damage permeates into the Shaoyang [meridian] but emerges from the external. That is why [they are] different."

Fenghou asked, "[Does it] transmit to the meridians?"

Qibo answered, "Damage by wind in winter transmits [in the meridians], [but] damage by wind in spring does not transmit [in the meridians]."

Fenghou asked, "Why [does it] not transmit?"

Qibo answered, "[If] damage is shallow, [it is] in the skin [and body] hair. Skin [and body] hair belong to the lung. That is why the lung is infected. [It is] not like deep damage [that] permeates into nutrient [Qi] and defense [Qi]."

Fenghou asked, "Damage by wind in spring [causes] headache,

岐伯曰：“胃为肺之母，见肺子之寒，必以热救之。夫胃之热，心火生之也。胃得心火之生，则胃土过旺，然助胃必克肺矣。火能刑金，故因益而反损也。”

风后曰：“呕吐者何也？”

岐伯曰：“此风伤于太阴也。风在地中，土必震动，水泉上溢则呕吐矣。散风，而土自安也。”

风后曰：“风邪入太阳头痛，何以有痛不痛之殊也。”

岐伯曰：“肺不移风于太阳，则不痛耳。”

风后曰：“风不入于太阳，头即不痛乎？”

岐伯曰：“肺通于鼻，鼻通于脑，风入于肺，自能引风入脑而作头痛。肺气旺，则风入于肺而不上走于脑，故不痛也。”

风后曰：“春伤于风，往来寒热，热结于里，何也？”

岐伯曰：“冬寒入于太阳，久则变寒；春风入于太阳，久则变热。寒则动传于脏，热则静结于腑。寒在脏，则阴与阳战而发热；热在腑，则阳与阴战而发寒。随脏腑之衰旺，分寒热之往来也。”

风后曰：“伤风自汗何也？”

岐伯曰：“伤寒之邪，寒邪也；伤风之邪，风邪也。寒邪入胃，胃恶寒而变热；风邪入胃，胃喜风而变温。温则不大热也，得风以扬之，火必外泄，故汗出矣。”

风后曰：“春伤于风，下血谵语，一似冬伤于寒之病，何也？”

岐伯曰：“此热入血室，非狂也。伤于寒者，热自入于血室之中，其热重；伤于风者，风祛热入于血室之内，其热轻也。”

stuffy nose and fever. [Is it] different from damage by cold in winter?"

Qibo answered, "[When] wind invades the lung, the nose becomes stuffy because the nose governs the lung. Since the lung is infected by evil, lung-Qi cannot effuse. [As a result,] the function of depuration is ceased and evil is inevitably transferred to the Taiyang [meridian]. The bladder fears evil and firmly closes its meridian, [consequently resulting in] inability of water to move upflaming of fire and headache. The head is the top of Yang [Qi]. [When the head is] occupied by evil fire, genuine Qi in the whole body all contends with evil, [leading to] fever in the body."

Fenghou asked, "The lung is the son of the stomach. [When] the lung is attacked by evil, [it] should be supported by the stomach. Why are there syndromes/patterns of aversion to heat and thirst [when] evil has invaded the lung? Isn't [it the one that] is produced by the lung but punishes the lung?"

Qibo answered, "The stomach is the mother of the lung. [When] seeing cold in the lung, [it] must rescue with heat. Heat in the stomach is produced by heart-fire. [When] the stomach is promoted by heart-fire, stomach-earth [will become] exuberant. Although [it] promotes stomach [-earth], [it will] certainly restrict lung [-metal]. [Since] fire can restrict metal, that is why [it] benefits [the stomach] but damages [the lung]."

Fenghou asked, "What is the cause of vomiting?"

Qibo answered, "This [is caused by] wind damaging the Taiyin [meridian]. [When] wind is in the earth, the earth must be shaken and water in the spring[1] will overflow, [consequently causing]

风后曰："谵语而潮热者,何也?"

岐伯曰："其脉必滑者也。"

风后曰："何也?"

岐伯曰："风邪入胃,胃中无痰则发大热,而谵语之声高;胃中有痰,则发潮热,而谵语之声低。潮热发谵语,此痰也。滑者,痰之应也。"

风后曰："春伤于风,发厥,心下悸,何也?"

岐伯曰："伤于寒者邪下行,伤于风者邪上冲也。寒乃阴邪,阴则走下;风乃阳邪,阳则升上。治寒邪,先定厥,后定悸;治风邪,先定悸,后定厥。不可误也!"

风后曰："伤于风而发热,如见鬼者,非狂乎?"

岐伯曰："狂乃实邪,此乃虚邪也。实邪从太阳来也,邪炽而难遏;虚邪从少阴来也,邪旺而将衰。实邪,火逼心君而外出,神不守于心也;虚邪,火引肝魂而外游,魄不守于肺也。"

风后曰："何论之神乎? 吾无测师矣!"

陈士铎曰："风与寒殊,故论亦殊,人当细观之。"

【今译】

风后请问岐伯："冬天遭受寒气的伤害与春天遭受寒气的伤害,是否有差异呢?"

岐伯说："春天遭受寒气伤害的,是风气而不是寒气。"

风后问："风气就是寒气,这到底有什么差异呢?"

vomiting. [When] wind is dissipated, the earth will be pacified. "

Fenghou asked, "[When] wind evil invades the Taiyang [meridian], [there will be] headache. Why is there pain and is there no pain?"

Qibo answered, "[If] the lung does not transfer wind to the Taiyang [meridian], there will be no pain. "

Fenghou asked, "Is there no headache [when] wind is not transferred to the Taiyang [meridian]?"

Qibo answered, "The lung is connected with the nose and the nose is connected with the brain. [When] wind has entered the lung, [the lung will] certainly lead wind into the brain and cause headache. [When] lung-Qi is exuberant, wind will enter the lung but will not move to the brain. That is why [the head is] not painful. "

Fenghou asked, "Damage by wind in spring [leads to] alternate cold and heat, [resulting in] heat binding in the internal. What is the reason?"

Qibo answered, "[When] cold in winter enters the Taiyang [meridian], [it will] cause cold [disease after] long-term [duration]. [When] wind in spring enters the Taiyang [meridian], [it will] cause heat [disease after] long-term [duration]. Cold [disease is] active and transmits to the Zang-organs [while] heat [disease is] static and binds in the Fu-organs. [When] cold [disease] is in the Zang-organs, Yin will fight [against] Yang and cause fever; [when] heat [disease] is in the Fu-organs, Yang will fight [against] Yin and cause chilliness. [Hence] with debilitation and exuberance of the Zang-organs and Fu-organs, [there will be]

岐伯说:"冬天的风则寒冷,春天的风则温暖。寒气对人的伤害比较深,风气对人的伤害则比较浅。伤害深的入少阳后即传于里,伤害浅的入少阳后则出于表,所以是有差异的。"

风后问:"会传经吗?"

岐伯说:"遭受冬季风寒伤害,就会传经;遭受春季风气伤害,就不会传经。"

风后问:"为什么不传经呢?"

岐伯说:"伤害浅的,伤在皮毛。皮毛属于肺,所以伤害由肺脏承受。这不像伤害深的,则会进入营卫。"

风后问:"春天遭受风气的伤害,会引起头痛鼻塞,身体也发热。这与冬天遭受寒气的伤害有什么差异吗?"

岐伯说:"寒风侵入肺中,鼻子就不通畅,因为鼻主肺。肺既然遭受了邪气的侵袭,肺气就不宣,失去了清肃之令,就必然会将邪气移入太阳。膀胱畏惧邪气,所以就会紧闭经络,水道因而就不能通行,水液不能向下排泄,火于是上炎,头就会疼痛。头是阳之首,但头被火邪所占据时,全身的真气都与邪气抗争,于是身体就会发热。"

风后问:"肺金是胃土之子,肺遭受了邪气的侵袭,胃理应救援,为什么邪气侵入肺后会出现恶热、口渴的症状呢? 这岂不是生肺的转而克肺了吗?"

岐伯说:"胃土是肺金之母,见到肺遭受寒气的侵袭,胃必然会用热来救援。胃中的热气,是由心火所生的,胃得到心火的救援,胃土就会过旺,虽然能够扶助胃土,但也必然会克伤肺金。火能克金,所以就

alternate cold and heat."

Fenghou asked, "Why [is there] spontaneous sweating [after] damage by wind?"

Qibo answered, "Evil in cold damage is cold evil; evil in wind damage is wind evil. [When] cold evil invades the stomach, the stomach fears cold and changes [it into] heat; [when] wind evil invades the stomach, the stomach likes wind and changes [it into] warmth. Warmth is not very hot and starts to spread [when] meeting with wind, [consequently leading to] leakage of fire. That is why there is sweating."

Fenghou asked, "Damage by wind in spring [will cause] blood in stool and delirium, similar to disease [caused by] cold damage in winter. What is the reason?"

Qibo answered, "This is heat entering the blood chamber[2], not mania. [When there is] damage by cold, heat will spontaneously enter the blood chamber and heat [in it will be] serious; [when there is] damage by wind, wind will dissipate, [but] heat will enter the blood chamber and heat [in it will be] light."

Fenghou asked, "Why is there delirium and tidal fever?"

Qibo answered, "The pulse must be slippery."

Fenghou asked, "Why?"

Qibo answered, "[When] wind evil invades the stomach, [there will be] great heat [if] there is no phlegm in the stomach. That is why the sound of delirium is high. [If] there is phlegm in the stomach, there will be tidal fever and the sound of delirium is low. Tidal fever with delirium indicates phlegm. Slippery [pulse] is the reaction of phlegm."

会由助益而造成损害了。"

风后问："为什么会呕吐呢？"

岐伯说："因为风气损伤了太阴。风在地中，土必然震动，水泉向上溢出，因此就导致呕吐了。驱散了风邪，土气自然就会安宁。"

风后问："风邪侵入太阳就会引起头痛，为什么会有痛与不痛之别呢？"

岐伯说："如果肺不将风气转移到太阳，就不会导致头痛。"

风后问："如果风气不进入太阳，头难道就不会痛吗？"

岐伯说："肺气上通于鼻，鼻上通于脑，风气进入肺中，自然能将风气引入脑中，从而导致头痛。如果肺气旺盛，风气进入于肺中，但不会上行于脑中，因此头就不会痛。"

风后问："春天遭受风气的伤害，会寒热往来，热结于里，这是为什么呢？"

岐伯说："冬天寒气侵入太阳，日久则变成寒证；春天风气侵入太阳，日久则变成热证。寒证因变动而传入脏，热证则静止而结于腑。寒气在脏，阴气与阳气相斗而发热；热结在腑，阳气与阴气相斗而发寒。根据脏腑的衰旺，可分出寒和热的往来。"

风后问："伤风后身体出汗，这是为什么呢？"

岐伯说："伤寒的邪气，是寒邪；伤风的邪气，是风邪。寒邪侵入胃，胃厌恶寒气而发热；风邪侵入胃，胃喜欢风气而变成暖，温暖但不太热。得到风气的传扬，火气必然外泄，所以就会出汗。"

风后问："春天遭受风气的伤害，就会引起下血和谵语的症状，就像冬天遭受寒气伤害而引起的病证，这是为什么呢？"

Volume 8

Fenghou asked, "Damage by wind in spring [causes] reversal cold of foot and palpitation. What is the reason?"

Qibo answered, "[When] damaged by cold, evil will move downwards; [when] damaged by wind, evil will rush up. Cold is Yin evil and Yin [evil] will run downwards; wind is Yang evil and Yang [evil] will rise up. To deal with cold evil, [measures should be taken] to resolve reversal cold first and then subside palpitation; to deal with wind evil, [measures should be taken] to subside palpitation first and then resolve reversal cold. No mistakes should be made."

Fenghou asked, "Damage by wind causes fever like meeting a ghost. Isn't it mania?"

Qibo answered, "Mania indicates excess-evil, [but] this is deficiency-evil. Excess-evil starts from Taiyang, intense and difficult to suppress; deficiency-evil starts from Shaoyin, effulgent but soon to debilitate. Excess-evil [refers to] fire [that] forces heart-monarch to move out, [and that is why] the spirit cannot stand fast at the heart; deficiency-evil [refers to] fire [that] leads the ethereal soul [in] the liver to fly outside, [and that is why] the corporeal soul cannot stand fast at the lung."

Fenghou asked, "What a marvelous discussion! I am unable to estimate [Celestial] Master."

Chen Shiduo's comment, "Wind and cold are different. So the discussion is also different. Readers should observe it carefully."

岐伯说："这是热气进入血室，不是狂证。因遭受寒气的伤害，热气就会进入血室，热势就比较重；因遭受风气的伤害，风邪就已散去，但热气则进入血室之内，热势则比较轻。"

风后问："有谵语且潮热的，又是什么原因呢？"

岐伯说："病人的脉象必然是滑的。"

风后问："为什么呢？"

岐伯说："风邪侵入胃，胃中没有痰就会产生大热，谵语的声音就会高；胃中如果有痰，则会发潮热，谵语的声音就会低。有潮热和发谵语，是因为有痰。滑脉，就是胃中有痰的表现。"

风后问："春天遭受风气的伤害，就会引起手足逆冷，心下悸动。这是为什么呢？"

岐伯说："遭受寒气伤害，邪气就会向下行走；遭受风气伤害，邪气就会向上逆冲。寒是阴邪，阴则向下行走；风是阳邪，阳则向上升起。治疗寒邪时，先要祛除逆冷，然后平息悸动；治疗风邪时，先要平息悸动，然后祛除逆冷，不能有任何失误啊！"

风后问："遭受风邪的伤害，身体就会发热，就像见到鬼一样，这难道不是狂证吗？"

岐伯说："狂证是实邪，而这则是虚邪。实邪从太阳来，邪气炽盛而难以遏止；虚邪从少阴来，邪气由旺而转衰。实邪为火气逼迫心君而外出，精神不能固守在心中；虚邪是火气引动肝魂而外游，魄不能固守于肺中。"

风后说："天师为什么论述得如此神妙啊？我无法测度天师了！"

陈士铎评论说："风与寒不同，所以论述也不同。读者应该仔细观察。"

Notes

[1] Please see [3] in Chapter 51.

[2] Blood chamber（血室）here refers to the uterus. In traditional Chinese medicine, blood chamber usually means three things, i.e. uterus, thoroughfare vessel（冲脉）and the liver.

阴寒格阳篇第七十一

【原文】

盘盂问于岐伯曰："大小便闭结不通,饮食辄吐,面赪唇焦,饮水亦呕,脉又沉伏,此何证也?"

岐伯曰："肾虚寒盛,阴格阳也。"

盘盂曰："阴何以格阳乎?"

岐伯曰："肾少阴经也,恶寒喜温。肾寒则阳无所附,升而不降矣!"

盘盂曰："其故何也?"

岐伯曰："肾中有水火存焉,火藏水中,水生火内,两相根而两相制也。邪入则水火相离,而病生矣!"

盘盂曰："何邪而使之离乎?"

岐伯曰："寒热之邪皆能离之,而寒邪为甚。寒感之轻,则肾中之虚阳上浮,不至格拒之至也。寒邪太盛,拒绝过坚,阳格阴而力衰,阴格阳而气旺,阳不敢居于下焦,冲逆于上焦矣。上焦冲逆,水谷入喉,安能下入于胃乎?"

盘盂曰："何以治之?"

岐伯曰："以热治之。"

盘盂曰："阳宜阴折,热宜寒折。今阳在上而作热,不用寒反用热,

Volume 8

【英译】

Chapter 71
Yin Cold Restricting Yang

Panyu asked Qibo, "[There are symptoms and signs of] constipation, anuresis, vomiting after taking food, red face, scorched lips, vomiting after drinking water, deep and hidden pulse. What disease is it?"

Qibo answered, "[This is a disease due to] deficiency of kidney, exuberance of cold and Yin expulsing Yang."

Panyu asked, "Why does Yin expulse Yang?"

Qibo answered, "The kidney is Shaoyin meridian, fearing cold and liking warmth. [If there is] cold [in] the kidney, there is no [place for] Yang to depend on, [therefore Yang can only] rise up but cannot descend."

Panyu asked, "What is the reason?"

Qibo answered, "[Because] there is water and fire in the kidney. [When] fire is stored in water, water is produced in fire, both [of which] depend on each other and control each other. Invasion of evil [leads to] separation of water and fire [which] causes disease."

Panyu asked, "What does evil make [water and fire] separate [from each other]?"

Qibo answered, "Both cold and heat evil can separate [water and fire], [especially] cold evil [which is more] serious. [If] cold

不治阴反治阳,岂别有义乎?"

岐伯曰:"上热者,下逼之使热也;阳升者,阴祛之使升也。故上热者,下正寒也,以阴寒折之转害之矣,故不若以阳热之品,顺其性而从治之,则阳回而阴且交散也。"

盘盂曰:"善。"

陈士铎曰:"阴胜必须阳折,阳胜必须阴折,皆从治之法也。"

【今译】

盘盂请问岐伯:"大小便闭结不通,饮食之后就呕吐,面赭色,唇干焦,饮水后就呕吐,脉象又沉伏,这是什么病证呢?"

岐伯说:"这是肾虚寒盛、阴气格拒阳气所致。"

盘盂问:"阴为什么会格拒阳呢?"

岐伯说:"肾为少阴经,所以有厌恶寒冷、喜欢温暖的表现。如果肾中寒冷,且阳气没有依附之处,就会升而不降。"

盘盂问:"这是什么原因呢?"

岐伯说:"肾中有水火存在,火藏在水中,水生于火内,两者相互为根,又互相制约。邪气侵入,导致水火二气分离,于是就导致了疾病的产生。"

盘盂问:"是什么邪气促使其分离呢?"

岐伯说:"寒热之邪都能使水火二气分离,寒邪更为严重。感染寒邪较轻的,肾中的虚阳就会上浮,不至于造成格拒。寒邪如果太过旺

evil is light, deficiency-Yang in the kidney will fly up, [but is] unapt to expulse [anything]. [If] cold evil is exuberant, [it will cause] severe expulsion. [In this case,] Yang will be debilitated because of expulsing Yin and Yin will be exuberant because of expulsing Yang. [As a result,] Yang dares not to stay in the lower energizer but rushes reversely to the upper energizer. [When] the upper energizer is rushed reversely, how can water and food in the throat descend and enter the stomach in the lower?"

Panyu asked, "How to treat it?"

Qibo answered, "[It can be] treated by [medicinals] heat [in property]."

Panyu asked, "Yang [disease] should [be treated by medicinals with] Yin [property] and heat [disease] should [be treated by medicinals with] cold [property]. Now Yang is in the upper and causes heat, [medicinals with] cold [property are] not used but [medicinals with] heat [property are] used. Yin is not treated but Yang is treated. Is there any special significance?"

Qibo answered, "Heat in the upper [energizer is caused by] force of the lower [energizer]; uprise of Yang is due to expelling of Yin. Hence heat in the upper [indicates] cold in the lower. [For this reason,] to reduce it [with medicinals with] Yin cold [property] will damage [it]. Thus it is better to use [medicinals with] Yang heat [property] to treat in complying with its tendency [to rise up]. [Such a way of treatment not only can] restore Yang [Qi] but [also] disperse Yin [cold]."

Panyu said, "Excellent [explanation]!"

盛,就会造成极度的格拒,阳气因极度的格拒阴邪而导致其力量的衰弱,而阴气则因为格拒阳气而变得旺盛,阳气因不敢处于下焦的位置,因而向上逆冲到上焦。上焦受到冲逆,水谷就会进入咽喉,怎么能够下行到胃呢?"

盘盂问:"怎么治疗呢?"

岐伯说:"用温热之法治疗。"

盘盂问:"阳病应用阴性药物消解,热性病应用寒凉药来消解,现在阳气在上焦造成热证,不用寒凉药反而用温热药治疗,不治阴反而治阳,难道有特别的意义吗?"

岐伯说:"上焦之所以有热证,是由于下焦的逼迫而使其发热;阳气之所以上升,是因为阴气的驱使使其上升。因此,上焦之所以发热,是由于下焦的虚寒,用寒凉的药物消解反而会导致伤害,所以不如用温热的药物治疗,以顺从其性与势而治疗。这样不仅可以回复阳气,而且也能消散阴寒。"

盘盂说:"好!"

陈士铎评论说:"阴胜必须要用阳来消解,阳胜必须用阴来消解。这都是从治的方法。"

Volume 8

Chen Shiduo's comment , "Prevailing of Yin must be rebated by Yang and prevailing of Yang must be rebated by Yin . [These are] all the methods for treatment ."

春温似疫篇第七十二

【原文】

风后问于岐伯曰："春日之疫,非感风邪成之乎?"

岐伯曰："疫非独风也。春日之疫,非风而何?"

风后曰："然则春温即春疫乎?"

岐伯曰："春疫非春温也。春温有方,而春疫无方也。"

风后曰："春疫无方,何其疾之一似春温也?"

岐伯曰："春温有方,而时气乱之,则有方者变而无方,故与疫气正相同也。"

风后曰："同中有异乎?"

岐伯曰："疫气热中藏杀,时气热中藏生。"

风后曰："热中藏生,何多死亡乎?"

岐伯曰："时气者,不正之气也。脏腑闻正气而阴阳和,闻邪气而阴阳乱。不正之气即邪气也,故闻之而辄病,转相传染也。"

风后曰："闻邪气而不病者,又何故欤?"

岐伯曰："脏腑自和,邪不得而乱之也。春温传染,亦脏腑之虚也。"

风后曰："脏腑实而邪远,脏腑空而邪中,不洵然乎!"

陈士铎曰："温似疫症,不可谓温即是疫,辨得明爽。"

Volume 8

【英译】

Chapter 72
Warmth[1] in Spring Like Pestilence

Fenghou asked Qibo, "Is pestilence in spring caused by infection of wind evil?"

Qibo answered, "Pestilence [is] not [only caused by] wind [evil]. [But] pestilence in spring [is only caused by] wind [evil]."

Fenghou asked, "But is warmth in spring [the same of] pestilence in spring?"

Qibo answered, "Pestilence in spring is not warmth in spring. There is orientation for warmth in spring, but there is no orientation for pestilence in spring."

Fenghou asked, "There is no orientation for pestilence in spring. [But] why is disease [caused by pestilence in spring] similar to warmth in spring?"

Qibo answered, "[Although] there is orientation for warmth in spring, Qi from seasonal climate disturbs it. [In this case, warmth in spring that] has an orientation will lose [its] orientation. That is why [it is] the same as pestilent Qi[2]."

Fenghou asked, "Is there any difference in the sameness?"

Qibo answered, "There is intention of killing in heat stored in pestilent Qi [while] there is vitality in heat stored in seasonal Qi."

Fenghou asked, "Vitality is stored in heat. [But] why do most of the patients die?"

【今译】

风后请问岐伯："春天的疫气难道不是感染风邪吗?"

岐伯说："疫气不只是风气所致。但春天的疫气不是风气所致又是什么呢?"

风后问："难道春天的温气就是春疫吗?"

岐伯说："春疫不是春温。春温是有方位,但春疫却没有方位。"

风后问："春疫没有方位,但为什么其疾病就像春温一样呢?"

岐伯说："春温有方位,但由于受时气的干扰,有方位的也会变得没有方位了,所以与疫气恰好相同。"

风后问："相同之中有无差异呢?"

岐伯说："疫气在温热中隐藏着杀机,时气在温热中隐藏着生机。"

风后问："既然温热中隐藏着生机,为什么多数病人会死亡呢?"

岐伯说："时气是四时中的不正之气。当脏腑感受到了正气,阴阳就会调和;当脏腑感染了邪气,阴阳就会紊乱。不正之气就是邪气,因此感染了邪气很快就会致病,并且转而引起互相传染。"

风后问："虽然感染了邪气但却没有引发疾病的产生,这又是什么原因呢?"

岐伯说："脏腑如果能够自然调和,就不会受到邪气的扰乱。春天的温疫传染,也是由于脏腑的空虚所致。"

风后说："如果脏腑充实,邪气就会远离;如果脏腑空虚,邪气就会感染。这不是自然而然的吗?"

陈士铎评论说："春温类似疫证,但不能说春温就是疫病。这里分辨得非常明确清楚。"

Qibo answered, "[Because] seasonal Qi is not the orthodoxical Qi [in the four seasons]. [When] the Zang-organs and Fu-organs are influenced by orthodoxical Qi, Yin and Yang will be in harmony; [when the Zang-organs and Fu-organs are] affected by evil Qi, Yin and Yang will be in disorder. Qi [that is] not orthodoxical is evil Qi. That is why [when] affected by [evil Qi], [people will] immediately contract disease [and consequently the disease will] become infectous."

Fenghou asked, "[Some people are] affected by evil Qi but seldom contract disease. What is the reason?"

Qibo answered, "[Because] the Zang-organs and Fu-organs can harmonize [each other] spontaneously and evil cannot harass them. Infection of warm [pestilence] in spring is also [due to] deficiency of the Zang-organs and Fu-organs."

Fenghou said, "[When] the Zang-organs and Fu-organs are strong, evil will be far away [from them]; [when] the Zang-organs and Fu-organs are weak, evil will invade [them]. This is certainly natural."

Chen Shiduo's comment, "Warm [disease] in spring seems to be pestilence, [but it] cannot be called pestilence. The analysis is clear and thorough."

Notes

[1] Warmth here means warm Qi in spring.

[2] Pestilent Qi (疫气) refers to disease caused by pestilence.

卷九

补泻阴阳篇第七十三

【原文】

雷公问于岐伯曰："人身阴阳分于气血，《内经》详之矣，请问其余。"

岐伯曰："气血之要，在气血有余不足而已。气有余则阳旺阴消，血不足则阴旺阳消。"

雷公曰："治之奈何?"

岐伯曰："阳旺阴消者，当补其血;阴旺阳消者，当补其气。阳旺阴消者，宜泻其气;阴旺阳消者，宜泻其血。无不足，无有余，则阴阳平矣。"

雷公曰："补血则阴旺阳消，不必再泻其气;补气则阳旺阴消，不必重泻其血也。"

岐伯曰："补血以生阴者，言其常补阴也;泻气以益阴者，言其暂泻阳也。补气以助阳者，言其常补阳也;泻血以救阳者，言其暂泻阴也。故新病可泻，久病不可轻泻也;久病宜补，新病不可纯补也。"

雷公曰："治血必当理气乎?"

岐伯曰："治气亦宜理血也。气无形，血有形。无形生有形者，变也;有形生无形者，常也。"

雷公曰："何谓也?"

岐伯曰："变治急，常治缓。势急不可缓，亟补气以生血;势缓不可

Volume 9

【英译】

Chapter 73
Supplementation and Purgation of Yin and Yang

Leigong asked Qibo, "Yin and Yang in the human body is divided into Qi and blood. [This is] described thoroughly in [*Yellow Emperor's*] *Internal Canon* [*of Medicine*]. Please explain the rest [issues]."

Qibo answered, "The essentials of Qi and blood are embodied in excess and insufficiency of Qi and blood. Excess of Qi [results in] exuberance of Yang and dispersion of Yin; insufficiency of blood [results in] exuberance of Yin and dispersion of Yang."

Leigong asked, "How to treat it?"

Qibo answered, "[To treat] exuberance of Yang and dispersion of Yin, the blood should be tonified first; [to treat] exuberance of Yin and dispersion of Yang, Qi should be tonified first. [To treat] exuberance of Yang and dispersion of Yin, Qi should be purged; [to treat] exuberance of Yin and dispersion of Yang, the blood should be purged. [Only when] there is no insufficiency [of the blood] and no excess [of Qi] can Yin and Yang be harmonized."

Leigong asked, "To tonify the blood makes Yin exuberant and Yang disperse, there is no need to purge Qi again; to tonify Qi makes Yang exuberant and Yin disperse, there is no need to purge the blood again."

急,徐补血以生气。"

雷公曰:"其故何也?"

岐伯曰:"气血两相生长,非气能生血,血不能生气也。第气生血者其效速,血生气者其功迟。宜急而亟者,治失血之骤也;宜缓而徐者,治失血之后也。气生血,则血得气而安,无忧其沸腾也;血生气,则气得血而润,无虞其干燥也。苟血失补血,则气且脱矣;血安补气,则血反动矣。"

雷公曰:"善。"

陈士铎曰:"气血俱可补也,当于补中寻其原,不可一味呆补为妙。"

【今译】

雷公请问岐伯:"人身的阴阳分为气和血,《内经》已经详细说明了,请谈谈其他相关问题吧。"

岐伯说:"气血的关键在于气血的有余与不足。气有余时则阳亢阴虚;血不足则阴盛阳虚。"

雷公问:"该如何治疗呢?"

岐伯说:"阳旺阴虚的,应当通过补血治疗;阴旺阳消的,要通过补气治疗。阳旺阴虚的,应当通过泻气治疗;阴旺阳消的,应当通过泻血治疗。如果气血没有不足,也没有多余,那么阴阳就平衡了。"

雷公说:"通过补血就可以使阴旺阳消,不需要再泻其气了;通过补气就可以使阳旺阴消,就不需要再泻其血了。"

岐伯说:"通过补血生阴的,指的是经常补阴;通过泻气益阴的,指的

Volume 9

Qibo answered, "Tonifying the blood to produce Yin means always tonifying Yin; purging Qi to replenish Yin means purging Yang for the time being. Tonifying Qi to assist Yang means always tonifying Yang; purging the blood to rescue Yang means purging Yin for the time being. Thence new disease can [be treated by] purgation, [but] chronic disease cannot rashly [be treated by] purgation. Chronic disease should [be treated by] tonification [while] new disease cannot simply [be treated by] tonification."

Leigong asked, "Is it necessary to treat the blood by regulating Qi?"

Qibo answered, "[It is] also appropriate to regulate the blood [in] treating Qi. Qi is invisible and the blood is visible. [When] the invisible produces the visible, [it is] the changeable [way]; [when] the visible produces the invisible, [it is] the natural [way]."

Leigong asked, "How to explain [it]?"

Qibo answered, "The changeable [way can be used] to treat emergency [while] the natural [way can be used] to treat chronic [disease]. Emergency cannot [be treated in a] chronic [way], [only when] Qi is immediately tonified can the blood be produced; chronic [disease] cannot [be treated in a] emergent [way], [only when] the blood is gently tonified can Qi be produced."

Leigong asked, "What is the reason?"

Qibo answered, "[Because] Qi and the blood promote each other. [So it does] not [mean that only] Qi can produce the blood [while] the blood cannot produce Qi. [The fact is that it is] rapid [when] Qi produces the blood [and it is] slow [when] the blood produces Qi. [The therapeutic method for] rescuing [purpose]

是暂时泻阳。通过补气来助阳的,指的是经常补阳;通过泻血来救阳的,指的是暂时泻阴。因此,新生病可以采用泻法治疗,慢性病就不能轻易用泻法治疗。慢性病应当采用补法治疗,新生病则不能单纯地用补法治疗。"

雷公问:"治血一定要理气吗?"

岐伯说:"治气也应该理血。气无形,血有形,以无形之气生有形之血,这就是变法;以有形之血生无形之气,这就是常法。"

雷公问:"怎么理解呢?"

岐伯说:"这就是所谓的以变法治疗急症,以常法治疗缓症。病势危急的不能用缓慢法治疗,要立即补气以生血;病势缓慢的不能用急法治疗,要通过缓慢补血以生气。"

雷公问:"其原因是什么呢?"

岐伯说:"这是因为气与血相互助长,并非气能生血而血不能生气。气生血的功效比较快速,而血生气的功效则比较迟缓。应急治的就要用急救的方法治疗,这是治疗失血的紧急措施;应缓慢治疗的就要用进补的方法治疗,以便能及时缓解失血造成的后果。气生血时,血得到气则安宁,就不用担忧会出现逆乱扰动的现象;血生气时,气得血而获得濡养,就不用担忧出现气枯燥的现象。如果因失血而单纯补充血液,就会造成气的虚脱;如果血液安平但却要补气,就会引起血液的妄行。"

雷公说:"好!"

陈士铎评论说:"气血都是可以补益的,但补益的时候要寻求其根源,不可一味地将单一的进补视为奇效。"

should [be used] to treat emergency, [this is the way for] treating massive bleeding; [the therapeutic method for] tonifying [purpose] should [be used] to treat chronic [disease], [this is the way for recuperating health] after treating bleeding. [In terms of] Qi producing the blood, [only when] the blood is assisted by Qi can [it be] harmonized [and only when the blood is harmonized] can there be no turbulent flow. [In terms of] the blood producing Qi, [only when] Qi is assisted by the blood can [it be] moistened and [only when Qi is moistened by the blood] can there be no dryness. If [measures are taken only for] tonifying the blood [because of] bleeding, [it will cause] collapse of Qi; [if measures are taken only for] tonifying Qi [when] the blood [is already] harmonized, [it will cause] wanton flow of the blood."

Leigong said, "Excellent [explanation]!"

Chen Shiduo's comment, "Qi and blood all can be tonified. The evidence [for tonifying treatment] can be found in [the therapeutic methods for] tonifying [purpose]. [Cares should be taken] to avoid rigid tonifying [practice]. [This is] the excellent [way in treating disease]."

善养篇第七十四

【原文】

雷公问于岐伯曰:"春三月谓之发陈,夏三月谓之蕃秀,秋三月谓之容平,冬三月谓之闭藏,天师详载《四气调神大论》中,然调四时则病不生,不调四时则病必作。所谓调四时者,调阴阳之时令乎?抑调人身阴阳之气乎?愿晰言之。"

岐伯曰:"明乎哉问也!调阴阳之气,在人不在时也。春三月,调木气也;调木气者,顺肝气也。夏三月,调火气也;调火气者,顺心气也。秋三月,调金气也;调金气者,顺肺气也。冬三月,调水气也;调水气者,顺肾气也。肝气不顺,逆春气矣,少阳之病应之。心气不顺,逆夏气矣,太阳之病应之。肺气不顺,逆秋气矣,太阴之病应之。肾气不顺,逆冬气矣,少阴之病应之。四时之气可不调乎?调之实难,以阴阳之气不易调也,故人多病耳。"

雷公曰:"人既病矣,何法疗之?"

岐伯曰:"人以胃气为本,四时失调,致生疾病,仍调其胃气而已。胃调脾自调矣,脾调而肝心肺肾无不顺矣!"

雷公曰:"先时以养阴阳,又何可不讲乎?"

岐伯曰:"阳根于阴,阴根于阳。养阳则取之阴也,养阴则取之阳也。以阳养阴,以阴养阳,贵养之于豫也,何邪能干乎?闭目塞兑,内观

Volume 9

【英译】

Chapter 74
Good [Way for] Cultivating [Health]

Leigong asked Qibo, "[In] the three months of spring, [all things in the natural world] begin to develop; [in] the three months of summer, [all things in the natural world] develop prosperously; [in] the three months of autumn, [all things in the natural world] stop growing; [in] the three months of winter, [all things in the natural world are] stored. [In the Chapter entitled] *Major Discussion of Spirit Regulation in the Four Seasons*, Celestial Master described [these issues] in details. [If Qi in] the four seasons is regulated [and harmonized], no disease will occur; [if Qi] in the four seasons is not regulated [and harmonized], disease will certainly occur. Does the so-called regulation of the four seasons [means] to regulate Qi of Yin and Yang in the four seasons or to regulate Qi of Yin and Yang in the human body? Please explain in detail."

Qibo answered, "What an excellent question! [The way] to regulate Qi of Yin and Yang [is related] to the human [body], not to the [four] seasons. [In] the three months of spring, wood-Qi is regulated and wood-Qi should be regulated according to [the circulation of] liver-Qi; [in] the three months of summer, fire-Qi is regulated and fire-Qi should be regulated according to [the circulation of] heart-Qi; [in] the three months of autumn, metal-Qi

心肾,养阳则漱津送入心也,养阴则漱津送入肾也,无他异法也。"

雷公曰:"善。"

天老问曰:"阴阳不违背而人无病,养阳养阴之法,止调心肾乎?"

岐伯曰:"《内经》一书,皆养阳养阴之法也。"

天老曰:"阴阳之变迁不常,养阴养阳之法,又乌可执哉?"

岐伯曰:"公言何善乎! 奇恒之病,必用奇恒之法疗之。豫调心肾,养阴阳于无病时也。然而病急不可缓,病缓不可急,亦视病如何耳。故不宜汗而不汗,所以养阳也;宜汗而急汗之,亦所以养阳也。不宜下而不下,所以养阴也;宜下而大下之,亦所以养阴也。岂养阳养阴,专尚补而不尚攻乎? 用攻于补之中,正善于攻也;用补于攻之内,正善补也。攻补兼施,养阳而不损于阴,养阴而不损于阳,庶几善于养阴阳者乎!"

天老曰:"善。"

陈士铎曰:"善养一篇,俱非泛然之论,不可轻用攻补也。"

【今译】

雷公问岐伯:"春天的三个月被称为发陈,夏天的三个月被称为蕃秀,秋天的三个月被称为容平,冬天的三个月被称为闭藏,在《素问·四气调神大论》中天师已经详细地作了记载。调和四时则疾病不会发生,不调和四时则疾病必然发生。所谓调和四时,是调节四时的阴阳之气吗? 抑或是调节人体的阴阳之气呢? 请予以详细说明。"

岐伯说:"这个问题问得很好啊! 调节阴阳之气,关键在于人体而

is regulated and metal-Qi should be regulated according to [the circulation of] lung-Qi; [in] the three months of winter, water-Qi is regulated and water-Qi should be regulated according to [the circulation of] kidney-Qi. [If] liver-Qi is abnormal [in circulation], [it runs] against Qi in spring and Shaoyang disease will occur accordingly; [if] heart-Qi is abnormal [in circulation], [it runs] against Qi in summer and Taiyang disease will occur accordingly; [if] lung-Qi is abnormal [in circulation], [it runs] against Qi in autumn and Taiyin disease will occur accordingly; [if] kidney-Qi is abnormal [in circulation], [it runs] against Qi in winter and Shaoyin disease will occur accordingly. How could Qi in the four seasons be not regulated? [It is] really difficult to regulate because Qi in Yin and Yang is not easy to regulate. That is why people tend to contract disease."

Leigong asked, "[When] people are ill, what [can therapeutic methods be used] to treat them?"

Qibo answered, "[In] the human [body], stomach-Qi is the root[1]. [If it runs] against [Qi of Yin and Yang in] the four seasons, [it will] cause disease. [Thus the most important thing is] still to regulate stomach-Qi. [When] stomach [-Qi] is regulated, spleen [-Qi] is also regulated spontaneously. [When] spleen [-Qi] is regulated, [Qi in] the liver, heart, lung and kidney is all normal."

Leigong asked, "[In every] season, [measures should be taken] to cultivate Yin and Yang first. [But] why [is it] not mentioned?"

Qibo answered, "Yang depends on Yin and Yin depends on Yang. [For the purpose of] cultivating Yang, [it must be] obtained from Yin; [for the purpose of] cultivating Yin, [it must be]

不在于四时。在春天的三个月里，需要调节的是木气；要调节木气，就要顺应肝气。在夏天的三个月里，需要调节的是火气；要调节火气，就要顺应心气。在秋天的三个月里，需要调节的是金气；要调节金气，就要顺应肺气。在冬天的三个月里，需要调节的是水气；要调节水气，就要顺应肾气。如果肝气不顺，就悖逆了春天的木气，少阳病就会因此而发生。心气不顺，就悖逆了夏天的火气，太阳病就会因此而发生；肺气不顺，就悖逆了秋天的金气，太阴病就会因此而发生。肾气不顺，就悖逆了冬天的水气，少阴病就会因此而发生。四时阴阳之气怎么能不调节呢？但调节确实很难，因为阴阳之气不易调节，这可就是为什么人会容易得病。"

雷公问："人们既然得病了，用什么方法来治疗呢？"

岐伯说："人以胃气为本，如果悖逆了四时阴阳之气而导致疾病的产生，仍然需要调理胃气而已。胃气调理好了，脾气也就自然调理好了。如果脾气得到了调节，肝、心、肺和肾就不会不顺畅了！"

雷公问："时令转变之前调养阴阳，又为什么不谈呢？"

岐伯说："阳以阴为其根，阴以阳为其根。养阳则需要从阴中求阳，养阴则需要从阳中取阴。以阳养阴，以阴养阳，贵在预先调养。如果这样做到了，还会有什么邪气入侵的呢？闭上眼睛，合上嘴巴，内观心肾，养阳就意味着将含漱津液送入胃脘中，养阴就意味着将含漱津液送入肾中，除此之外没有其他特别方法可以使用。"

雷公说："好。"

天老问："阴阳相互不背离，人就不会生病，养阳养阴的方法，只是

obtained from Yang. [Obviously,] cultivation of Yang depends on Yin and cultivation of Yin depends on Yang. [Hence it is] very important to cultivate in advance. [If it is well cultivated in advance,] how can evil invade [the body]? [To achieve such a goal, you should] close [your] eyes and mouth and internally observe [your own] heart and kidney. [In this way,] lucid liquid will enter the heart[2] [when] cultivating Yang and lucid liquid will enter the kidney [when] cultivating Yin. No other special methods [can be used]."

Leigong said, "Excellent [explanation]!"

Tianlao asked, "[When] Yin and Yang do not run against [each other], people will not contract disease. [Is] the method [for] cultivating Yang and cultivating Yin used just for regulating the heart and kidney?"

Qibo answered, "[What mentioned in] the book [entitled *Yellow Emperor's*] *Internal Canon* [*of Medicine*] is all about [how] to cultivate Yang and [how] to cultivate Yin."

Tianlao asked, "The changes of Yin and Yang are complicated. [But] why is the method for cultivating Yin and cultivating Yang unchangeable?"

Qibo answered, "What an excellent question! Unusual disease must be treated with unusual methods. To regulate the heart and kidney in advance [means] to cultivate Yin and Yang before occurrence of disease. However, emergency cannot [be treated with] chronic [methods] and chronic disease cannot [be treated with] emergent [method], [indicating that treatment should be] decided according to [the condition of] disease. Hence, [in dealing

靠调养心肾吗?"

岐伯说:"《内经》一书所强调的就是养阳和养阴的方法。"

天老问:"阴阳的变化复杂无常,养阴养阳的方法又怎么会一成不变的呢?"

岐伯说:"你问的问题很好啊! 奇异的病,必须用奇异的方法来治疗。预先调养心肾,就是在没有发病之前对阴阳的调养。但是病情急重的不能缓慢地进行调养,病情缓慢的不需要采取急治之法治疗,也需要根据疾病的实际情况来进行。所以不适宜发汗就不能使用发汗法治疗,这就是为了养阳;适宜发汗就立刻使用发汗法治疗,这也是为了养阳。不适宜攻下就不能使用攻下法治疗,这就是为了养阴;适宜攻下的就应立即使用攻下法治疗,这也是为了养阴。而养阴养阳,又怎么能只重视补而不重视攻呢? 将攻法纳入补法之中,正是善于运用攻法;将补法纳入攻法之中,也正是善于运用补法。兼顾使用了攻法和补法,养阳就不会损伤阴,养阴就不会损伤阳,这才是善于调养阴阳的方略啊!"

天老说:"好!"

陈士铎评论说:"《善养》这一章节,完全不是泛泛而谈,在实际应用中不可轻率使用攻补之法。"

with the disease that is] inappropriate [to be treated by] sweating [therapy], diaphoresis cannot [be used] because [it concentrates on] cultivating Yang; [in dealing with the disease that is] appropriate [to be treated by] sweating [therapy], diaphoresis [should be used] immediately because [it] also [concentrates on] cultivating Yang; [in dealing with the disease that is] inappropriate [to be treated by] purgative [therapy], purgation cannot [be used] because [it concentrates on] cultivating Yin; [in dealing with the disease that is] appropriate [to be treated by] purgative [therapy], purgation [should be used] immediately because [it] also [concentrates on] cultivating Yin. [Thus in] cultivating Yang and cultivating Yin, how [can it] just [focus on] tonification but not [on] purgation? To adopt purgation in tonification is good at [applying] purgation [while] to adopt tonification in purgation is good at [applying] tonification. Concurrent application of purgation and tonification will not damage Yin in cultivating Yang and will not damage Yang in cultivating Yin. This is just the right way to cultivate Yin and Yang."

Tianlao said, "Excellent [explanation]!"

Chen Shiduo's comment, " This chapter about excellent cultivation is not discussed in general. Purgation and tonification cannot be used at random."

Notes

[1] Root here means very important.

[2] Heart here refers to the stomach.

亡阴亡阳篇第七十五

【原文】

鸟师问于岐伯曰："人汗出不已，皆亡阳也？"

岐伯曰："汗出不已，非尽亡阳也。"

鸟师曰："汗证未有非热也，热病即阳病矣，天师谓非阳，何也？"

岐伯曰："热极则阳气难固，故汗泄亡阳。溺属阴，汗属阳。阳之外泄，非亡阳而何？谓非尽亡阳者，以阳根于阴也。阳之外泄，由于阴之不守也。阴守其职，则阳根于阴，阳不能外泄也。阴失其职，则阴欲自顾不能，又何能摄阳气之散亡乎？故阳亡本于阴之先亡也。"

鸟师曰："阴亡则阴且先脱，何待阳亡而死乎？"

岐伯曰："阴阳相根，无寸晷之离也。阴亡而阳随之即亡，故阳亡即阴亡也，何分先后乎？"

鸟师曰："阴阳同亡，宜阴阳之共救矣！乃救阳则汗收而可生，救阴则汗止而难活，又何故乎？"

岐伯曰："阴生阳则缓，阳生阴则速。救阴而阳之绝不能遽回，救阳而阴之绝可以骤复，故救阴不若救阳也。虽然，阴阳何可离也？救阳之中附以救阴之法，则阳回而阴亦自复也。"

鸟师曰："阴阳之亡，非旦夕之故也，曷不于未亡之前先治之？"

岐伯天师曰："大哉言乎！亡阴亡阳之证，皆肾中水火之虚也。阳

Volume 9

【英译】

Chapter 75
Collapse of Yin and Collapse of Yang

Niaoshi asked Qibo, "[When] a person is constantly sweating, is [it] collapse of Yang?"

Qibo answered, "Constant sweating does not only mean collapse of Yang."

Niaoshi asked, "There is no absence of heat in disease [with] sweating and heat disease is certainly Yang disease. [But] Celestial Master have said [that it is] not only Yang [disease]. Why?"

Qibo answered, "[When] heat [has increased to] the extreme, Yang Qi is difficult to be stable. That is why sweating causes collapse of Yang. Urine belongs to Yin [while] sweating belongs to Yang. [If] external leakage of Yang is not collapse of Yang, what is it then? [I have] said [that it is] not just collapse of Yang, because Yang depends on Yin. External leakage of Yang is due to failure of Yin to hold its ground. [Only when] Yin fulfils its duty can Yang depend on Yin and will not leak. [When] Yin fails to fulfil its duty, Yin is unable to defend itself. How can [it] protect Yang Qi [and prevent it] from collapse? Hence collapse of Yang is caused by collapse of Yin."

Niaoshi asked, "Collapse of Yin means loss of Yin [fluid] first. [But] why [only when] collapse of Yang occurs does death [happen]?"

虚,补火以生水,阴虚,补水以制火,可免两亡矣!"

鸟师曰:"善。"

陈士铎曰:"阴阳之亡,由于阴阳之两不可守也,阳摄于阴,阴摄于阳。本于水火之虚,虚则亡,又何疑哉?"

【今译】

鸟师问岐伯:"人不停地出汗,这都是亡阳的表现吗?"

岐伯说:"人汗出不停,不一定都是亡阳所致。"

鸟师问:"汗证没有不发热的,这说明热病就是阳病。为什么天师说不全是阳病呢?"

岐伯说:"热到极点阳气就难以稳固,所以出汗过多就会亡阳。尿属阴,汗属阳。阳气外泄,不是亡阳又是什么呢? 之所以说其不全是亡阳,是因为阳以阴为其根。阳气外泄,是因为阴气不能固守的缘故。如果阴气恪守其职,阳就会以阴为根,阳气就不会外泄。如果阴气失其职,阴气就自顾不能,哪又怎么能够固摄阳气并使之不亡呢? 所以阳亡的根源是阴的先亡。"

鸟师问:"阴亡后阴液应先脱,为什么要等到阳亡了才会导致死亡呢?"

岐伯说:"阴阳互根,彼此之间没有片刻的分离。阴亡了阳就会随之而亡,因此阳亡就是阴亡,什么要分其先后呢?"

鸟师问:"既然阴和阳是同时消亡的,那么就应该同时救护阳和阴

Qibo answered, "Yin and Yang depend on each other and never separate [from each other]. [When] Yin collapses, Yang [will also] collapse accordingly. Thus collapse of Yang indicates collapse of Yin. Why should there be order of priority?"

Niaoshi asked, "[When] both Yin and Yang collapse, [it is] appropriate to rescue Yin and Yang at the same time. To rescue Yang, sweating will stop and [the patient] will be cured. To rescue Yin, sweating will stop but [the patient is] difficult to survive. What is the reason?"

Qibo answered, "[When] Yin is produced, Yang [develops] slowly; [when] Yang is produced, Yin [develops] rapidly. [Thus when] Yin is rescued, collapse of Yang cannot be restored immediately; [when] Yang is rescued, collapse of Yin can be restored immediately. Hence to rescue Yin is not better than to rescue Yang. Nevertheless, how can Yin and Yang be separated [from each other]? [In] rescuing Yang, the method for rescuing Yin [should be] adopted. [In this case, when] Yang is restored, Yin is also restored."

Niaoshi asked, "Collapse of Yin and Yang is not caused in a short while. Why is treatment not taken before collapse occurs?"

Celestial Master Qibo said, "What a great question! Disease [with] collapse of Yin and collapse of Yang is all caused by deficiency of water and fire in the kidney. [For] Yang deficiency, fire [should be] tonified to produce water; [for] Yin deficiency, water [should be] tonified to control fire. [Such a way of treatment] can avoid collapse of both."

Niaoshi said, "Excellent [explanation]!"

啊！救阳时出汗就会停止，而人能因此而生存。救阴时出汗也会停止，但人却因此而难以生存，这又是什么原因呢？"

岐伯说："阴生阳则比较缓慢，阳生阴则比较迅速。救阴不能立即挽回阳的消亡，救阳则可以立即恢复阴气，所以救阴不如救阳。虽然如此，阴和阳又怎么会分离呢？如果救阳之中附加使用救阴之方，那么阳气回复的同时阴气也就能自行恢复。"

鸟师问："阳阴之亡并非旦夕所致，为什么不在未亡之前就预先采取措施进行治疗呢？"

岐伯天师说："问得很好啊！亡阴亡阳之证，都是因为肾中水火虚衰所致。如果阳虚，通过补火就能生水；如果阴虚，通过补水就能生火。这样就能避免阴阳两亡了！"

鸟师说："好！"

陈士铎评论说："阴阳的消亡是由于阴阳相互不能固守的缘故。阳固摄阴，阴固摄阳。疾病的发生源自于肾脏中水火的亏虚，其亏虚则导致阴阳的亡失。这又有什么可以质疑的呢？"

Volume 9

Chen Shiduo's comment, "Collapse of Yin and Yang is due to failure of Yin and Yang to protect each other. [As a result,] Yang checks Yin and Yin checks Yang. [Occurrence of disease is] due to deficiency of water and fire [in the kidney], and deficiency [inevitably] leads to collapse. How could there be doubt [about it]?"

昼夜轻重篇第七十六

【原文】

雷公问于岐伯曰:"昼夜可辨病之轻重乎?"

岐伯曰:"病有重轻,宜从昼夜辨之。"

雷公曰:"辨之维何?"

岐伯曰:"阳病昼重,阴病昼轻,阳病夜轻,阴病夜重。"

雷公曰:"何谓也?"

岐伯曰:"昼重夜轻,阳气旺于昼,衰于夜也;昼轻夜重,阴气旺于夜,衰于昼也。"

雷公曰:"阳病昼轻,阴病夜轻,何故乎?"

岐伯曰:"此阴阳之气虚也。"

雷公曰:"请显言之。"

岐伯曰:"阳病昼重夜轻,此阳气与病气交旺,阳气未衰也,正与邪斗,尚有力也,故昼反重耳;夜则阳衰矣,阳衰不与邪斗,邪亦不与正斗,故夜反轻耳。阴病昼轻夜重,此阴气与病气交旺,阴气未衰也,正与邪争,尚有力也,故夜反重耳;昼则阴衰矣,阴衰不敢与邪争,邪亦不与阴争,故昼反轻耳。"

雷公曰:"邪既不与正相战,宜邪之退舍矣,病犹不瘥,何也?"

岐伯曰:"重乃真重,轻乃假轻。假轻者,视之轻而实重,邪且重入

Volume 9

【英译】

Chapter 76
Severity and Lightness of [Disease in the Day and Night]

Leigong asked Qibo, "Can the severity and lightness of disease be differentiated in the daytime and at night?"

Qibo answered, "Disease is either severe or light. [It] should be differentiated from daytime and night."

Leigong asked, "What is the standard to differentiate?"

Qibo answered, "Yang disease is severe in the daytime [while] Yin disease is light in the daytime; Yang disease is light at night [while] Yin disease is severe at night."

Leigong asked, "What is the reason?"

Qibo answered, "[Yang disease is] severe in the daytime and light at night [because] Yang Qi is exuberant in the daytime and debilitated at night; [Yin disease is] light in the daytime and severe at night [because] Yin Qi is exuberant at night and debilitated in the daytime."

Leigong asked, "Why Yang disease is light in the daytime and Yin disease is light at night?"

Qibo answered, "This [is because of] deficiency of Qi in Yin and Yang."

Leigong asked, "Please explain clearly."

Qibo answered, "Yang disease is severe in the daytime and light at night, because Yang Qi and disease Qi are all exuberant. [At this

矣,乌可退哉? 且轻重无常,或昼重夜亦重,或昼轻夜亦轻,或时重时轻,此阴阳之无定,昼夜之难拘也。"

雷公曰:"然则,何以施疗乎?"

岐伯曰:"昼重夜轻者,助阳气以祛邪;昼轻夜重者,助阴气以祛邪,皆不可专祛其邪也。昼夜俱重,昼夜俱轻,与时重时轻,峻于补阴,佐以补阳,又不可泥于补阳而专于祛邪也。"

陈士铎曰:"昼夜之间,轻重自别。"

【今译】

雷公问岐伯:"可以通过白天和夜晚辨别疾病的轻重吗?"

岐伯说:"病情有重有轻,应当通过白天和夜晚进行辨别。"

雷公问:"辨别的原则是什么?"

岐伯说:"阳病白天重,阴病白天轻;阳病夜晚轻,阴病夜晚重。"

雷公问:"什么道理呢?"

岐伯说:"阳病之所以白天重而晚间轻,是因为阳气在白天旺而在夜晚衰;阴病之所以白天轻而夜间重,是因为阴气在夜晚旺而在白天衰。"

雷公问:"阳病白天轻,阴病晚间轻,是什么原因呢?"

岐伯说:"这是阴阳气虚的原因。"

雷公说:"请予详细说明。"

岐伯说:"阳病白天重而晚间轻,这是因为阳气与病气在白天都很

time,] Yang Qi is not debilitated and healthy [Qi] is still strong [when] fighting with evil [Qi]. That is why [Yang disease is] severe in the daytime. At night Yang is debilitated and will not fight with evil Qi. [In this case,] evil [Qi] will not also fight with healthy [Qi]. That is why [Yang disease is] light at night. Yin disease is light in the daytime and severe at night because Yin Qi and disease Qi are all exuberant. [At this time,] Yin Qi is not debilitated and healthy [Qi] is still strong [when] fighting with evil [Qi]. That is why [Yin disease is] severe at night. At night Yin is debilitated and will not fight with evil [Qi]. [In this case,] evil [Qi] will not also fight with Yin [Qi]. That is why [Yin disease is] light in the daytime. "

Leigong asked,"Now that evil [Qi] will not fight with healthy [Qi] and should retreat far away, [but] the disease still does not heal. What is the reason?"

Qibo answered, "Severe [disease] is really severe and light [disease] is falsely light. [The so-called] falsely light [disease] seems to be light but is actually severe. [In this case,] invasion of evil Qi is more serious, how could [it] retreat? Furthermore, severity and lightness [of disease is] not regular. [It may be] severe in the daytime and also severe at night, or light in the daytime and also light at night, or now severe and then light. This [is due to] instability of Yin and Yang [which makes it] difficult to be managed in the daytime and at night. "

Leigong asked,"Since it is so, how to treat it then?"

Qibo answered, "[The disease that is] severe in the daytime and light at night [can be treated by] assisting Yang Qi to eliminate

旺盛,阳气没有衰微,正气与邪气争斗,因为还有力量,所以白天病症反而较重。晚间阳气衰微,阳气衰微就不能与邪气争斗,而邪气也不与正气争斗,所以晚间病症反而较轻。阴病白天轻而晚间重,因为阴气和病气在晚间都比较旺盛,阴气没有衰微,正气与邪气争斗,因为还有力量,所以夜间病症反而较重。白天阴气衰微,阴气衰微就无力与邪气争斗,而邪气也不与阴气争斗,这就是为什么病症在白天反而较轻。"

雷公问:"病邪既然不与正气相争,邪气就应当退避,可是疾病仍然不愈,这又是为什么呢?"

岐伯说:"病症重的确实是重,而病症轻的则并非真轻。并非真轻的,是看起来轻而实际上重,邪气侵入后则更为严重,怎么会退避呢?至于那些轻重无常的病症,有的白天重而晚间也重,有的白天轻晚间也轻,有的时重时轻,这是阴阳不定所造成的,所以难以受昼夜变化的制约。"

雷公问:"既然这样,那该怎么治疗呢?"

岐伯说:"白天重而夜间轻的,可通过助长阳气以祛除邪气;白天轻夜间重的,可通过助长阴气以祛除邪气,都不能专门去攻伐邪气。白天晚间都重的,或者白天夜间都轻的,或者时重时轻的病症,其治疗的关键都在于补阴,同时辅以补阳,不可拘泥于专门通过补阳以祛除邪气。"

陈士铎评论说:"昼夜之间,病症的轻重自然是有区别的。"

evil [Qi]; [the disease that is] light in the daytime and severe at night [can be treated by] assisting Yin Qi to eliminate evil [Qi]. [In both cases, trials] cannot [be made] just for eliminating evil [Qi]. [For treating disease] severe both in the daytime and at night, or light both in the daytime and at night, or now severe and then light, the key point is to tonify Yin [with] supplementary [efforts] to tonify Yang, avoiding rigidly adhering to tonification of Yang and elimination of evil [Qi]."

Chen Shiduo's comment, "In the daytime and at night, [disease is] certainly either light or severe."

解阳解阴篇第七十七

【原文】

奢龙问于岐伯曰："阳病解于戌,阴病解于寅,何也?"

岐伯曰："阳病解于戌者,解于阴也;阴病解于寅者,解于阳也。然解于戌者,不始于戌;解于寅者,不始于寅。不始于戌者,由寅始之也;不始于寅者,由亥始之也。解于戌而始于寅,非解于阴乃解于阳也;解于寅而始于亥,非解于阳乃解于阴也。"

奢龙曰："阳解于阳,阴解于阴,其义何也?"

岐伯曰："十二经均有气旺之时,气旺则解也。"

奢龙曰："十二经之旺气,可得闻乎?"

岐伯曰："少阳之气,旺寅卯辰;太阳之气,旺巳午未;阳明之气,旺申酉戌;太阴之气,旺亥子丑;少阴之气,旺子丑寅;厥阴之气,旺丑寅卯也。"

奢龙曰："少阴之旺何与各经殊乎?"

岐伯曰："少阴者,肾水也。水中藏火,火者阳也。子时一阳生,丑时二阳生,寅时三阳生,阳进则阴退,故阴病遇子丑寅而解者,解于阳也。"

奢龙曰："少阴解于阳,非解于阴矣!"

岐伯曰："天一生水,子时水生,即是旺地,故少阴遇子而渐解也。"

Volume 9

【英译】

Chapter 77
Relief of Yang [Disease] and Relief of Yin [Disease]

Shelong asked Qibo, "Why is Yang disease relieved in [the time of] Xu (19:00 - 21:00) and Yin disease relieved in [the time of] Yin (3:00 - 5:00)?"

Qibo answered, "Yang disease [that is] relieved in [the time of] Xu (19:00 - 21:00) [means] to relieve [in the time of] Yin, and Yin disease [that is] relieved in [the time of] Yin [1] (3:00 - 5:00) [means] to relieve [in the time of] Yang. However, to relieve [in the time of] Xu (19:00 - 21:00) does not [mean that the disease] starts [to be relieved from the time of] Xu (19:00 - 21:00); to relieve [in the time of] Yin (3:00 - 5:00) does not [mean that the disease] starts [to be relieved from the time of] Yin (3:00 - 5:00). [The disease that] does not begin [to be relieved from the time of] Xu (19:00 - 21:00) [actually] starts [from the time of] Yin (3:00 - 5:00); [the disease that] does not begin [to be relieved from the time of] Yin (3:00 - 5:00) [actually] starts [from the time of] Hai (21:00 - 23:00). [The disease that is] relieved in [the time of] Xu (19:00 - 21:00) and starts from [the time of] Yin (3:00 - 5:00) is not relieved in [the time of] Yin but relieved in [the time of] Yang. [The disease that is] relieved in [the time of] Yin (3:00 - 5:00) and starts from [the time of] Hai (21:00 - 23:00) is not relieved in [the time of] Yang but relieved in [the time of] Yin."

奢龙曰:"少阳之解,始于寅卯,少阴、厥阴之解,终于寅卯,又何也?"

岐伯曰:"寅为生人之首,卯为天地门户。始于寅卯者,阳得初之气也;终于寅卯者,阴得终之气也。"

奢龙曰:"三阳之时旺,各旺三时,三阴之时旺,连旺三时,又何也?"

岐伯曰:"阳行健,其道长,故各旺其时;阴行钝,其道促,故连旺其时也。"

奢龙曰:"阳病解于夜半,阴病解于日中,岂阳解于阳,阴解于阴乎?"

岐伯曰:"夜半以前者,阴也;夜半以后者,阳也;日中以后者,阴也;日中以前者,阳也。阳病必于阳旺之时先现解之机,至夜半而尽解也。阴病必于阴旺之时先现解之兆,至日中而尽解也。虽阳解于阳,实阳得阴之气也;虽阴解于阴,实阴得阳之气也。此阳根阴,阴根阳之义耳。"

奢龙曰:"善。"

陈士铎曰:"阳解于阴,阴解于阳,自有至义,非泛说也。"

【今译】

奢龙请问岐伯:"阳病缓解于戌时,阴病缓解于寅时,这是为什么呢?"

Shelong asked, "Yang [disease is] relieved in [the time of] Yang and Yin [disease is] relived in [the time of] Yin. What does it mean?"

Qibo answered, "Qi in all the twelve meridians is exuberant at a certain time. [When] Qi [in the meridians is] exuberant, [the disease will be] relieved. "

Shelong asked, "Can [I] know [when] Qi in the twelve meridians is exuberant?"

Qibo answered, "Qi in Shaoyang [meridian] is exuberant [in the time of] Yin (3:00 - 5:00), Mao (5:00 - 7:00) and Chen (7:00 - 9:00); Qi in Taiyang [meridian] is exuberant [in the time of] Si (9:00 - 11:00), Wu (11:00 - 13:00) and Wei (13:00 - 15:00); Qi in Yangming [meridian] is exuberant [in the time of] Shen (15:00 - 17:00), You (17:00 - 19:00) and Xu (19:00 - 21:00); Qi in Taiyin [meridian] is exuberant [in the time of] Hai (21:00 - 23:00), Zi (23:00 - 1:00) and Chou (1:00 - 3:00); Qi in Shaoyin [meridian] is exuberant [in the time of] Zi (23:00 - 1:00), Chou (1:00 - 3:00) and Yin (3:00 - 5:00); Qi in Jueyin [meridian] is exuberant [in the time of] Chou (1:00 - 3:00), Yin (3:00 - 5:00) and Mao (5:00 - 7:00). "

Shelong asked, "Why is the exuberance of Shaoyin [meridian] different from [that of] other meridians?"

Qibo answered, "Shaoyin [meridian belongs to] kidney-water. In water there stores fire and fire is Yang. [In] the time of Zi (23:00 - 1:00), one [kind of] Yang is produced; [in] the time of Chou (1:00 - 3:00), two [kinds of] Yang are produced; [in] the time of Yin (3:00 - 5:00), three [kinds of] Yang are produced. [When] Yang progresses, Yin retreats. That is why Yin disease is relieved in [the time of] Zi (23:00 - 1:00), Chou (1:00 - 3:00) and Yin (3:00 - 5:00), [being] relieved in [the time of] Yang. "

岐伯说："阳病缓解于戌时,也就是缓解于阴时;阴病缓解于寅时,也就是缓解于阳时。但缓解于戌时的,并不是从戌时开始;而缓解于寅时的,也并不是从寅时开始。不是开始于戌时的,必然从寅时开始;不是开始于寅时的,当然从亥时开始。缓解于戌时而开始于寅时的,并非缓解于阴时,而是缓解于阳时;缓解于寅时而开始于亥时的,并不是缓解于阳时,而是缓解于阴时。"

奢龙问:"阳病缓解于阳时,阴病缓解于阴时,其含义是什么呢?"

岐伯说:"十二经都有气旺的时候,当经气旺盛的时候疾病就会因之而缓解了。"

奢龙问:"十二经的旺气,能否讲给我听听呢?"

岐伯说:"少阳经之气,旺于寅卯辰这三个时辰;太阳经的气,旺于巳午未这三个时辰;阳明经的气,旺于申酉戌这三个时辰;太阴经的气,旺于亥子丑这三个时辰;少阴经的气,旺于子丑寅这三个时辰,厥阴经的气,旺于丑寅卯这三个时辰。"

奢龙问:"少阴经气的旺盛,为什么与其它经络不同呢?"

岐伯说:"少阴经属于肾水,水中藏有火,火就是阳,子时一阳生,丑时二阳生,寅时三阳生,阳进则阴退,所以阴病在子丑寅这三个时辰就能得到缓解,而缓解的根本在于阳时。"

奢龙说:"少阴病缓解于阳时,并非缓解于阴时。"

岐伯说:"天一生水,子时水生,这就是水旺之地,因此少阴病遇到子时就会逐渐缓解。"

奢龙问:"少阳病的缓解从寅卯二时开始,少阴、厥阴病的缓解则

Volume 9

Shelong said, "Shaoyin [disease is] relieved in [the time of] Yang, not in [the time of] Yin."

Qibo answered, "The sky produces water[2]. Water is produced [in] the time of Zi (23:00 – 1:00), [which] is also the place [where water is] exuberant. That is why Shaoyin [disease] is gradually relieved [in] the time of Zi (23:00 – 1:00)."

Shelong asked, "Relief of Shaoyang [disease] begins in [the time of] Yin (3:00 – 5:00) and Mao (5:00 – 7:00). Relief of Shaoyin [disease] and Jueyin [disease] ends at [the time of] Yin (3:00 – 5:00) and Mao (5:00 – 7:00). What is the reason?"

Qibo answered, "Yin (3:00 – 5:00) is [the time when] man was born and Mao (5:00 – 7:00) is the gate of the sky and earth. [The relief of a disease] begins in [the time of] Yin (3:00 – 5:00) and Mao (5:00 – 7:00) [indicates that] Yang has obtained initial Qi; [the relief of a disease] ends at [the time of] Yin (3:00 – 5:00) and Mao (5:00 – 7:00) [indicates that] Yin has met final Qi."

Shelong asked, "[When Qi in] the three Yang [meridians is] exuberant, [it is] exuberant [in] three periods; [when Qi in] the three Yin [meridians is] exuberant, [it is] exuberant [in] three periods. What is the reason?"

Qibo answered, "Yang [Qi is] strong [when it] moves and the road [along which it moves is] long. That is why [Qi in the three Yang meridians is] exuberant in three periods. Yin [Qi is] slow [when it] moves and the road [along which it moves is] short. That is why [Qi in the three Yin meridians is] exuberant in three periods."

Shelong asked, "Yang disease is relieved at midnight [while] Yin disease is relieved at the noon. Does [it mean that] Yang [disease is] relieved in [the time of] Yang and Yin [disease is]

在寅卯二时结束,这又是为什么呢?"

岐伯说:"寅是生人的开始,卯是天地的门户。开始于寅卯之时的,阳就得到了初生之气;终止于寅卯之时的,就是阴遇到了终结之气。"

奢龙问:"三阳经气的旺盛,分别旺盛于三个不同的时辰。而三阴经气的旺盛,则连续旺盛在三个时辰,这又是为什么呢?"

岐伯说:"阳气因为运行而刚健,其路径较长,因此其经气旺盛在不同的时辰;阴气运行迟缓,期路径较短,所以连续旺盛在三个时辰。"

奢龙问:"阳病缓解于夜半,阴病缓解于日中,这难道不是阳病缓解于阳时而阴病缓解于阴时吗?"

岐伯说:"夜半之前的时辰属阴,夜半之后的时辰属阳;日中之后的时辰属阴,日中之前的时辰属阳。因此阳病必然在阳气旺盛的时候先表现出缓解的迹象,而到了夜半之时则全部得以消除;而阴病必然在阴气旺盛的时候先表现出缓解的征兆,到日中之时就将全部消解。虽然阳病缓解于阳时,实际上是阳得益于阴气而缓解;虽然阴病缓解于阴时,实际上是阴得益于阳气而缓解。其实际含义就是阳以阴为根、阴以阳为根。"

奢龙说:"好!"

陈士铎评论说:"阳病缓解于阴时,阴病缓解于阳时,含义至为深刻,并非泛泛而论。"

relieved in [the time of] Yin?"

Qibo answered, "[The time] before midnight is Yin [while the time] after midnight is Yang; [the time] after the noon is Yin [while the time] before the noon is Yang. [In terms of] Yang disease, there must be the opportunity to relieve [when] Yang [Qi] is exuberant and [it will be] completely relieved in [the time of] midnight; [in terms of] Yin disease, there must be the chance to relieve [when] Yin [Qi] is exuberant and [it will be] completely relieved in [the time of] the noon. Although [it seems that] Yang [disease is] relieved in [the time of] Yang, in fact [it depends on] Yang obtaining Qi from Yin. Although [it seems that] Yin [disease is] relieved in [the time of] Yin, in fact [it depends on] Yin obtaining Qi from Yang. That is what Yang depends on Yin and Yin depends on Yang means."

Shelong said, "Excellent [explanation]!"

Chen Shiduo's comment, "Yang [disease is] relieved in [the time of] Yin and Yin [disease is] relieved in [the time of] Yang. The meaning is unique. [Such an] analysis [is certainly] not in general."

Notes

[1] "Yin" here refers to the Chinese concept 寅, the third sign of the ten Earthly Branches, the pronunciation of which is similar to 阴, but the meaning of which is quite different from 阴.

[2] This is an ancient Chinese concept based on observation of celestial phenomana, indicating combination of water star (Mercury) with the sun and the moon. The original Chinese characters in this concept are "Tian (天, sky) Yi (一, one) Sheng (生, produce) Shui (水, water)".

真假疑似篇第七十八

【原文】

雷公问曰："病有真假，公言之矣。真中之假，假中之真，未言也。"

岐伯曰："寒热虚实尽之。"

雷公曰："寒热若何?"

岐伯曰："寒乃假寒，热乃真热。内热之极，外现假寒之象，此心火之亢也。火极似水，治以寒则解矣。热乃假热，寒乃真寒，下寒之至，上发假热之形，此肾火之微也。水极似火，治以热则解矣。"

雷公曰："虚实若何?"

岐伯曰："虚乃真虚，实乃假实，清肃之令不行，饮食难化，上越中满，此脾胃假实，肺气真虚也，补虚则实消矣。实乃真实，虚乃假虚，疏泄之气不通，风邪相侵，外发寒热，此肺气假虚，肝气真实也，治实则虚失矣。"

雷公曰："尽此乎?"

岐伯曰："未也。有时实时虚，时寒时热，状真非真，状假非假，此阴阳之变，水火之绝也。"

雷公曰："然则，何以治之?"

岐伯曰："治之早则生，治之迟则死。"

雷公曰："将何法早治之?"

Volume 9

【英译】

Chapter 78
True or False Manifestations

Leigong asked, "You have mentioned [that the manifestation of] disease is either true or false. [But] false [manifestation] in true [disease] and true [manifestation] in false [disease] are not mentioned yet."

Qibo answered, "[In some cases,] cold, heat, deficiency and excess are all mentioned."

Leigong asked, "What about cold and heat?"

Qibo answered, "[In some cases,] cold is false cold [but] heat is true heat. [When] internal heat [increases to] the extreme, [there will be] manifestation of false cold in the external, indicating hyperactivity of heart-fire. [When] heat [increases to] the extreme, [it appears] like water [and can be] relieved by treating [with medicinals] cold [in property]. [In other cases,] heat is false heat [but] cold is true cold. [When] cold [Qi in] the lower [increases to] the extreme, [there will be] manifestation of false heat in the upper, indicating faint fire in the kidney. [When] water [increases to] the extreme, [it appears] like fire [and can be] relieved by treating [with medicinals] heat [in property]."

岐伯曰："救胃肾之气,则绝者不绝,变者不变也。"

雷公曰："水火各有其假,而火尤难辨,奈何?"

岐伯曰："真火每现假寒,假火每现真热,然辨之有法也。真热者,阳证也。真热现假寒者,阳证似阴也,此外寒内热耳。真寒者,阴证也。真寒现假热者,阴证似阳也,此外热内寒耳。"

雷公曰："外寒内热,外热内寒,水火终何以辨之?"

岐伯曰："外寒内热者,真水之亏,邪气之胜也;外热内寒者,真火之亏,正气之虚也。真水真火,肾中水火也。肾火得肾水以相资,则火为真火,热为真热;肾火离肾水以相制,则火为假火,热成假热矣! 辨真辨假,以外水试之,真热得水则解,假热得水则逆也。"

雷公曰："治法若何?"

岐伯曰："补其水则假火自解矣。"

雷公曰："假热之证,用热剂而瘥者,何也?"

岐伯曰："肾中之火,喜阴水相济,亦喜阴火相引,滋其水矣。用火引之,则假火易藏,非舍水竟用火也。"

雷公曰："请言治火之法。"

岐伯曰："补真水则真火亦解也。虽然,治火又不可纯补水也,祛热于补水之中,则假破真现矣。"

雷公曰："善。"

陈士铎曰："不悟真,何知假? 不悟假,何知真? 真假之间,亦水火之分也。识破水火之真假,则真假何难辨哉?"

Leigong asked,"How about deficiency and excess?"

Qibo answered, "[In some cases,] deficiency is true deficiency [but] excess is false excess. [If] the function of depuration cannot be performed, food is difficult to digest, [causing] vomiting in the upper and fullness in the middle, indicating false excess in the spleen and stomach and true deficiency of lung-Qi. [When] deficiency is tonified, excess will disappear. [In other cases,] excess is true excess [but] deficiency is false deficiency, [causing] obstruction of Qi for dispersing [evil], invasion of wind-evil and manifestation of cold and heat in the external, indicating false deficiency of liver-Qi and true excess of liver-Qi. [When] excess [disease is] treated, deficiency [disease will be] eliminated."

Leigong asked,"That's all?"

Qibo answered, "No. [It is] sometimes of excess, sometimes of deficiency, sometimes of cold and sometimes of heat. [Sometimes] the manifestation [seems] true, [but in fact it is] not true; [sometimes] the manifestation [seems] false, [but in fact is] not false. This indicates changes of Yin and Yang [as well as] exhaustion of water and fire."

Leigong asked,"But how to treat it?"

Qibo answered, "Early treatment rescues life [while] delayed treatment leads to death."

Leigong asked,"How to treat it earlier?"

Qibo answered, "[When] Qi in the stomach and kidney is

【今译】

雷公问:"病有真假,您已经讲了。但真中之假象与假中之真象,还没有谈到啊。"

岐伯说:"寒热虚实可以说详尽地谈谈。"

雷公问:"寒热是怎样的呢?"

岐伯说:"寒可以是假寒,但热却可以是真热。体内热到极点,体外则表现出假寒的症状,这是心火亢进的原因。火旺盛到极点就像水一样,因此用寒凉之法予以治疗就会消解。同时,热也会是假热,寒也会是真寒。如果下面的寒气发展到了极点,上面就会出现假热的症状,这是肾火衰微所致。水旺到极点就会像火一样,用热法予以治疗就会得以消解。"

雷公问:"虚实又是怎样的呢?"

岐伯说:"虚可以是真虚,但实却可能是假实。如果清肃的功能失调,饮食就难以消化,于是就会出现呕吐、中脘胀满的症状,这是脾胃假实、肺气真虚的缘故。如果用补益虚症之法治疗,实证就会消除。实是真实,而虚则是假虚。如果疏泄之气不通,风邪侵入,体表就会出现时寒时热的症状,这就是肺气假虚、肝气真实的缘故。通过治疗实证,虚证就会消失。"

雷公问:"要讲解的就是这些吗?"

岐伯说:"我还没有讲完呢。还有时实时虚、时寒时热,症状的表现似乎是真的,但其实却不是真的,症状的表现似乎是假的,但其实却不是假的,这是阴阳的变化以及水火二气将绝的缘故。"

rescued, [Qi that is] lost [will be] restored and [Qi that has] changed [will] stop changing."

Leigong asked, "[There are] false [manifestations in] water and fire respectively. [But the false manifestation of] fire is especially difficult to differentiate. How [to deal with it]?"

Qibo answered, "[There are] often [manifestations of] false cold in true fire and true heat in false fire. However, there are ways to differentiate. True heat is Yang syndrome/pattern. [When there is] manifestation of false cold in true heat, Yang syndrome/pattern seems to be Yin, indicating [that there is] external cold and internal heat. True cold is Yin syndrome/pattern. [When there is] manifestation of false heat in true cold, Yin syndrome/pattern seems to be Yang, indicating [that there is] external heat and internal cold."

Leigong asked, "How to differentiate external cold and internal heat [as well as] external heat and internal cold through water and fire?"

Qibo answered, "[The case with] external cold and internal heat [indicates] depletion of true water and domination of evil-Qi; [the case with] external heat and internal cold [indicates] depletion of true fire and deficiency of healthy Qi. True water and true fire [refer to] water and fire in the kidney. [When] kidney-fire is supported by kidney-water, fire is true fire and heat is true heat; [when] kidney-fire estranges from restriction of kidney-water, fire

雷公问："那么,该如何治疗呢?"

岐伯说："预先治疗就可以生存,而治疗晚了就会导致死亡。"

雷公问："该用何法予以及时治疗呢?"

岐伯说："如果救援了胃肾之气,行将断绝之气就能得以恢复,变化了的就不会再变化了。"

雷公问："水火各有假症,而火的假症尤其难以辨别,该怎么应对呢?"

岐伯说："真火经常表现为假寒,假火经常表现为真热,但还是有办法对其予以辨别的。真热是阳证。真热证表现为假寒象的,为阳证表现为阴证,这是外寒内热的原因。真寒是阴证。但真寒证却表现为假热象的,为阴证表现为阳证,这是外热内寒的缘故。"

雷公问："外寒内热,外热内寒,究竟该如果通过水火来辨别呢?"

岐伯说："外寒内热,是真水亏虚,邪气旺盛的缘故;外热内寒,是真火亏虚,正气不足的缘故。真水真火,是肾中的水火。肾火得到肾水的资助,火就是真火,热也是真热;肾火离开了肾水的制约,那火就变成了假火,热也就变成假热了。辨别真假,可以用外水来试,因为真热遇到冷水就会缓解,假热遇到冷水则会加剧。"

雷公问："治疗之法是什么呢?"

岐伯说："通过补益肾水,假火就会自行消解。"

雷公问："假热病症可用温热的方剂治愈,这是为什么呢?"

岐伯说："肾中的火,喜欢用阴水来相济,也喜欢得到阴火的引导,所以可滋养肾水。用阴火引导肾水,假火就容易伏藏,但这并不是舍弃

becomes false fire and heat changes into false heat. True [heat] and false [heat] can be differentiated through the test of external fire. True heat will be resolved [when] meeting [with external] water and false heat will be worsened [when] meeting [with external] water."

Leigong asked,"What method [can be used to] treat [it]?"

Qibo answered, "[When kidney-] water is tonified, false fire will resolve spontaneously."

Leigong asked,"Why can false heat syndrome/pattern be cured by heat formula?"

Qibo answered, "Fire in the kidney likes to be supported by Yin-water and also likes to be guided by Yin-fire, [both of which all can] enrich water [in the kidney]. [When] guided by fire, false fire is easy to hide. [This is] not to abandon water and directly use fire."

Leigong asked,"Please explain how to treat fire."

Qibo answered, "[When] true water is tonified, true fire is also resolved. However, to treat fire is not simply to tonify water. In tonifying water, [measures should also be taken] to eliminate heat. [In this way] false [manifestation will be] removed and true [condition will be] revealed."

Leigong said,"Excellent [explanation]!"

Chen Shiduo's comment, "[*If one*] *cannot understand* [*what*

肾水而直接用火。"

雷公问:"请介绍治热的方法。"

岐伯说:"补益了真水,真火也就解除了。虽然如此,治火又不可单纯补水,在补水的同时也要用祛热之法,这样假相就会被攻破,真相就会显现出来。"

雷公说:"好!"

陈士铎评论说:"不懂得真相,又怎么能知道假相呢?不懂得假相,又怎么能知道真相呢?真假之间,也就是水火之分。懂得了破解水火的真假,真假之相又怎么会难以分辨呢?"

is] true, how [*can he*] know [*what is*] false? [*If one*] cannot understand [*what is*] false, how [*can he*] know [*what is*] true? [*The difference*] between true and false is also [*the same as that*] between water and fire. [*If*] true and false water and fire are differentiated, how could it be difficult to differentiate true and false [*phenomena*]?"

从逆窥源篇第七十九

【原文】

应龙问曰："病有真假,证有从逆,予知之矣,但何以辨其真假也?"

岐伯曰："寒热之证,气顺者多真,气逆者多假。凡气逆者,皆假寒假热也。知其假,无难治真矣!"

应龙曰："请问气逆也,何证也?"

岐伯曰："真阴之虚也。"

应龙曰："真阴之虚,何遂成气逆乎?"

岐伯曰："真阴者,肾水也。肾水之中有火存焉,火得水而伏,火失水而飞。凡气逆之证,皆阴水不能制阴火也。"

应龙曰："予闻阴阳则两相配也,未闻阴与阴而亦合也。"

岐伯曰："人身之火不同,有阴火阳火。阳火得阴水而制者,阴阳之顺也;阴火得阴水而伏者,阴阳之逆也。"

应龙曰："阴阳逆矣,何以伏之?"

岐伯曰："此五行之颠倒也。逆而伏者,正顺而治之也。"

应龙曰："此则龙之所不识也。"

岐伯曰："肾有两岐,水火藏其内。无火而水不生,无水而火不长,不可离也。火在水中,故称阴火。其实水火自分阴阳也。"

应龙曰："阴火善逆,阴水亦易逆,何故?"

【英译】

Chapter 79
Origin of Normality and Counterflow

Yinglong asked, "I know [that] disease is either true or false and syndrome/pattern is either normal or reverse. But how to differentiate [whether it is] true or false?"

Qibo answered, "Cold and heat syndrome/pattern [is] usually true [when] Qi is normal and false [when] Qi is in counterflow. Once [when] Qi is in counterflow, all cold and heat are false. [When one has] known [what is] false, [it is] not difficult to treat true [disease or syndrome/pattern]."

Yinglong asked, "What is the syndrome/pattern [related to] counterflow of Qi?"

Qibo answered, "It is syndrome/pattern of genuine Yin deficiency."

Yinglong asked, "Why does syndrome/pattern of genuine Yin deficiency cause counterflow of Qi?"

Qibo answered, "Genuine Yin is kidney-water and there is fire in kidney-water. [When] meeting with water[1], fire [will] hide; [when] losing water, fire will fly away[2]. Syndrome/pattern of Qi counterflow is all [caused by] failure of Yin-water to control Yin-fire."

岐伯曰："此正显水火之不可离也。火离水而逆，水离火亦逆也。

应龙曰："水火相离者，又何故欤？"

岐伯曰："人节欲少而纵恣多，过泄其精，则阴水亏矣。水亏则火旺，水不能制火而火逆矣。"

应龙曰："泄精损水，宜火旺不宜火衰也，何火有时而寒乎？"

岐伯曰："火在水中，水泄而火亦泄也。泄久则阴火亏矣，火亏则水寒，火不能生水而水逆也。故治气逆者，皆以补肾为主。水亏致火逆者，补肾则逆气自安；火亏致水逆者，补肾而逆气亦安。"

应龙曰："不足宜补，有余宜泻，亦其常也。何治肾水之火，不尚泻尚补乎？"

岐伯曰："肾中水火，各脏腑之所取资也，故可补不可泻，而水尤不可泻也。各脏腑有火无水，皆肾水滋之，一泻水则各脏腑立槁矣。气逆之证，虽有水火之分，而水亏者多也。故水亏者补水，而火亏者亦必补水，水旺则火衰，水生则火长也。"

应龙曰："补水而火不衰，补水而火不长，又奈何？"

岐伯曰："补水以衰火者，益水之药宜重；补水以长火者，益水之药宜轻也。"

应龙曰："善。"

陈士铎曰："人身之逆，全在肾水之不足。故补逆必须补水，水足，而逆者不逆也。"

Volume 9

Yinglong asked, "I have heard [that] Yin and Yang coordinate with each other, [but I] have never heard [that] Yin can coordinate with Yin."

Qibo answered, "Fire [in] the human body is different, either Yin-fire or Yang-fire. Yang-fire [will be] controlled [when] meeting with Yin-fire, [and therefore ensuring] normality of Yin and Yang; Yin-fire [will be] subdued [when] meeting with Yin-water, [and therefore causing] counterflow of Yin and Yang."

Yinglong asked, "How to subdue counterflow of Yin and Yang?"

Qibo answered, "This is reversal of the five elements. [Thus,] counterflow [indicates rebellion in the five elements and makes Yin-fire] hidden. [In this case, it is] appropriate to treat it according to its tendency."

Yinglong asked, "This is what I do not know."

Qibo answered, "There are two ways in the kidney, water and fire are stored in [it]. [If] there is no fire, water cannot be produced; [if] there is no water, fire cannot be promoted. [Hence, water and fire] cannot separate [from each other]. [Since] fire exists in [kidney-] water, so [it is] called Yin-fire. In fact water and fire are spontaneously divided into Yin and Yang."

Yinglong asked, "Yin-fire tends to counterflow and so does Yin-water. What is the reason?"

Qibo answered, "This just indicates [that] water and fire cannot separate [from each other]. [When] fire is separate from

【今译】

应龙问："病有真假,证有顺逆,我已经知道了,但如何才能辨别其真假呢?"

岐伯说："对于热证和寒证来说,气顺的多为真,气逆的多为假。凡是气逆的,都是假寒假热。知道了何为假证,就不难治疗真证了。"

应龙问："请问气逆的是什么证?"

岐伯说："是真阴虚弱。"

应龙问："真阴虚弱,怎么就造成气上逆了呢?"

岐伯说："真阴就是肾水。肾水之中蕴藏着火,火得到水的制约就会伏藏,火失去肾水就会飞散。凡是气逆之证,都是因为阴水不能制约阴火的缘故。"

应龙说："我只听说阴阳相配,从没听说阴阴相合。"

岐伯说："人身上的火彼此不同,有阴火和阳火之别。阳火得到阴水就会受到制约,阴阳就会因此而和顺;阴火受到阴水就会受到压制,阴阳就会因此而悖逆。"

应龙问："阴阳发生悖逆,如何才能制伏?"

岐伯说："这就属于颠倒五行了。上逆属于藏伏,正应顺其性而治疗。"

应龙问："这是我所不了解的。"

岐伯说："肾有两径,水火各藏在其中。没有火的资助水就不能发生,没有水的滋养火就不能生发,两者不能分离。火存在于肾水之中,所以称为阴火。其实水火已经自行分为阴阳了。"

water, [it tends] to counterflow; [when] water is separate from fire, [it] also [tends] to counterflow."

Yinglong asked, "Why water and fire are separate from each other?"

Qibo answered, "[When] a person indulges in erotism, seminal emission [will be] serious and Yin-water [will be] deficient. [When] water [is] deficient, fire [will be] exuberant. [If] water cannot control fire, fire [will] counterflow."

Yinglong asked, "Seminal emission damages water. [In this case,] fire should be exuberant but not debilitated. Why is sometimes there cold [manifestation] in fire?"

Qibo answered, "[Since] fire is stored in water, emission of water [will certainly cause] emission of fire. Long-term emission [of water will result in] depletion of Yin-fire. [When] fire is depleted, water [will become] cold. [If] fire cannot promote water, [it will cause] counterflow of water. Therefore treatment of counterflow of Qi all focuses on tonifying the kidney. [To treat] counterflow of fire caused by depletion of water, tonification of the kidney will spontaneously normalize counterflow of Qi; [to treat] counterflow of water caused by depletion of fire, tonification of the kidney will also normalize counterflow of Qi."

Yinglong asked, "[Cases of] insufficiency should [be treated by] tonification [while cases of] excess should [be treated by] purgation. [This is] the normal [way of treatment]. To treat [counterflow of] fire [caused by insufficiency of] kidney-water,

应龙问："阴火善于上逆,阴水也易于上逆,这是什么原因呢?"

岐伯说："这正是对水火不能分离的显示。如果火离开了水的节制,就会上逆;如果水离开了火的滋养,也会上逆。"

应龙问："水火互相分离,这又是什么原因呢?"

岐伯说："人们想节制的少,想放纵的多。如果过多地排泄了精气,就会造成阴水亏虚。如果阴水亏虚了,火就会旺盛。如果水不能制约火,火就会上逆。"

应龙问："泄泻了精气就会损伤水,火应当旺而不应当衰,但为什么火气有时会出现寒象呢?"

岐伯说："火藏在水中,水泄了火也会泄,水泄久了就会导致阴火亏虚。火亏虚了水就会变寒,火也就不能资助水了,水因而就开始上逆了。所以治疗气逆的,都应以补肾为主。水亏虚而导致火上逆的,通过补肾就可以使逆气自安。火亏虚而导致水上逆的,补肾也可以使逆气安静。"

应龙问："不足的应当予以补充,有余的应当予以排泻,这是常规疗法。为什么治疗肾水不足而引起的火逆,不强调泻法而重视补法呢?"

岐伯说："肾中的水火是各个脏腑获取资助的来源,所以只能补而不能泄,水尤其不能泻。如果各脏腑都有火而无水,都需要用肾水予以滋养。一旦将水泻了,各脏腑马上就会干枯。气逆之证,虽然有水火之分,但更多的还是水亏所致。所以水亏的就要补水,而火亏的也同样需要补水,只有水旺了火才会衰微,只有水得以滋生火才会生发。"

why is purgation not used [but] tonification [of the kidney] is used?"

Qibo answered, "Water and fire in the kidney are the resources for all the Zang-organs and Fu-organs [to take]. That is why [the kidney] can only be tonified [but] cannot be purged, especially water [in the kidney which] can never be purged. [In] all the Zang-organs and Fu-organs, there is fire [but] no water. [So they] all [depend on] kidney-water to nourish. Once [when] water is purged, all the Zang-organs and Fu-organs [will become] dry. Although in the syndrome/pattern of Qi counterflow there is difference [between] water and fire, the frequently [encountered problem is] water depletion. That is why water depletion [is treated by] tonifying water and fire depletion [is] also [treated by] tonifying water. [When] water is exuberant, fire [will be] debilitated; [when] water promotes, fire [will] increase."

Yinglong asked, "Water is tonified but fire is not debilitated; water is tonifed but fire does not increase. How to deal with [it then]?"

Qibo answered, "To debilitate fire through tonifying water, more medicinals for replenishing water should [be used]; to promote fire through tonifying water, less medicinals for replenishing water should [be used]."

Yinglong said, "Excellent [explanation]!"

Chen Shiduo's comment, "Counterflow [of water and fire in]

应龙问："补水而火不衰，补水而火不长，这该怎么办呢？"

岐伯说："通过补水可以削弱火势，所以益水的药物应当重用；通过补水可以助长火势，因此益水的药物应当少用。"

应龙说："好！"

陈士铎评论说："人体发生的各种逆证，都是肾水不足所致。所以必须通过补益肾水治疗上逆之证。肾水足了，上逆的就不会继续上逆了。"

the human body is all [due to] insufficiency of kidney-water. Therefore counterflow must be treated by tonifying water. [When] water is sufficient, counterflow [will certainly] cease."

Notes

[1] Meeting with water here means to be controlled by water.

[2] To fly away here means to flame up or to blaze.

移寒篇第八十

【原文】

应龙问曰："肾移寒于脾,脾移寒于肝,肝移寒于心,心移寒于肺,肺移寒于肾,此五脏之移寒也。脾移热于肝,肝移热于心,心移热于肺,肺移热于肾,肾移热于脾,此五脏之移热也。五脏有寒热之移,六腑有移热无移寒,何也?"

岐伯曰："五脏之五行正也,六腑之五行副也。五脏受邪,独当其胜;六腑受邪,分受其殃。且脏腑之病,热居十之八,寒居十之二也。寒易回阳,热难生阴,故热非一传而可止。脏传未已,又传诸腑,腑又相传。寒则得温而解,在脏有不再传者,脏不遍传,何至再传于腑乎? 此六腑所以无移寒之证也。"

应龙曰："寒不移于腑,独不移于脏乎?"

岐伯曰："寒入于腑而传于腑,甚则传于脏,此邪之自传也,非移寒之谓也。"

应龙曰："移之义若何?"

岐伯曰："本经受寒,虚不能受,移之于他脏腑,此邪不欲去而去之,嫁其祸也。"

应龙曰："善。"

Volume 9

【英译】

Chapter 80
Transference of Cold

Yinglong asked, "The kidney transfers cold to the spleen, the spleen transfers cold to the liver, the liver transfers cold to the heart, the heart transfers cold to the lung and the lung transfers cold to the kidney. This [is how] the five Zang-organs transfer cold. The spleen transfers heat to the liver, the liver transfers heat to the heart, the heart transfers heat to the lung, the lung transfers heat to the kidney and the kidney transfers heat to the spleen. This [is how] the five Zang-organs transfer heat. [In] the five Zang-organs, there is transference of cold and heat; [in] the six Fu-organs, there is transference of heat but no transference of cold. What is the reason?"

Qibo answered, "The five movements of the five Zang-organs are orthodoxical [while] the five movements of the six Fu-organs are subsidiary. [When] invaded by evil, the five Zang-organs depend on their own energy to defend; [when] invaded by evil, the six Fu-organs endure suffering respectively. Besides, [in] the diseases of the five Zang-organs and six Fu-organs, about eighty percent are heat [diseases] and twenty percent are cold [diseases].

陈士铎曰:"六腑有移热,而无移寒,以寒之不移也,独说得妙,非无征之文。"

【今译】

应龙问道:"肾转移寒于脾,脾转移寒于肝,肝转移寒于心,心转移寒于肺,肺转移寒于肾,这是五脏转移寒邪的规律。脾转移热于肝,肝转移热于心,心转移热于肺,肺转移热于肾,肾转移热于脾,这是五脏转移热邪的规律。为什么五脏有寒热的转移,而六腑却只有移热而没有移寒呢?"

岐伯说:"在五脏中,五行处于正位;在六腑中,五行则处于附属之位。所以五脏受到邪气的侵犯,就完全依靠自身的力量予以抵御;而六腑受到邪气的侵犯,则只能承受邪气的伤害。而且脏腑的疾病,热证占十分之八,寒证占十分之二。寒证容易回复阳气,而热证则难以滋生阴气,所以热证并非一传就止。病症在五脏中的转移没有停止时,又传移到六腑,在六腑间又相互传移。寒证得到温煦就能解除,在五脏间就不再传移了。既然五脏之间不再传移了,为什么还会再传移到六腑呢?这就是寒证不再转移于六腑中的主要原因。"

应龙问:"寒邪不转移到六腑,是否也不转移到五脏?"

岐伯说:"寒邪入侵六腑后,又在六腑间转移,甚至还会转移到五脏。这是邪气的自行传变,不可称为寒证的转移。"

应龙问:"转移是什么意思呢?"

岐伯说:"本经遭受寒邪的入侵,该脏因虚弱而不能承受寒邪的侵

[In] cold [disease], Yang is easy to restore; [in] heat [disease], Yin is difficult to promote. Thus heat [disease] cannot stop right [after being] transferred [to the meridian]. Before transferring to all the Zang-organs, [the disease is already] transferred to the concerned Fu-organ and begins to transfer among the Fu-organs. [When] warmed [by Yang Qi], cold [disease will be] relieved and stop transferring among the Zang-organs. [When it] stops transferring in the Zang-organs, how can [it] transfer to the Fu-organs? This [is why] there is no cold syndrome/pattern to be transferred in the six Fu-organs."

Yinglong asked, "Cold [evil] will not transfer to the Fu-organs. [Does it] also not transfer to the Zang-organs?"

Qibo answered, "[When] cold [evil] invades the Fu-organs, [it will] transfer in the Fu-organs, or even transfer to the Zang-organs. This [is] spontaneous transference of evil, not transference of cold [disease]."

Yinglong asked, "What is the meaning of transference?"

Qibo answered, "[When] this meridian is invaded by cold, [it] cannot endure [because of] deficiency. [That is why it] transfers [cold] to other Zang-organs and Fu-organs. [Although] evil is unwilling to retreat, [it has to be] transferred [under such a condition]. [This is how evil] shifts its disaster."

Yinglong said, "Excellent [explanation]!"

袭,因而将其转移给其他脏腑,寒邪因此而不想退去而不得不退去,从而将其祸害予以转嫁。"

应龙说:"好!"

陈士铎评论说:"六腑只能转移热邪而不能转移寒邪,因为寒邪不能转移。论述独特奇妙,这并非不是没有实际验证的文字。"

Volume 9

Chen Shiduo's comment, "[In] the six Fu-organs, there is only transference of heat [evil], no transference of cold [evil] because cold [evil] cannot be transferred. [Such an] analysis is excellent, not an article without verification."

寒热舒肝篇第八十一

【原文】

雷公问曰："病有寒热,皆成于外邪乎?"

岐伯曰："寒热不尽由于外邪也。"

雷公曰："斯何故欤?"

岐伯曰："其故在肝。肝喜疏泄,不喜闭脏。肝气郁而不宣,则胆气亦随之而郁,胆木气郁,何以生心火乎?故心之气亦郁也。心气郁则火不遂,其炎上之性,何以生脾胃之土乎?土无火养则土为寒土,无发生之气矣。肺金无土气之生,则其金不刚,安有清肃之气乎?木寡于畏,反克脾胃之土,土欲发舒而不能,土木相刑,彼此相角,作寒作热之病成矣。正未尝有外邪之干,乃五脏之郁气自病。徒攻其寒而热益盛,徒解其热而寒益猛也。"

雷公曰："合五脏以治之,何如?"

岐伯曰："舒肝木之郁,诸郁尽舒矣!"

陈士铎曰："五郁发寒热,不止木郁也。而解郁之法独责于木,以木郁解而金土水火之郁尽解,故解五郁惟尚解木郁也,不必逐经解之。"

Volume 9

【英译】

Chapter 81
To Soothe the Liver with Cold and Heat

Leigong asked, "Is disease with cold and heat caused by external evil?"

Qibo answered, "[Disease with] cold and heat is not simply caused by external evil."

Leigong asked,"What is the reason?"

Qibo answered, "The cause is in the liver. The liver likes depuration and dislikes storage. [When] liver-Qi is stagnated and unable to effuse, gallbladder-Qi is also stagnated accordingly. [When] Qi in gallbladder-wood is stagnated, how [can it] produce heart-fire? That is why heart-Qi is also stagnated. [When] heart-Qi is stagnated, fire [-Qi] cannot rise up [although it tends] to flame up. [In such a case,] how can [it] produce earth in the spleen and stomach? [If] there is no fire to nourish earth, earth becomes cold earth without vital Qi. [If] lung-metal is not promoted by earth-Qi, its metal is not hard. [Under such a circumstance,] how could there be Qi for depuration? [If] wood is not enough, [it] fears [metal] and, on the countrary, restricts earth in the spleen and stomach. [In this case,] earth desires to stretch but fails. [As a result,] earth and wood restrict each other and contend with each other, [consequently] causing disease with cold and heat [symptoms and signs]. [Such a disease is] certainly not caused by invasion of

【今译】

雷公问："病有寒有热,都是由外邪所引起的吗?"

岐伯说："寒热之病并不全是由外邪所引起的。"

雷公问："是什么原因呢?"

岐伯说："原因在肝。肝喜欢疏泄,不喜欢闭藏。如果肝气郁闭而得不到宣发,胆气也将随之郁闭,胆木之气郁闭,怎么能够生发心火呢?所以心气也将因此而郁闭。心气郁闭则会导致火气不能上达,而火性则为炎上,这又怎么能够资生脾胃之土呢? 土若失去了火的资养,土将变为寒土,也就因此而失去了发生之气。肺金失去了土气的生发,其金性就不再刚硬,怎么还会保持有清肃之气呢? 木少了就会畏惧金,反而克制脾胃之土。在这种情况下,土本想舒发而不能,土与木就相互刑伐,彼此相互争斗,从而引发了时寒时热的病症。这显然是没有外邪的干扰,而是五脏之郁气自行引发的病变。如果只攻伐其寒,热就会更加旺盛;如果只消解其热,寒证也会更加凶猛。"

雷公问："如何才能配合好五脏来治疗呢?"

岐伯说："只要舒发消散了肝木的郁气,其他各种郁证都可得以舒发消散。"

陈士铎评论说："五种郁闭情况均可引发寒证和热证,并非只有木郁才会引发。消解郁闭之法只有依赖肝木。木郁解除了,金、土、水、火之郁也就随之而完全解除。所以要解除五种郁闭之证,关键在于解除木郁,根本不需要逐经消解。"

external evil, but caused spontaneously by stagnated Qi in the five Zang-organs. [If treatment] only [focuses on] attacking cold, heat [will be] more exuberant; [if treatment] only [focuses on] resolving heat, cold [will become] more severe."

Leigong asked, "How to treat it in cooperation with the five Zang-organs?"

Qibo answered, "[When] stagnated [Qi] in liver-wood is soothed, stagnated [Qi in] all [Zang-organs and Fu-organs] will be soothed."

Chen Shiduo's comment, "*Five [kinds of] stagnation [all can] cause [disease with] cold and heat, not just wood stagnation. However, resolution of stagnation must start from wood. Because [when] wood stagnation is resolved, stagnation of metal, earth, water and fire all can be resolved. Thus resolution of five [kinds of] stagnation depends only on resolution of wood stagnation. [Hence it is] unnecessary to resolve [stagnation] along each meridian.*"

图书在版编目(CIP)数据

黄帝外经英译:英文/(远古)岐伯天师论述;(明)陈士铎评述;刘希茹今译;李照国英译.—上海:上海三联书店,2022.8
(国学经典外译丛书.第一辑)
ISBN 978 - 7 - 5426 - 7800 - 3

Ⅰ.①黄… Ⅱ.①岐…②陈…③刘…④李… Ⅲ.①医经一英文 Ⅳ.①R22

中国版本图书馆 CIP 数据核字(2022)第 142548 号

国学经典外译丛书 · 第一辑

黄帝外经英译

论　　述 / (远古)岐伯天师

评　　述 / (明)陈士铎

今　　译 / 刘希茹

英　　译 / 李照国

责任编辑 / 杜　鹃

装帧设计 / 徐　徐

监　　制 / 姚　军

责任校对 / 王凌霄

出版发行 / 上海三联书店

(200030)中国上海市漕溪北路 331 号 A 座 6 楼

邮　　箱 / sdxsanlian@sina.com

邮购电话 / 021 - 22895540

印　　刷 / 上海颛辉印刷厂有限公司

版　　次 / 2022 年 8 月第 1 版

印　　次 / 2022 年 8 月第 1 次印刷

开　　本 / 640mm×960mm　1/16

字　　数 / 620 千字

印　　张 / 40.5

书　　号 / ISBN 978 - 7 - 5426 - 7800 - 3/R · 126

定　　价 / 130.00 元

敬启读者,如发现本书有印装质量问题,请与印刷厂联系 021 - 56152633